# DRUGS IN PREGNANCY

*A Handbook for Pharmacists and Physicians*

# DRUGS IN PREGNANCY

*A Handbook for Pharmacists and Physicians*

**Radhwan Nidal Al-Zidan**

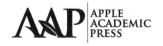

Apple Academic Press Inc.
4164 Lakeshore Road
Burlington ON L7L 1A4
Canada

Apple Academic Press, Inc.
1265 Goldenrod Circle NE
Palm Bay, Florida 32905
USA

© 2021 by Apple Academic Press, Inc.

*Exclusive worldwide distribution by CRC Press, a member of Taylor & Francis Group*

No claim to original U. S. Government works

International Standard Book Number-13: 978-1-77188-895-0 (Hardcover)
International Standard Book Number-13: 978-1-00301-910-7 (eBook)

**Library and Archives Canada Cataloguing in Publication**

Title: Drugs in pregnancy : a handbook for pharmacists and physicians / Radhwan Nidal Al-Zidan.
Names: Al-Zidan, Radhwan Nidal, author.
Description: Includes bibliographical references and index.
Identifiers: Canadiana (print) 20200221590 | Canadiana (ebook) 20200221833 |
    ISBN 9781771888950 (hardcover) | ISBN 9781003019107 (ebook)
Subjects: LCSH: Obstetrical pharmacology—Handbooks, manuals, etc. | LCGFT: Handbooks
    and manuals.
Classification: LCC RG528 .A4 2020 | DDC 615/.766—dc23

CIP data on file with US Library of Congress

Apple Academic Press also publishes its books in a variety of electronic formats. Some content that appears in print may not be available in electronic format. For information about Apple Academic Press products, visit our website at **www. appleacademicpress. com** and the CRC Press website at **www. crcpress. com**

# About the Author

**Radhwan Nidal Al-Zidan, BSc Pharm, MSc**
*Department of Pharmaceutics, College of Pharmacy, Mosul University, Mosul, Iraq*

Radhwan Al-Zidan is a specialized pharmacist with more than 10 years of professional experience from working as a hospital pharmacist, community pharmacist, and from his current position in academia. Radhwan started his professional career as a trainee pharmacist in the teaching hospitals of Mosul city. He honored his role within the clinical team; he actively participated in shaping the clinical decisions and, at the same time, in educating patients. Thanks to his dedication to work, Radhwan obtained three "letters of appreciation" from the general manager of Nineveh Health Directorate during his work as a hospital pharmacist. Moreover, Radhwan's position as manager of Royaa Pharmacy, one of the largest private pharmacies in Mosul city, put him in daily contact with many patients who sought advice and consultation.

Radhwan's passion for teaching and disseminating medical knowledge drove him back to the academia, where he worked, initially, as a demonstrator in teaching labs. After specializing in medical biotechnology, Radhwan was promoted to assistant lecturer in the College of Pharmacy/ University of Mosul. Attributable to his merit in work, Radhwan obtained two "letters of appreciation" from the President of Mosul University, and now he is the rapporteur of the Department of Pharmaceutics. Furthermore, he has been selected as a member of the Scientific Committee of the Iraqi Syndicate of the Pharmacists-Nineveh branch.

Radhwan has distinctive academic achievements. He won the prize of "Academic Excellence" from the Ministry of Higher Education and Scientific Research (MOHESR) in Iraq for graduating third of all graduating Iraqi pharmacists in 2010. Additionally, Radhwan received a scholarship, in 2014, from the Higher Committee for Education Development (HCED) in Iraq to study for a master's degree in the United Kingdom. During his study in the UK, he won the Medical Elective & Summer Placement Award Scheme (MESPAS) award from the British Society for Immunology (BSI). In addition, Radhwan graduated first on his peers in the masters and won the "Class Medal" from Edinburgh Napier University.

Radhwan's professional positions as a hospital pharmacist, community pharmacist, lab demonstrator, and presently, assistant lecturer were instrumental to helping him to create a unique source of information for healthcare professionals who are seeking accurate, succinct, and easy-to-read handbook.

# Contents

# Abbreviations

| | |
|---|---|
| AUC | area under the curve |
| BSA | body surface area |
| CMV | cytomegalovirus |
| DMARDs | disease-modifying anti-rheumatic drugs |
| FDA | Food and Drug Administration |
| HPA axis | hypothalamic-pituitary-adrenal axis |
| IUGR | intrauterine growth restriction |
| MRHD | maximum recommended human dose |
| OTC | over-the-counter |
| PLLR | pregnancy and lactation labeling rule |
| RANKL | RANK ligand |
| RDA | recommended daily allowance |
| SABs | spontaneous abortions |
| TGA | Therapeutic Goods Administration |

# Disclaimer

The knowledge in the field of pharmacology is increasing rapidly, and it is constantly changing. As newly published scientific research widens our understanding, changes in drug treatment or professional practices may become essential. Therefore, healthcare providers must regularly rely on their knowledge and experience in assessing and using any information described herein. In using such information, healthcare providers should be vigilant of the safety of their patients.

Regarding any drug or products described in this handbook, healthcare providers are urged to check the most up-to-date information provided by the manufacturer of each drug/product to be administered. It is the sole responsibility of the healthcare providers to choose the best drug, dose, and/or formula for their patients.

To the fullest extent of the law, neither the authors nor the publisher, or the reviewers, accept any responsibility for any injury and/or damage to persons from any use of any information contained in the handbook.

# Acknowledgments

It is a pleasure to acknowledge the tremendous efforts and the helpful comments of the book reviewers: Dr. Harith Alqazaz (BSc Pharm, MSc, PhD in Clinical Pharmacy), Dr. Fawaz Alassaf (BSc Pharm, MSc, PhD in Medical Physiology and Pharmacology), Dr. Mohannad Qazzaz (BSc Pharm, MSc, PhD in Pharmacology), Dr. Mohammed Najem (BSc Pharm, MSc, PhD in Pharmacology), Dr. Mahmood Hashim (BSc Pharm, MSc, PhD in Drug Design), Waqar Qidar (Clinical Pharmacist), and as well as Khubeeb Mohammed (Community Pharmacist). I also am pleased to thank my current student, Shahad Muthana, for the creative graphic used on the book's cover.

Also, I want to thank all the lovely people who believed in me and continuously encouraged me over the last two years spent in writing this book. At the outset, all of my family members, particularly my mother, Yusra Hashim, and my wife, Aseel Abdulah. Also, my dear colleagues, Dr. Moataaz Alsalman and Dr. Hasan Aldewachy.

Last but not least, I would like to thank all of the great people who enlightened me over the last 26 years. Commencing from my first teacher, Ms. Molkia Abdullah, who taught me how to write my name—and not ending with my master's supervisor, Dr. Graham Wright.

# Preface

The principal motivation that drove me to write *Drugs in Pregnancy: A Handbook for Pharmacists and Physicians* was the countless number of times when my colleagues, pharmacists, and physicians asked me about the safety of using certain drugs during pregnancy. Moreover, from my personal experience, I know that every community pharmacist needs to use such a handbook, possible on a daily basis, to confidently answer the questions of the worried pregnant mothers seeking consultation from their community pharmacist. In addition, the recent reforms in the labeling of drugs in pregnancy imposed by the U.S. Food and Drug Administration (FDA) requires all the manufacturers of the FDA approved drugs to remove the labeling of the old A, B, C, D, & X letter categorization of drugs use during pregnancy that has been used since 1979. Instead, the manufacturers are required to provide the information mentioned in the newly approved "pregnancy and lactation labeling rule (PLLR)." Many experts around the globe, pointed out that the abrupt switch from the widely used FDA letter categorization system to the new labeling required by the PLLR will negatively impact the decisions of healthcare providers regarding the prescription of drugs to pregnant women. Therefore, it is crucial to provide healthcare providers with a credible source of information that connects the old-fashioned FDA letter classification and the new requirements of the PLLR rule.

This handbook is the first of its kind in the category of books interrogating the issue of drugs and pregnancy. The information provided for each drug uses the FDA letter categorization and PLLR systems for rating drug risks in pregnancy. To enable the reader to develop a well-informed opinion about a drug safety profile during pregnancy, three sections of data have been provided for each drug (i.e., FDA Category, Risk Summary, and Further Reading).

The scope of this manuscript is wide as it includes anti-infective, cardiovascular, hematologic, dermatologic drugs and drugs affecting endocrine, central, autonomic, gastrointestinal, musculoskeletal systems in addition to herbs and vitamin and dietary supplements.

This handbook is easy to use and will save the precious time of the healthcare providers by enabling them to promptly locating the drug(s) in question. Additionally, the handbook will enable healthcare providers to

compare the safety profile of the desired drug with its counterparts within
the same pharmacological group—at the same time.

I hope you find this handbook helpful!

**—Radhwan N. Al-Zidan**

# CHAPTER 1

# Introduction

## 1.1 HISTORICAL BACKGROUND

Humans have a long history of using different chemicals and herbs in treating a variety of medical conditions in both genders. The use of such compounds for pregnant women was not an exception. There is a translated Assyrian Script, dating back 3500 years, which describes three different prescriptions to relieve abdominal cramps in pregnant women [1]. However, the concern about the safety of chemical agents (drugs and herbs) given to females during pregnancy was not raised until the tragedy of the thalidomide. In 1957, thalidomide gained marketing approval as a safe over-the-counter (OTC) drug for treating insomnia in pregnant women. Unfortunately, a few years later case reports of phocomelia (malformation of the limbs) began to accumulate. With thousands of children born with tragic limb deformities, the health care providers and the public around the world were shocked by the unforeseen relationship of thalidomide use in pregnant women and the development of serious birth defects in the newborns.

The moral impact of the thalidomide tragedy and subsequent demands of the public in the mid-1960s were the driving force for the researchers and health care professionals to better scrutinize the potential effects of a drug on both the conceptus and the mother. Furthermore, the governmental regulations of drugs approval around the globe became more restricted as to thoroughly examine the safety profile of the drug use in pregnancy before granting marketing approval. In addition, the pharmaceutical companies became obliged to provide enough data, within the patient information leaflet, about the use of their drug in pregnant women.

Aiming to make it easier for the health care providers to deal with the safety of drug use in pregnancy, a number of classification systems were adopted in different countries around the globe. The United States Food and Drug Administration (FDA) letter categorization system (A, B, C, D, and

X) was the most commonly used one since 1979. However, in December 2014, the FDA replaced the old categorization system with a completely different *pregnancy and lactation labeling rule* (PLLR), which became effective in mid-2015. By the year 2020, all the manufacturers of the FDA approved prescription drugs and biologic products are required to comply with the PLLR rule obligations [2]. Therefore, the need for books like this one became inevitable to bridge the gap between the outdated FDA categorization system, which has been used for more than three decades, and the considerably different style of information provided in accordance with the PLLR rule. The FDA is changing the regulations and by 2020 the letter categorization, which has been used for more than three decades, will be removed from all of the FDA approved prescription drugs and biologic products. Therefore, physicians and pharmacists urgently need a book that merges the old categorization system with a considerably different style of information provided in accordance with the PLLR rule.

## 1.2   SCOPE OF THE PROBLEM

Women can be prescribed a variety of drugs for treating a medical condition or a disease without considering the possibility of pregnancy. For example, a sexually-active young female suffering from recurrent convulsions are usually prescribed an antiepileptic drug—to be taken continuously. It is quite possible for such a woman to become pregnant while taking the antiepileptic drug. Since most of the antiepileptic drugs are teratogenic, serious damage to the conceptus as well as a significant psychological burden on the mother may occur.

The previous case-scenario is not uncommon. For instance, a multinational, cross-sectional study performed by Lupattelli [3] found that 81.2% of women have taken at least one drug (prescribed or OTC) during pregnancy. Sedgh [4] estimated that only in 2012 there were nearly 213 million pregnancies world-widely. Therefore, it is reasonable to anticipate that every year there are, at least, tens of millions of pregnant women around the globe who are being exposed to medications. Some of these medications could be extremely harmful to the development of the fetus and could lead to loss of the conceptus. For example, a cohort study conducted in Finland on 43,470 pregnant women found that 20.4% of the sample bought at the minimum one drug classified as possibly harmful during conception, and 3.4% bought at the minimum one drug categorized as clearly harmful [5].

Accurate numbers of birth defects due to the intake of drugs by pregnant women has not been determined, yet, for many reasons. First of all, there is a global lack of well-designed cohort studies, which are the most reliable source of information regarding drug safety in pregnancy, to exactly determine the negative effect(s) of each drug given during pregnancy. Secondly, it is not uncommon for addicted mothers to avoid mentioning the intake of alcohol or illicit drugs to their general practitioners, which makes it even harder to determine the true cause of birth defects in the newborns. However, not all birth defects are caused by drugs. A study found that 4% of newborns in the U.S. suffer from birth defects, and that approximately only 1% of those neonates were born to mothers who have ingested harmful drug(s) during pregnancy [6].

## 1.3   CRITICAL TIME PERIODS DURING PREGNANCY

In general, the anticipated effect(s) of a given drug during pregnancy can be divided according to the fetal age, as follows:

- **From the 1st day until the 20th day after fertilization:** Interestingly, teratogenesis is unlikely to occur during this period. However, the effect(s) of any harmful drug given during this period could lead either to the death of the conceptus or to no adverse effects at all, which is commonly known as the all-or-nothing effect.
- **From the 21st day until the 56th day after fertilization:** The hallmark of this fetal period is characterized by organogenesis. Therefore, teratogenesis is most likely to occur at this stage of conception. The spectrum of harmful effects of a drug given during this period could range from spontaneous abortion, through teratogenicity (revealed as a gross anatomical defect), to a hidden embryopathy (like a permanent subtle functional or metabolic defect that may become noticeable later in life). Furthermore, the harmful effect(s) of the given drug may result in increased rates of childhood malignancies (for example, a child of a mother treated, during pregnancy, with radioactive iodine for thyroid malignancy).
- **From the start of the 2nd trimester till delivery:** The exposure of the conceptus to a drug during this period is unlikely to cause teratogenic effects because the stage of fetal organogenesis has completed. However, the exposure of the fetus to certain drugs during this period may lead to a change in the growth and/or function of the normally

formed fetal tissues and organs. It is worth mentioning that at this stage, the contribution of the placenta in the metabolism of drugs rises. Therefore, for fetal toxicity to occur, higher doses are required to be used by the mother.

In general, the developmental and reproductive toxicological effects of a drug on the conceptus vary depending on multiple factors. The fetal age at the time of exposure, which is described above, represents only one of the factors that determine the effect of the given drug on the fetus. Another important factor is related to the given drug itself, in terms of the dose, the duration, and the route of administration. In addition, the factors related to the mother also play crucial roles in governing the occurrence and/or the severity of adverse events in the conceptus. For example, nausea, and vomiting associated with pregnancy may decrease the absorption and bioavailability of drugs taken orally. Therefore, the same dose of a certain drug that is ingested by two different women, at the same gestational age, could lead to the development of adverse event(s) in one fetus but not the other.

## 1.4   CLINICAL TOOLS FOR EVALUATING DRUGS' SAFETY IN PREGNANCY

In general, the available sources of drug information regarding their safety during pregnancy are mainly obtained from animal and human studies. Although animal tests are extensively used in the study of drugs' safety during pregnancy, they are considered weak predictors of whether a drug is harmful or has a teratogenic effect in humans. The specificity and sensitivity of animal models as predictors of human teratogenicity is determined by the relative proximity of the used animal species to Homo sapiens. For example, it is known that the sensitivity and specificity of rodent studies are less than 60% [7]. There are a number of explanations to describe the differences in the response to the same drug by different species, such as the dissimilarities in the pharmacodynamics and pharmacokinetics of the same drug in different species. Additionally, there are variations in the placentation and embryonic development timing of the conceptus.

On the other hand, more accurate and realistic data, regarding the safety of drugs during pregnancy, are obtained from case reports, case-control studies, and cohort studies that have been conducted in humans [8]. The case reports are crucial in raising the causal hypothesis, which appeals to the health care providers and clinical researchers to carry out more sophisticated epidemiological studies. The case-control and cohort studies are more informative, than case reports, and have a higher degree of accuracy. Case-control studies examine the frequencies of exposure to the drug before the delivery between children having or lacking certain birth defect, whereas cohort studies examine the frequencies of anomalies in the females' youngsters who were exposed to a drug in comparison to youngsters of women who were not exposed to the drug of interest.

The discovery of the teratological effects of carbamazepine, the anti-epileptic drug, gave a hint about the significance of the epidemiological studies in discovering the toxic effects of drugs given during pregnancy. For years, carbamazepine was considered safer than phenytoin in the treatment of epilepsy during pregnancy. However, in 1989 Jones [9] published a retrospective case-control study that linked the use of carbamazepine during pregnancy with increased frequency of birth defects. This case-control study paved the way for conducting further epidemiological studies regarding carbamazepine over the next decades [10]. Sequentially, in 2006 the relationship of exposure to carbamazepine during the early stages of conception, with the increased risk of neural tube defect was established as causal.

The epidemiological studies have a number of advantages such as the higher specificity and sensitivity, and the significant ability to detect the teratological effects of drugs given during pregnancy. However, they suffer from a number of weaknesses. False associations frequently occur because many epidemiologists lack the proper medical knowledge and training, and fail to analyze their statistical causal for biological plausibility. Another common problem is the inappropriate sample size used by many epidemiological studies, which makes the conclusion of those studies questionable.

## 1.5   CLASSIFICATION SYSTEMS FOR DRUGS IN PREGNANCY

The pharmaceutical companies always tried to protect themselves from legal prosecution, especially after the thalidomide disaster. Therefore, when it comes to the use of the drugs during pregnancy, particularly before the 1980s, it is common to read disclaim sentences, such as "safe use in pregnancy has not been established" or "should not be used in pregnant women unless, in the judgment of the physician, the potential benefits outweigh the possible hazards." These sentences were intentionally stated to protect the pharmaceutical companies in the courtroom and to put the responsibility on the prescribers and dispensers without providing them with sufficient scientific information about the drug use in pregnant women.

Around the globe, the health care providers and the general public have urged the legislators to put suitable regulations in order to oblige the pharmaceutical companies to change the labeling of the manufactured drugs. Consequently, a number of classification systems for drug safety during pregnancy were developed and adopted in different countries, and the pharmaceutical companies were required to use the classification systems.

The widely known classification systems are the United States FDA classification system, the Australian Therapeutic Goods Administration (TGA) classification system, as well as the Swedish Catalogue of Approved Drugs Swedish (FASS). However, there are significant differences between these classification systems. For instance, Addis [11] found that only 25% of drugs mutual to all three classification systems have the same risk factor. The differences were mainly attributed to dissimilarity in definitions. This variation is an indicator of the presence of a real problem in those classification systems. Accordingly, health care providers would be confused by the different, and sometimes, contradictory classification of the same drug by the different classification systems. That could lead to a misled medical decision.

Nonetheless, the FDA classification system is widely known and commonly used in the Middle East and the rest of the world. Therefore, it will be discussed briefly in this chapter to give the reader a glimpse about the fundamentals of the FDA letter categorization system. The pros and cons of this system, and the shortcomings that pushed the FDA, recently, to replace this system will be explained. The old-fashioned FDA letter categorization system rates medication risk using categories (A, B, C, D, and X), depending on the available data from human and animal studies, as described below:

- **Category A:** Controlled studies in humans fail to demonstrate a risk to the fetus in the first trimester, there is no proof of a risk in later trimesters, AND the possibility of fetal harm appears remote.
- **Category B:** Either animal-reproduction studies have revealed an adverse effect that was not confirmed in controlled studies in humans OR animal-reproduction studies have not proved a fetal risk but there are no controlled studies in humans.
- **Category C:** Either studies in animals have shown adverse effects on the conceptus (embryocidal, teratogenic or other) and there are no controlled studies in humans OR studies in humans and animals are not available. These drugs should be used only if the potential benefit outweighs the potential risk to the fetus.

- **Category D:** There is positive evidence of human fetal hazard, however, the benefits from use in pregnant women may be adequate despite the risk (e.g., for a serious disease for which safer drugs are ineffective OR if the drug is needed in a life-threatening condition).
- **Category X:** Studies in humans and animals have confirmed fetal abnormalities AND/OR there is a sign of fetal risk based on human experience AND the risk of the usage of the drug in pregnant females undoubtedly outweighs any potential benefit. Such drugs are contra-indicated in women who are or want to become pregnant.
- **Category N:** It is a non-official FDA letter categorization. However, it has been used in this handbook to indicate the drug in question has not been assigned with a corresponding letter by the FDA.

The FDA letter categorization has been used, in different countries worldwide, for more than 30 years. The health care professionals found this classification system simple and easy to memorize. However, since its adoption by the FDA in 1979, the FDA letter categorization system has received a body of criticism, which is summarized below:

1. The FDA letter categorization system is over-simplistic.
2. It provides insufficient information for health care professionals to accurately counsel pregnant women in the event of unintentional fetal drug exposures.
3. The highest numbers of drugs included in the FDA letter categorization system are classified as Category "C," which is not quite helpful for the health care providers who need to make well-informed medical decisions [12].
4. There are a great number of drugs that have not been assigned a suitable pregnancy risk category.
5. Some clinicians, mistakenly, use the FDA categorization as a grading system for drugs safety during pregnancy.

## 1.6   PREGNANCY AND LACTATION LABELING RULE (PLLR)

The PLLR labeling changes became effective on 30 June 2015. All the biologic products and prescription drugs applications submitted after 30 June 2015, should use the new PLLR format immediately. Whereas, labeling of the prescription medications approved after 30 June 2001 will be phased in gradually. However, by 2020, the manufacturers of all the FDA approved prescription drugs and biologic products are required to comply with the PLLR rule obligations.

The PLLR rule involves changes to the format and content of information presented in the prescription drug labeling to assist the health care providers in assessing benefit against risk and in the subsequent steps of counseling the pregnant. Most importantly, the PLLR rule implementation removes the pregnancy letter categories-A, B, C, D, and X. The PLLR rule also needs the label to be updated when information becomes out-of-date.

Figure 1.1 shows a comparison between the existing prescription drugs labeling with the new PLLR rule labeling requirements.

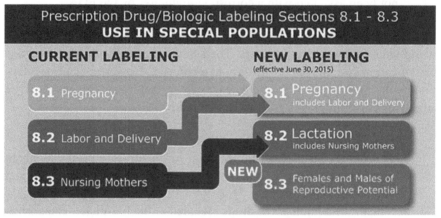

**FIGURE 1.1**    The effect of the new PLLR rule on the Labeling Sections (8.1–8.3) of the Prescription Drug & Biologic Products. The left side of the figure shows the old-fashioned labeling, whereas the right side of the figure represents the newly approved structuring of the sections (8.1–8.3). Reprinted from the U.S. Food and Drug Administration [13].

The "pregnancy" subsection (8.1) of the drug labeling, according to the PLLR rule, contains four headings, as follows:

- Pregnancy exposure registry;
- Risk summary*;
- Clinical considerations;
- Data.
  (*) Mandatory heading.

The Pregnancy Exposure Registry collects and maintains data on the effects of approved medications that are prescribed to pregnant women. *The*

*Pregnancy Exposure Registry* includes specific contact information, like the phone number and the website of the registry. The enclosure of information about the presence of any pregnancy registry in drug labeling has been recommended but not required until now. However, according to the PLLR rule, the Pregnancy Exposure Registry heading is optional unless there is an available pregnancy exposure registry [2].

The Risk Summary is a mandatory heading within the "Pregnancy" subsection (8.1). The information in this heading depends on the ability of the given drug to reach the systemic circulation or not. For example, heading of the *Risk Summary* for a drug with no systemic absorption is expected to have the following description:

"[TRADE NAME] is not absorbed systemically following (route of administration) and maternal use is not expected to result in fetal exposure to the drug." Whereas, the *Risk Summary* for drugs having the ability to reach the systemic absorption should consider the following points [2]:

- When the use of a drug is contraindicated during pregnancy, this must be stated first in the Risk Summary
- Risk statement based on human data*
- Risk statement based on animal data*
- Risk statement based on pharmacology
- Background risk information in general population*
- Background risk information in the disease population
  (*) Mandatory.

To get a clearer overview of the content of the *Risk Summary* heading, the reader is advised to look at the example below:

---

## 8.1 PREGNANCY

***Risk Summary:*** There are no adequate and well-controlled studies of [TRADENAME] in pregnant women. The limited available information on [TRADENAME] use during pregnancy is not sufficient to inform a drug-associated risk of major birth defects or miscarriage. In animal reproduction studies, oral administration of [drug name] to pregnant rats and rabbits during the period of organogenesis at doses up to 40 and 20 times the maximum recommended human dose (MRHD), respectively, resulted in decreased fetal body weight gain and delayed skeletal ossification but no teratogenic effects were observed. Decreased fetal body weight and delayed skeletal ossification were not observed at doses up to 10 and 5 times the MRHD in rats and rabbits, respectively [*see Data*]. The estimated background risk of major birth defects and miscarriage for the indicated population is unknown. In the U.S. general population, the estimated background risks of major birth defects and miscarriage in clinically recognized pregnancies are 2–4% and 15–20%, respectively" [2].

The clinical considerations heading is optional. This heading deals with the following aspects:

- The disease-related maternal and/or embryo/fetal risk;
- Dose modifications during pregnancy and the postpartum period;
- Adverse reactions on the mother;
- Adverse reactions on the fetus/neonate;
- Labor and delivery.

Finally, the *Data* heading provides a meticulous description of the 0information that provides the scientific foundation for the summary information offered in the *Risk Summary* and *Clinical Considerations* headings. The applicant delivers to the FDA a comprehensive review of related published articles, their pharmacovigilance record, and pregnancy exposure registry (if one is available) to maintain an updated language of the *"Pregnancy"* section of the labeling.

Section 8.2 *"Lactation"* and Section 8.3 *"Females and Males of Reproductive Potential,"* of the drug labeling according to the PLLR rule, are out of the scope of this handbook.

---

## 1.7   ABOUT THIS HANDBOOK

For decades, millions of healthcare providers, around the globe, were depending solely on the FDA letter labeling of the drugs in pregnancy. However, the dramatic change in the information provided regarding the use of drugs in pregnancy, brought by the implementation of the PLLR rule, is expected to have a substantial restrictive impact on the decision of the healthcare providers. Interestingly, in May 2018 Robinson et al. published a randomized study showing that removal of the FDA letter categorization, suddenly, will have a negative impact on the medical decisions of the physicians. The study forecasted that by removing the pregnancy letter category, healthcare providers are less likely to prescribe category B and C drugs, which are the most common medications used during pregnancy [14].

Therefore, it is crucial to provide the healthcare providers with a reliable source of information that combines the old-fashioned FDA letter classification and the new requirements of the PLLR rule. This book is the first of its kind, in the category of books dealing with the use of drugs during pregnancy, because the information provided for each drug will be a perfect combination between the old-fashioned FDA letter categorization and the "risk summary" that is required by the newly approved PLLR rule of the FDA.

The information regarding each drug, described in this handbook, follows the style of the monograph books. Therefore, there is a uniformed structure in which the information is presented to the reader. In order to enable the reader to develop a well-informed opinion about a drug safety profile during pregnancy, three sections of data have been provided for each drug (i.e., FDA Category, Risk Summary, and Further Reading).

The reader is advised to have a look at the following example of warfarin that has been shown in Figure 1.2:

The first set of information is represented by the old-fashioned FDA letter categorization of the drug which is intended to interconnect the health care providers, who have used this categorization system for decades, with the new style of information that will be provided in the drug information leaflets—in accordance with the new requirements of the PLLR rule.

Secondly, a summarization of the available human and/or animal studies that have been performed to examine the safety of using the drug during pregnancy is provided to the reader. The section of *Risk Summary* will help the health care providers to develop a well-informed opinion on the safety level of using the drug during pregnancy.

Regarding the data description of the animal reproduction studies, it is noteworthy to mention the definition of the following expressions:

- **Animal Data Has Shown Low Risk:** At doses ≤10 folds the human dose, based on area under the curve (AUC) or body surface area (BSA), the drug in question does not cause developmental toxicity (structural anomalies, growth restriction, behavioral/functional deficits, or death) in all the studied animal species.

### 4.1.9  WARFARIN

- **FDA Category**: D (for women with mechanical heart valves)
- **FDA Category**: X (all other indications)
- *Risk Summary:* It is generally contraindicated during pregnancy, especially during the 1ˢᵗ trimester, because of the high incidence of fetal warfarin syndrome. However, it could be used only for women with mechanical heart valves, who are at elevated risk of thromboembolism, and for whom the advantages of this drug might surpass the risks.

### FURTHER READING:

- Baillie, M., Allen, E. D., & Elkington, A. R., (1980). The congenital warfarin syndrome: A case report. *Br. J. Ophthalmol., 64,* 633–635.
- Kaplan, L. C., Anderson, G. G., & Ring, B. A., (1982). Congenital hydrocephalus and dandy-walker malformation associated with warfarin use during pregnancy. *Birth Defects, 18,* 79–83.
- Lee, P. K., Wang, R. Y. C., Chow, J. S. F., Cheung, K. L., Wong, V. C. W., & Chan, T. K., (1986). Combined use of warfarin and adjusted subcutaneous heparin during pregnancy in patients with an artificial heart valve. *J. Am. Coll. Cardiol., 8,* 221–224.
- Ruthnum, P., & Tolmie, J. L., (1987). Atypical malformations in an infant exposed to warfarin during the first trimester of pregnancy. *Teratology, 36,* 299–301.

**FIGURE 1.2**   The style used in the handbook for displaying the drug information. Three layers of information are provided to the reader; the FDA Category, Risk Summary, and the Further Reading sections.

- **Animal Data Has Shown Moderate Risk:** At doses ≤10 folds the human dose, based on AUC or BSA, the drug in question causes developmental toxicity (structural anomalies, growth restriction, behavioral/functional deficits, or death) in one of the studied animal species.

- **Animal Data Has Shown Risk:** At doses ≤10 folds the human dose, based on AUC or BSA, the drug in question causes developmental toxicity (structural anomalies, growth restriction, behavioral/functional deficits, or death) in two of the studied animal species.
- **Animal Data Has Shown High Risk:** At doses ≤10 folds the human dose, based on AUC or BSA, the drug in question causes developmental toxicity (structural anomalies, growth restriction, behavioral/functional deficits, or death) in three or more of the studied animal species.

Finally, the section of *Further Reading* contains a list of resources to support the readers, who are looking for more in-depth information, via providing them with the references to the most relevant articles, official websites, and/or textbooks.

The handbook is composed of fifteen chapters which contain the commonly used drugs for the treatment of most diseases and clinical conditions. The drugs are distributed to the corresponding chapters based on the physiological system affected by their main pharmacological action(s). For instance, all the drugs with an anti-infective activity are collected within Chapter 2 of this handbook. Within Chapter 2, there are different sections (for example; Antibacterial drugs, Antiviral drugs, etc.) and each section has subsections and subsubsections.

The main reason for choosing this unique classification system is to enable the pharmacists and the physicians to compare the drug in question with other drugs that have the same pharmacological action(s). Consequently, the health care provider will be able to instantly compare the safety profile of the drug of interest with those of comparable indication(s) and to choose the safest one.

With respect to the resources used in this handbook, the official website of the U.S. FDA was the main source of information. The FDA information vis-à-vis the pregnancy letter category (A, B, C, D, and X) of each drug, and the available human and/or animal studies were obtained by searching through the list of the FDA Approved Drug Products, available at the following website (https://www.accessdata.fda.gov/scripts/cder/daf/). Whereas, the resources in the section of *Further Reading* were chosen based on the opinion and experience of the author—regarding the most relevant references that could be of assistance to the readers.

## KEYWORDS

- area under the curve
- body surface area
- Food and Drug Administration
- maximum recommended human dose
- over-the-counter
- pregnancy and lactation labeling rule

## REFERENCES

1. Lambert, W. G., (1969). *A Middle Assyrian Medical Text* (Vol. 31, No. 1, pp. 28–39). Iraq, Cambridge University Press.

2. *Pregnancy and Lactation Labeling Rule*, (2014). [Internet]. Food and Drug Administration; [cited 20 February 2019]. Available from: https://www.fda.gov/drugs/labeling-information-drug-products/pregnancy-and-lactation-labeling-drugs-final-rule (accessed on 30 January 2020).

3. Lupattelli, A., Spigset, O., Twigg, M. J., Zagorodnikova, K., Mårdby, A. C., Moretti, M. E., Drozd, M., et al., (2014). Medication use in pregnancy: A cross-sectional, multinational web-based study. *BMJ Open, 4*(2), e004365.

4. Sedgh, G., Singh, S., & Hussain, R., (2014). Intended and unintended pregnancies worldwide in 2012 and recent trends. *Studies in Family Planning, 45*(3), 301–314.

5. Malm, H., Martikainen, J., Klaukka, T., & Neuvone, P. J., (2004). Prescription of hazardous drugs during pregnancy. *Drug Safety, 27*(12), 899–908.

6. Polifka, J. E., & Friedman, J. M., (2002). Medical genetics. 1. Clinical teratology in the age of genomics. *CMAJ, 167,* 265–273.

7. Schardein, J. L., (2000). *Chemically Induced Birth Defects* (3rd edn.). New York: Marcel Dekker.

8. Shepard, T. H., (2004). *Catalog of Teratogenic Agents* (11th edn.). Baltimore: Johns Hopkins University Press.

9. Jones, K. L., Lacro, R. V., Johnson, K. A., & Adams, J., (1989). Pattern of malformations in the children of women treated with carbamazepine during pregnancy. *New England Journal of Medicine, 320*(25), 1661–1666.

10. Little, B. B., Santos-Ramos, R., Newell, J. F., & Maberry, M. C., (1993). Megadose carbamazepine during embryogenesis. *Obstet. Gynecol., 82,* 705–708.

11. Addis, A., Sharabi, S., & Bonati, M., (2000). Risk classification systems for drug use during pregnancy. Are they a reliable source of information? *Drug Saf., 23,* 245–253.

12. Uhl, K., Kennedy, D. L., & Kweder, S. L., (2002). Risk management strategies in the Physicians' Desk Reference product labels for pregnancy category X drugs. *Drug Saf., 25,* 885–892.

13. U.S. Food and Drug Administration, (2018). *A Comparison of the Current Prescription Drug Labeling with the New PLLR Labeling Requirements [Internet].* Available from: https://www.fda.gov/vaccines-blood-biologics/biologics-rules/pregnancy-and-lactation-labeling-final-rule (accessed on 30 January 2020).
14. Robinson, A., Atallah, F., Weedon, J., Chen, Y. J., Apostol, R., & Minkoff, H., (2018). Effect of removal of pregnancy category on prescribing in pregnancy: A randomized [5op]. *Obstetrics and Gynecology, 131,* 2S.

# CHAPTER 2

# Anti-Infective Agents

## 2.1 ANTIBACTERIAL DRUGS

### 2.1.1 PENICILLINS

#### 2.1.1.1 PENICILLIN G, PROCAINE PENICILLIN G, AND BENZATHINE PENICILLIN G

**FDA Category: B**
***Risk Summary:*** The reproduction studies in animals have shown no evidence of fetal harm or impaired fertility. The pregnancy experience in humans is adequate to exhibit that the embryo-fetal risk is nonexistent or very low.

**Further Reading:**
- *Drug Information.* Bicillin, L. A. Wyeth-Ayerst Pharmaceuticals.
- *Drug Information.* Pfizerpen. Pfizer.
- Hutter, A., & Parks, J., (1945). The transmission of penicillin through the placenta. A preliminary report. *Am. J. Obstet. Gynecol., 49,* 663–665.
- Ravid, R., & Toaff, R., (1972). On the possible teratogenicity of antibiotic drugs administered during pregnancy: a prospective study. In: Klingberg, M., Abramovici, A., Chemki, J., (eds.), *Drugs and Fetal Development* (pp. 505–510). New York, NY: Plenum Press.

#### 2.1.1.2 NAFCILLIN

**FDA Category: B**
***Risk Summary:*** The reproduction studies in animals have shown no evidence of fetal harm or impaired fertility. The pregnancy experience in humans is adequate to exhibit that the embryo-fetal risk is nonexistent or very low.

**Further Reading:**
- Heinonen, O. P., Slone, D., & Shapiro, S., (1977). *Birth Defects and Drugs in Pregnancy*. Littleton, MA: Publishing Sciences Group.

## 2.1.1.3   OXACILLIN

**FDA Category: B**
***Risk Summary:*** The reproduction studies in animals have shown no evidence of fetal harm or impaired fertility. The pregnancy experience in humans is adequate to exhibit that the embryo-fetal risk is nonexistent or very low.

**Further Reading:**
- Czeizel, A. E., Rockenbauer, M., Sorensen, H. T., & Olsen, J., (1999). Teratogenic evaluation of oxacillin. *Scan. J. Infect Dis.*, *31*, 311, 312.
- Heinonen, O. P., Slone, D., & Shapiro, S., (1977). *Birth Defects and Drugs in Pregnancy*. Littleton, MA: Publishing Sciences Group.
- Prigot, A., Froix, C., & Rubin, E., (1962). Absorption, diffusion, and excretion of new penicillin, oxacillin. *Antimicrob. Agents Chemother.*, 402–410.

## 2.1.1.4   CLOXACILLIN

**FDA Category: B**
***Risk Summary:*** The pregnancy experience in humans is adequate to exhibit that the embryo-fetal risk is nonexistent or very low.

**Further Reading:**
- Heinonen, O. P., Slone, D., & Shapiro, S., (1977). *Birth Defects and Drugs in Pregnancy.* Littleton, MA: Publishing Sciences Group.

## 2.1.1.5   DICLOXACILLIN

**FDA Category: B**
***Risk Summary:*** The pregnancy experience in humans is adequate to exhibit that the embryo-fetal risk is nonexistent or very low.

**Further Reading:**
- Heinonen, O. P., Slone, D., & Shapiro, S., (1977). *Birth Defects and Drugs in Pregnancy.* Littleton, MA: Publishing Sciences Group.

## 2.1.1.6 *AMPICILLIN AND SULBACTAM/AMPICILLIN*

**FDA Category: B**
*Risk Summary:* The pregnancy experience in humans suggests risk in 1st Trimester. There is some indication that use of ampicillin during organogenesis is linked with oral clefts.

**Further Reading:**
- Czeizel, A. E., Rockenbauer, M., Sorensen, H. T., & Olsen, J., (2001). A population-based case-control teratologic study of ampicillin treatment during pregnancy. *Am. J. Obstet. Gynecol., 185*, 140–147.
- Rothman, K. J., Fyler, D. C., Goldblatt, A., & Kreidberg, M. B., (1979). Exogenous hormones and other drug exposures of children with congenital heart disease. *Am. J. Epidemiol., 109*, 433–439.
- Zierler, S., (1985). Maternal drugs and congenital heart disease. *Obstet. Gynecol., 65*, 155–165.

## 2.1.1.7 *AMOXICILLIN AND AMOXICILLIN/CLAVULANIC ACID*

**FDA Category: B**
*Risk Summary:* The pregnancy experience in humans suggests risk in 1st and 3rd Trimesters. There is some indication that use of amoxicillin during organogenesis is linked with oral clefts. Furthermore, one study reported a link between amoxicillin-clavulanic acid and necrotizing enterocolitis when the combination was used near preterm birth. Both of these associations need verification.

**Further Reading:**
- Berkovitch, M., Diav-Citrin, O., Greenberg, R., Cohen, M., Bulkowstein, M., Shechtman, S., Bortnik, O., Arnon, J., & Ornoy, A., (2004). First-trimester exposure to amoxicillin/clavulanic acid: A prospective, controlled study. *Br. J. Clin. Pharmacol., 58*, 298–302.
- *Drug Information*. Amoxil. SmithKline Beecham Pharmaceuticals.
- Lin, K. J., Mitchell, A. A., Yau, W. P., Louik, C., & Hernandez-Diaz, S., (2012). Maternal exposure to amoxicillin and the risk of oral clefts. *Epidemiology, 23*, 699–705.

## 2.1.1.8   CARBENICILLIN

**FDA Category: B**
*Risk Summary:* The reproduction studies in animals have shown no evidence of fetal harm or impaired fertility. The pregnancy experience in humans is adequate to exhibit that the embryo-fetal risk is nonexistent or very low.

**Further Reading:**
- *Drug Information.* Geocillin. Pfizer.
- Heinonen, O. P., Slone, D., & Shapiro, S., (1977). *Birth Defects and Drugs in Pregnancy.* Littleton, MA: Publishing Sciences Group.

## 2.1.1.9   PIPERACILLIN

**FDA Category: B**
*Risk Summary:* The reproduction studies in animals have shown no evidence of fetal harm or impaired fertility. The pregnancy experience in humans is adequate to exhibit that the embryo-fetal risk is nonexistent or very low.

**Further Reading:**
- *Drug Information.* Pipracil. Lederle Laboratories.
- Heikkilä, A., Erkkola, R., (1991). Pharmacokinetics of piperacillin during pregnancy. *J. Antimicrob. Chemother., 28*, 419–423.
- Lockwood, C. J., Costigan, K., Ghidini, A., Wein, R., Cetrulo, C., Alvarez, M., & Berkowitz, R. L., (1993). Double-blind, placebo-controlled trial of piperacillin sodium in preterm membrane rupture (abstract). *Am. J. Obstet. Gynecol., 168*, 378.

## 2.1.1.10   TICARCILLIN AND TICARCILLIN/CLAVULANIC ACID

**FDA Category: B**
*Risk Summary:* The reproduction studies in animals have shown no evidence of fetal harm or impaired fertility. The pregnancy experience in humans is adequate to exhibit that the embryo-fetal risk is nonexistent or very low.

**Further Reading:**
- *Drug Information.* Ticar. SmithKline Beecham Pharmaceuticals.

- Heinonen, O. P., Slone, D., & Shapiro, S., (1977). *Birth Defects and Drugs in Pregnancy*. Littleton, MA: Publishing Sciences Group.

## 2.1.2  CEPHALOSPORINS

### 2.1.2.1  CEFADROXIL (FIRST GENERATION)

**FDA Category: B**
*Risk Summary:* The reproduction studies in animals have shown no evidence of fetal harm or impaired fertility. The pregnancy experience in humans is adequate to exhibit that the embryo-fetal risk is nonexistent or very low.

**Further Reading:**
- Czeizel, A. E., Rockenbauer, M., Sorensen, H. T., & Olsen, J., (2001). Use of cephalosporins during pregnancy and in the presence of congenital abnormalities: A population-based, case-control study. *Am. J. Obstet. Gynecol., 184*, 1289–1296.
- *Drug Information*. Duricef. Bristol-Myers Squibb Company.
- Nathorst-Boos, J., Philipson, A., Hedman, A., & Arvisson, A., (1995). Renal elimination of ceftazidime during pregnancy. *Am. J. Obstet. Gynecol., 172*, 163–166.
- Takase, Z., Shirafuji, H., & Uchida, M., (1980). Experimental and clinical studies of cefadroxil in the treatment of infections in the field of obstetrics and gynecology. *Chemotherapy (Tokyo), 28*(2), 424–431.

### 2.1.2.2  CEFAZOLIN (FIRST GENERATION)

**FDA Category: B**
*Risk Summary:* The reproduction studies in animals have shown no evidence of fetal harm or impaired fertility. The pregnancy experience in humans is adequate to exhibit that the embryo-fetal risk is nonexistent or very low.

**Further Reading:**
- Cho, N., Ito, T., Saito, T., et al., (1970). Clinical studies on cefazolin in the field of obstetrics and gynecology. *Chemotherapy (Tokyo), 18*, 770–777.
- Czeizel, A. E., Rockenbauer, M., Sorensen, H. T., & Olsen, J., (2001). Use of cephalosporins during pregnancy and in the presence

of congenital abnormalities: A population-based, case-control study. *Am. J. Obstet. Gynecol., 184*, 1289–1296.
- *Drug Information*. Ancef. SmithKline Beecham Pharmaceuticals.
- Sanchez-Ramos, L., McAlpine, K. J., Adair, C. D., Kaunitz, A. M., Delke, I., & Briones, D. K., (1995). Pyelonephritis in pregnancy: Once-a-day ceftriaxone versus multiple doses of cefazolin. *Am. J. Obstet. Gynecol., 172*, 129–133.

## 2.1.2.3  CEPHALEXIN (FIRST GENERATION)

**FDA Category: B**
*Risk Summary:* The reproduction studies in animals have shown no evidence of fetal harm or impaired fertility. The pregnancy experience in humans is adequate to exhibit that the embryo-fetal risk is nonexistent or very low.

**Further Reading:**
- Campbell-Brown, M., & McFadyen, I. R., (1983). Bacteriuria in pregnancy treated with a single dose of cephalexin. *Br J. Obstet. Gynaecol., 90*, 1054–1059.
- Czeizel, A. E., Rockenbauer, M., Sorensen, H. T., & Olsen, J., (2001). Use of cephalosporins during pregnancy and in the presence of congenital abnormalities: A population-based, case-control study. *Am. J. Obstet. Gynecol., 184*, 1289–1296.
- *Drug Information*. Keflex. Dista Products.

## 2.1.2.4  CEFACLOR (SECOND GENERATION)

**FDA Category: B**
*Risk Summary:* The reproduction studies in animals have shown no evidence of fetal harm or impaired fertility. The pregnancy experience in humans is adequate to exhibit that the embryo-fetal risk is nonexistent or very low.

**Further Reading:**
- Czeizel, A. E., Rockenbauer, M., Sorensen, H. T., & Olsen, J., (2001). Use of cephalosporins during pregnancy and in the presence of congenital abnormalities: A population-based, case-control study. *Am. J. Obstet. Gynecol., 184*, 1289–1296.
- *Drug Information*. Ceclor. Eli Lilly and Company.

- Takase, Z., Shirafuji, H., & Uchida, M., (1979). Clinical and laboratory studies of cefaclor in the field of obstetrics and gynecology. *Chemotherapy (Tokyo), 27,* 666–672.

## 2.1.2.5  CEFOTETAN (SECOND GENERATION)

**FDA Category: B**
*Risk Summary:* The reproduction studies in animals have shown no evidence of fetal harm or impaired fertility. The pregnancy experience in humans is adequate to exhibit that the embryo-fetal risk is nonexistent or very low.

**Further Reading:**
- Czeizel, A. E., Rockenbauer, M., Sorensen, H. T., & Olsen, J., (2001). Use of cephalosporins during pregnancy and in the presence of congenital abnormalities: A population-based, case-control study. *Am. J. Obstet. Gynecol., 184,* 1289–1296.
- *Drug Information.* Cefotetan. Zeneca Pharmaceuticals.
- Takase, Z., Fujiwara, M., Kawamoto, Y., Seto, M., Shirafuji, H., & Uchida, M., (1982). Laboratory and clinical studies of cefotetan (YM09330) in the field of obstetrics and gynecology (English abstract). *Chemotherapy (Tokyo), 30*(1), 869–881.

## 2.1.2.6  CEFOXITIN (SECOND GENERATION)

**FDA Category: B**
*Risk Summary:* The reproduction studies in animals have shown no evidence of fetal harm or impaired fertility. The pregnancy experience in humans is adequate to exhibit that the embryo-fetal risk is nonexistent or very low.

**Further Reading:**
- Czeizel, A. E., Rockenbauer, M., Sorensen, H. T., & Olsen, J., (2001). Use of cephalosporins during pregnancy and in the presence of congenital abnormalities: A population-based, case-control study. *Am. J. Obstet. Gynecol., 184,* 1289–1296.
- *Drug Information.* Mefoxin. Merck & Company.
- Matsuda, S., Tanno, M., Kashiwakura, T., & Furuya, H., (1978). Laboratory and clinical studies on cefoxitin in the field of obstetrics and gynecology. *Chemotherapy (Tokyo), 26*(1), 460–467.

### 2.1.2.7  CEFPROZIL (SECOND GENERATION)

**FDA Category: B**

*Risk Summary:* The reproduction studies in animals have shown no evidence of fetal harm or impaired fertility. The pregnancy experience in humans is adequate to exhibit that the embryo-fetal risk is nonexistent or very low.

**Further Reading:**
- Czeizel, A. E., Rockenbauer, M., Sorensen, H. T., & Olsen, J., (2001). Use of cephalosporins during pregnancy and in the presence of congenital abnormalities: A population-based, case-control study. *Am. J. Obstet. Gynecol., 184*, 1289–1296.
- *Drug Information.* Cefzil. Bristol-Myers Squibb Company.

### 2.1.2.8  CEFUROXIME (SECOND GENERATION)

**FDA Category: B**

*Risk Summary:* The reproduction studies in animals have shown no evidence of fetal harm or impaired fertility. The pregnancy experience in humans is adequate to exhibit that the embryo-fetal risk is nonexistent or very low.

**Further Reading:**
- Bousfield, P., Browning, A. K., Mullinger, B. M., & Elstein, M., (1981). Cefuroxime: Potential use in pregnant women at term. *Br. J. Obstet. Gynaecol., 88*, 146–149.
- Czeizel, A. E., Rockenbauer, M., Sorensen, H. T., & Olsen, J., (2001). Use of cephalosporins during pregnancy and in the presence of congenital abnormalities: A population-based, case-control study. *Am. J. Obstet. Gynecol., 184*, 1289–1296.
- *Drug Information.* Ceftin. Glaxo Wellcome.
- Faro, S., Pastorek, J. G. II, Plauche, W. C., Korndorffer, F. A., & Aldridge, K. E., (1984). Short-course parenteral antibiotic therapy for pyelonephritis in pregnancy. *S. Med. J., 77*, 455–457.

### 2.1.2.9  CEFDINIR (THIRD GENERATION)

**FDA Category: B**

*Risk Summary:* The reproduction studies in animals have shown no evidence of fetal harm or impaired fertility. The pregnancy experience in humans is adequate to exhibit that the embryo-fetal risk is nonexistent or very low.

**Further Reading:**
- Czeizel, A. E., Rockenbauer, M., Sorensen, H. T., & Olsen, J., (2001). Use of cephalosporins during pregnancy and in the presence of congenital abnormalities: A population-based, case-control study. *Am. J. Obstet. Gynecol., 184*, 1289–1296.
- *Drug Information.* Omnicef. Abbott Laboratories.

### 2.1.2.10   CEFIXIME (THIRD GENERATION)

**FDA Category: B**
*Risk Summary:* The reproduction studies in animals have shown no evidence of fetal harm or impaired fertility. The pregnancy experience in humans is adequate to exhibit that the embryo-fetal risk is nonexistent or very low.

**Further Reading:**
- *Drug Information.* Suprax. Lupin Pharma.
- Kigozi, G. G., Brahmbhatt, H., Wabwire-Mangen, F., Wawer, M. J., Serwadda, D., Sewankambo, N., & Gray, R. H., (2003). Treatment of Trichomonas in pregnancy and adverse outcomes of pregnancy: A subanalysis of a randomized trial in Rakai, Uganda. *Am. J. Obstet. Gynecol., 189*, 1398–1400.
- Ramus, R. M., Sheffield, J. S., Mayfield, J. A., & Wendel, G. D. Jr., (2001). A randomized trial that compared oral cefixime and intramuscular ceftriaxone for the treatment of gonorrhea in pregnancy. *Am. J. Obstet. Gynecol., 185*, 629–632.

### 2.1.2.11   CEFOPERAZONE (THIRD GENERATION)

**FDA Category: B**
*Risk Summary:* The reproduction studies in animals have shown no evidence of fetal harm or impaired fertility. The pregnancy experience in humans is adequate to exhibit that the embryo-fetal risk is nonexistent or very low.

**Further Reading:**
- Chow, A. W., & Jewesson, P. J., (1985). Pharmacokinetics and safety of antimicrobial agents during pregnancy. *Reviews of Infectious Diseases, 7*(3), 287–313.

- Czeizel, A. E., Rockenbauer, M., Sorensen, H. T., & Olsen, J., (2001). Use of cephalosporins during pregnancy and in the presence of congenital abnormalities: A population-based, case-control study. *Am. J. Obstet. Gynecol., 184,* 1289–1296.
- Strausbaugh, L. J., & Llorens, A. S., (1983). Cefoperazone therapy for obstetric and gynecologic infections. *Rev. Infect. Dis., 5*(1), S154–S160.

## 2.1.2.12   CEFOTAXIME (THIRD GENERATION)

**FDA Category: B**
***Risk Summary:*** The reproduction studies in animals have shown no evidence of fetal harm or impaired fertility. The pregnancy experience in humans is adequate to exhibit that the embryo-fetal risk is nonexistent or very low.

**Further Reading:**
- Chow, A. W., & Jewesson, P. J., (1985). Pharmacokinetics and safety of antimicrobial agents during pregnancy. *Reviews of Infectious Diseases, 7*(3), 287–313.
- Czeizel, A. E, Rockenbauer, M., Sorensen, H. T., & Olsen, J., (2001). Use of cephalosporins during pregnancy and in the presence of congenital abnormalities: A population-based, case-control study. *Am. J. Obstet. Gynecol., 184,* 1289–1296.
- *Drug Information.* Claforan. Hoechst Marion Roussel.

## 2.1.2.13   CEFPODOXIME PROXETIL (THIRD GENERATION)

**FDA Category: B**
***Risk Summary:*** The reproduction studies in animals have shown no evidence of fetal harm or impaired fertility. The pregnancy experience in humans is adequate to exhibit that the embryo-fetal risk is nonexistent or very low.

**Further Reading:**
- Chow, A. W., & Jewesson, P. J., (1985). Pharmacokinetics and safety of antimicrobial agents during pregnancy. *Reviews of Infectious Diseases, 7*(3), 287–313.
- Czeizel, A. E., Rockenbauer, M., Sorensen, H. T., & Olsen, J., (2001). Use of cephalosporins during pregnancy and in the presence

of congenital abnormalities: A population-based, case-control study. *Am. J. Obstet. Gynecol., 184*, 1289–1296.
- *Drug Information*. Vantin. Pharmacia & Upjohn Company.


## 2.1.2.14   CEFTAZIDIME (THIRD GENERATION)

**FDA Category: B**
***Risk Summary:*** The reproduction studies in animals have shown no evidence of fetal harm or impaired fertility. The pregnancy experience in humans is adequate to exhibit that the embryo-fetal risk is nonexistent or very low.

**Further Reading:**
- Cho, N., Suzuki, H., Mitsukawa, M., Tamura, T., Yamaguchi, Y., Maruyama, M., Aoki, K., Fukunaga, K., & Kuni, K., (1983). Fundamental and clinical evaluation of ceftazidime in the field of obstetrics and gynecology (English abstract). *Chemotherapy (Tokyo), 31*(3), 772–782.
- Chow, A. W., & Jewesson, P. J., (1985). Pharmacokinetics and safety of antimicrobial agents during pregnancy. *Reviews of Infectious Diseases, 7*(3), 287–313.
- Czeizel, A. E., Rockenbauer, M., Sorensen, H. T., & Olsen, J., (2001). Use of cephalosporins during pregnancy and in the presence of congenital abnormalities: A population-based, case-control study. *Am. J. Obstet. Gynecol., 184*, 1289–1296.
- *Drug Information*. Fortaz. Glaxo Wellcome.


## 2.1.2.15   CEFTIBUTEN (THIRD GENERATION)

**FDA Category: B**
***Risk Summary:*** The reproduction studies in animals have shown no evidence of fetal harm or impaired fertility. The pregnancy experience in humans is adequate to exhibit that the embryo-fetal risk is nonexistent or very low.

**Further Reading:**
- Chow, A. W., & Jewesson, P. J., (1985). Pharmacokinetics and safety of antimicrobial agents during pregnancy. *Reviews of Infectious Diseases, 7*(3), 287–313.
- *Drug Information*. Cedax. Schering Corporation.

## 2.1.2.16  *CEFTIZOXIME (THIRD GENERATION)*

**FDA Category: B**
*Risk Summary:* The reproduction studies in animals have shown no evidence of fetal harm or impaired fertility. The pregnancy experience in humans is adequate to exhibit that the embryo-fetal risk is nonexistent or very low.

**Further Reading:**
- Blanco, J., Iams, J., Artal, R., Baker, D., Hibbard, J., McGregor, J., & Cetrulo, C., (1993). Multicenter double-blind prospective random trial of ceftizoxime vs. placebo in women with preterm premature ruptured membranes (PPROM). *Am. J. Obstet. Gynecol., 168,* 378.
- *Drug Information.* Cefizox. Fujisawa USA.

## 2.1.2.17  *CEFTRIAXONE (THIRD GENERATION)*

**FDA Category: B**
*Risk Summary:* The reproduction studies in animals have shown no evidence of fetal harm or impaired fertility. The pregnancy experience in humans is adequate to exhibit that the embryo-fetal risk is nonexistent or very low.

**Further Reading:**
- Chow, A. W., & Jewesson, P. J., (1985). Pharmacokinetics and safety of antimicrobial agents during pregnancy. *Reviews of Infectious Diseases, 7*(3), 287–313.
- Czeizel, A. E., Rockenbauer, M., Sorensen, H. T., & Olsen, J., (2001). Use of cephalosporins during pregnancy and in the presence of congenital abnormalities: A population-based, case-control study. *Am. J. Obstet. Gynecol., 184,* 1289–1296.
- *Drug Information.* Rocephin. Roche Laboratories.
- Sanchez-Ramos, L., McAlpine, K. J., Adair, C. D., Kaunitz, A. M., Delke, I., & Briones, D. K., (1995). Pyelonephritis in pregnancy: Once-a-day ceftriaxone versus multiple doses of cefazolin. *Am. J. Obstet. Gynecol., 172,* 129–133.

## 2.1.2.18  *CEFEPIME (FOURTH GENERATION)*

**FDA Category: B**
*Risk Summary:* The reproduction studies in animals have shown no evidence of fetal harm or impaired fertility. The pregnancy experience in humans is adequate to exhibit that the embryo-fetal risk is nonexistent or very low.

**Further Reading:**
- Chow, A. W., & Jewesson, P. J., (1985). Pharmacokinetics and safety of antimicrobial agents during pregnancy. *Reviews of Infectious Diseases, 7*(3), 287–313.
- Czeizel, A. E., Rockenbauer, M., Sorensen, H. T., & Olsen, J., (2001). Use of cephalosporins during pregnancy and in the presence of congenital abnormalities: A population-based, case-control study. *Am. J. Obstet. Gynecol., 184,* 1289–1296.
- *Drug Information.* Maxipime. Bristol-Myers Squibb Company.
- Ozyuncu, O., Nemutlu, E., Katlan, D., Kir, S., & Beksac, M. S., (2010). Maternal and fetal blood levels of moxifloxacin, levofloxacin, cefepime, and cefoperazone. *Int. J. Antimicrob. Agents, 36,* 175–178.

## 2.1.2.19 CEFTAROLINE FOSAMIL (FOURTH GENERATION)

**FDA Category: B**
*Risk Summary:* The reproduction studies in animals suggest a low risk. The pregnancy experience in humans is not available.

**Further Reading:**
- Chow, A. W., & Jewesson, P. J., (1985). Pharmacokinetics and safety of antimicrobial agents during pregnancy. *Reviews of Infectious Diseases, 7*(3), 287–313.
- Czeizel, A. E., Rockenbauer, M., Sorensen, H. T., & Olsen, J., (2001). Use of cephalosporins during pregnancy and in the presence of congenital abnormalities: A population-based, case-control study. *Am. J. Obstet. Gynecol., 184,* 1289–1296.
- *Drug Information.* Teflaro. Forest Pharmaceuticals.

## 2.1.3 CARBAPENEMS

### 2.1.3.1 IMIPENEM-CILASTATIN

**FDA Category: C**
*Risk Summary:* The reproduction studies in animals suggest a low risk. The pregnancy experience in humans is not available.

**Further Reading:**
- Cho, N., Fukunaga, K., Kunii, K., Kobayashi, I., & Tezuka, K., (1988). Studies on imipenem/cilastatin sodium in the perinatal period. *Jpn. J. Antibiot.*, *11*, 1758–1773.
- *Drug Information*. Primaxin. Merck & Co.
- Ryo, E., Ikeya, M., & Sugimoto, M., (2005). Clinical study of the effectiveness of imipenem/cilastatin sodium as the antibiotics of the first choice in the expectant management of patients with preterm premature rupture of membranes. *J. Infect. Chemother.*, *11*, 32–36.

### 2.1.3.2   MEROPENEM

**FDA Category: B**
***Risk Summary:*** The reproduction studies in animals suggest a low risk. The pregnancy experience in humans is not available.

**Further Reading:**
- *Drug Information*. Meropenem. APP Pharmaceuticals.
- Shea, K., Hilburger, E., Baroco, A., & Oldfield, E., (2008). Successful treatment of vancomycin-resistant Enterococcus faecium pyelonephritis with daptomycin during pregnancy. *Ann. Pharmacother.*, *42*, 722–725.
- Yoshida, M., Matsuda, H., & Furuya, K., (2013). Successful prognosis of brain abscess during pregnancy. *J. Reprod. Infertil.*, *14*, 152–155.

### 2.1.3.3   ERTAPENEM

**FDA Category: B**
***Risk Summary:*** The reproduction studies in animals showed mild fetal toxicity at a dose close to that used in human, however, these studies failed to show any teratogenicity in two animal species. The pregnancy experience in humans is not available.

**Further Reading:**
- *Drug Information*. Invanz. Merck & Company.

## 2.1.3.4   DORIPENEM

**FDA Category: B**
*Risk Summary:* The reproduction studies in animals showed no teratogenicity in two animal species. The pregnancy experience in humans is not available.

**Further Reading:**
- *Drug Information*. Doribax. Ortho-McNeil Pharmaceutical.

## 2.1.4   GLYCOPEPTIDES

### 2.1.4.1   VANCOMYCIN

**FDA Category: B**
*Risk Summary:* The pregnancy experience in humans is adequate to exhibit that the embryo-fetal risk is nonexistent or very low.

**Further Reading:**
- *Drug Information*. Vancocin. Eli Lilly.
- Gouyon, J. B., & Petion, A. M., (1990). Toxicity of vancomycin during pregnancy. *Am. J. Obstet. Gynecol., 163*, 1375–1376.
- Reyes, M. P., Ostrea, E. M. Jr., Cabinian, A. E., Schmitt, C., & Rintelmann, W., (1989). Vancomycin during pregnancy: Does it cause hearing loss or nephrotoxicity in the infant? *Am. J. Obstet. Gynecol., 161*, 977–981.

### 2.1.4.2   TEICOPLANIN

**FDA Category: C**
*Risk Summary:* The pregnancy experience in humans is inadequate for a risk assessment.

**Further Reading:**
- Peters, P. W., Miller, R. K., Schaefer, C., & Schaefer, C., (2015). *Drugs During Pregnancy and Lactation: Treatment Options and Risk Assessment* (3rd edn.). Academic Press.

### 2.1.4.3   TELAVANCIN

**FDA Category: C**
*Risk Summary:* No human data is available and the animal data suggest low risk.

**Further Reading:**
  • *Drug Information*. Vibativ. Astellas Pharma, U.S.A.


## 2.1.5   LIPOPEPTIDE

### 2.1.5.1   DAPTOMYCIN

**FDA Category: B**
*Risk Summary:* There is limited human data and the animal data suggest low risk

**Further Reading:**
  • Cunha, B. A., Hamid, N., Kessler, H., & Parchuri, S., (2005). Daptomycin cure after cefazolin treatment failure of methicillin-sensitive Staphylococcus aureus (MSSA) tricuspid valve acute bacterial endocarditis from a peripherally inserted central catheter (PICC) line. *Heart Lung, 34*, 442–447.
  • *Drug Information*. Cubicin. Cubist Pharmaceuticals.
  • Liu, S. L., Howard, L. C., Van Lier, R. B. L., & Markham, J. K., (1988). Teratology studies with daptomycin administered intravenously (IV) to rats and rabbits (abstract). *Teratology, 37*, 475.
  • Stroup, J. S., Wagner, J., & Badzinski, T., (2010). Use of daptomycin in a pregnant patient with *Staphylococcus aureus* endocarditis. *Ann. Pharmacother, 44*, 746–749.


## 2.1.6   MONOBACTAMS

### 2.1.6.1   AZTREONAM

**FDA Category: B**
*Risk Summary:* No human data is available and the animal data suggest low risk

**Further Reading:**
- Cho, N., Fukunaga, K., Kunii, K., & Kobayashi, I., (1990). Studies on aztreonam in the perinatal period. *Jpn. J. Antibiot.*, *43*,706–718.
- Furuhashi, T., Ushida, K., Kakei, A., & Nakayoshi, H., (1985). Toxicity study on azthreonam: Perinatal and postnatal study in rats. *Chemotherapy*, *33*, 219–231. As cited in Shepard, T. H., (1989). *Catalog of Teratogenic Agents* (6ᵗʰ edn., p. 66). Baltimore, MD: Johns Hopkins University Press.
- Furuhashi, T., Ushida, K., Sato, K., & Nakayoshi, H., (1985). Toxicity study on azthreonam: Teratology study in rats. *Chemotherapy*, *33*, 203–218. As cited in Shepard, T. H., (1989). *Catalog of Teratogenic Agents* (6ᵗʰ edn., p. 66). Baltimore, MD: Johns Hopkins University Press.

## 2.1.7 FOSFOMYCIN

**FDA Category: B**
*Risk Summary:* The reproduction studies in animals have shown no evidence of fetal harm or impaired fertility. The pregnancy experience in humans is adequate to exhibit that the embryo-fetal risk is nonexistent or very low.

**Further Reading:**
- Falagas, M. E., Vouloumanou, E. K., Togias, A. G., Karadima, M., Kapaskelis, A. M., Rafailidis, P. I., & Athanasiou, S. (2010). Fosfomycin versus other antibiotics for the treatment of cystitis: a meta-analysis of randomized controlled trials. *Journal of Antimicrobial Chemotherapy*, *65*(9), 1862–1877.
- *Drug Information*. Monurol. Forest Laboratories.
- Keating, G. M. (1994). Fosfomycin trometamol single-dose in the treatment of uncomplicated urinary tract infections in cardiac pregnant or nonpregnant women: A controlled study. *J. Bras Ginec, 104*, 345–351.

## 2.1.8 TETRACYCLINES

This group of antibiotics includes tetracycline, minocycline, doxycycline, oxytetracycline, and demeclocycline, and tigecycline.

**FDA Category: D**
*Risk Summary:* They are contraindicated in the 2nd and 3rd Trimesters. They are contraindicated after the 15th week of gestation due to their interference with the bone mineralization of the foetus.

**Further Reading:**
- Cohlan, S. Q., Bevelander, G., & Bross, S., (1961). Effect of tetracycline on bone growth in premature infant. *Antimicrob Agents Chemother*, 340–347.
- Czeizel, A. E., & Rockenbauer, M., (1997). Teratogenic study of doxycycline. *Obstet. Gynecol., 89*, 524–528.
- Czeizel, A. E., & Rockenbauer, M., (2000). A population-based case-control teratologic study of oral oxytetracycline treatment during pregnancy. *Eur. J. Obstet. Gynecol Reprod Biol, 88*, 27–33.
- Douglas, A. C., (1963). The deposition of tetracycline in human nails and teeth: A complication of long term treatment. *Br. J. Dis. Chest, 57*, 44–47.
- *Drug Information.* Tygacil. Wyeth Pharmaceuticals.
- Hunt, M. J., Salisbury, E. L. C., Grace, J., & Armati, R., (1996). Black breast milk due to minocycline therapy. *Br. J. Dermatol, 134*, 943–944.
- Pride, G. L., Cleary, R. E., & Hamburger, R. J., (1973). Disseminated intravascular coagulation associated with tetracycline-induced hepatorenal failure during pregnancy. *Am. J. Obstet. Gynecol., 115*, 585–586.

### 2.1.9   MACROLIDES

### 2.1.9.1   ERYTHROMYCIN

**FDA Category: B (Excluding the Estolate Salt)**
*Risk Summary:* The reproduction studies in animals have shown no evidence of fetal harm or impaired fertility. The pregnancy experience in humans is adequate to exhibit that the embryo-fetal risk is nonexistent or very low. The estolate salt of erythromycin has been identified to induce hepatotoxicity in the pregnant patients.

**Further Reading:**
- Czeizel, A. E., Rockenbauer, M., Sørensen, H. T., & Olsen, J., (1999). A population-based case-control teratologic study of oral erythromycin treatment during pregnancy. *Repro Toxicol, 13*, 531–536.
- *Drug Information*. Ery-Tab. Abbott Laboratories.
- Fenton, L. J., & Light, L. J., (1976). Congenital syphilis after maternal treatment with erythromycin. *Obstet. Gynecol., 47*, 492–494.
- McCormack, W. M., George, H., Donner, A., Kodgis, L. F., Albert, S., Lowe, E. W., & Kass, E. H., (1977). Hepatotoxicity of erythromycin estolate during pregnancy. *Antimicrob Agents Chemother, 12*, 630–635.
- Sorensen, H. T., Skriver, M. V., Pedersen, L., Larsen, H., Ebbesen, F., & Schonheyder, H. C., (2003). Risk of infantile hypertrophic pyloric stenosis after maternal postnatal use of macrolides. *Scand J. Infect. Dis., 35*, 104–106.

## 2.1.9.2 CLARITHROMYCIN

**FDA Category: C**
***Risk Summary:*** The animal reproduction information propose great risk, nevertheless the existing human pregnancy experience proposes that the risk is low.

**Further Reading:**
- Andersen, J. T., Petersen, M., Jimenez-Solem, E., Broedbaek, K., Andersen, N. L., Torp-Pedersen, C., Keiding, N., & Poulsen, H. E., (2013). Clarithromycin in early pregnancy and the risk of miscarriage and malformation: A register-based nationwide cohort study. *PLoS One, 8*, e53327. doi: 10.1371/journal.pone.0053327. Epub 2013 Jan 2.
- *Drug Information*. Biaxin. Abbott Laboratories.
- Escobar, L. F., & Weaver, D. D., (1990). Charge association. In: Buyse, M. L., (ed.), *Birth Defects Encyclopedia* (Vol. 1, pp. 308–309). Dover, MA: Center for Birth Defects Information Services.
- Schick, B., Hom, M., Librizzi, R., & Donnenfeld, A., (1996). Pregnancy outcome following exposure to clarithromycin (abstract). Abstracts of the Ninth International Conference of the Organization of Teratology Information Services, Salt Lake City, Utah. *Reprod Toxicol, 10*, 162.

## 2.1.9.3    AZITHROMYCIN

**FDA Category: B**
*Risk Summary:* The reproduction studies in animals have shown no evidence
of fetal harm or impaired fertility. The pregnancy experience in humans is
adequate to exhibit that the embryo-fetal risk is nonexistent or very low.

**Further Reading:**
- Bar-Oz, B., Weber-Schoendorfer, C., Berlin, M., Clementi, M., Di
  Gianantonio, D., De Vries, L., et al., (2012). The outcomes of preg-
  nancy in women exposed to the new macrolides in the first trimester: A
  prospective, multicentre, observations study. *Drug Saf.*, *35*, 589–598.
- *Drug Information.* Zithromax. Pfizer Labs.
- Edwards, M., Rainwater, K., Carter, S., Williamson, F., & Newman,
  R., (1994). Comparison of azithromycin and erythromycin for Chla-
  mydia cervicitis in pregnancy (abstract). *Am. J. Obstet. Gynecol.,*
  *170*, 419.

## 2.1.9.4    TELITHROMYCIN

**FDA Category: C**
*Risk Summary:* No human data is available and the reproduction studies in
animals have shown low risk.

**Further Reading:**
- *Drug Information.* Ketek. Sanofi-Aventis U.S.
- Ross, D. B., (2007). The FDA and the case of Ketek. *N. Engl. J. Med.,*
  *356*, 1601–1604.

## 2.1.10    LINCOSAMIDE

## 2.1.10.1    CLINDAMYCIN

**FDA Category: B**
*Risk Summary:* The reproduction studies in animals have shown no
evidence of fetal harm or impaired fertility. The pregnancy experience in
humans is adequate to exhibit that the embryo-fetal risk is nonexistent or
very low.

**Further Reading:**
- *Drug Information*. Cleocin. Pharmacia & Upjohn.
- Rehu, M., & Jahkola, M., (1980). Prophylactic antibiotics in cesarean section: Effect of a short preoperative course of benzylpenicillin or clindamycin plus gentamicin on postoperative infectious morbidity. *Ann. Clin. Res.*, *12*, 45–48.

## 2.1.10.2   LINCOMYCIN

**FDA Category: C**
*Risk Summary:* The reproduction studies in animals have shown no evidence of fetal harm or impaired fertility. The pregnancy experience in humans is adequate to exhibit that the embryo-fetal risk is nonexistent or very low.

**Further Reading:**
- Duignan, N. M., Andrews, J., & Williams, J. D., (1973). Pharmacological studies with lincomycin in late pregnancy. *Br. Med. J., 3*, 75–78.
- Medina, A., Fiske, N., Hjelt-Harvey, I., Brown, C. D., & Prigot, A., (1963). Absorption, diffusion, and excretion of a new antibiotic, lincomycin. *Antimicrob Agents Chemother*, 189–196.
- Mickal, A., & Panzer, J. D., (1975). The safety of lincomycin in pregnancy. *Am. J. Obstet. Gynecol., 121*, 1071–1074.

## 2.1.11   STREPTOGRAMINS

### 2.1.11.1   QUINUPRISTIN-DALFOPRISTIN

**FDA Category: B**
*Risk Summary:* The reproduction studies in animals have shown no evidence of fetal harm or impaired fertility. The pregnancy experience in humans is limited. Since the indication for the combination encompasses probably life-threatening infections, the maternal benefit of the therapy appears to prevail over the unknown fetal or embryo risk.

**Further Reading:**
- Bergeron, M., & Montay, G., (1997). The pharmacokinetics of quinupristin/dalfopristin in laboratory animals and in humans. *J. Antimicrob Chemother*, *39*(A), 129–138.

• *Drug Information*. Synercid. Aventis Pharmaceuticals.

### 2.1.12   OXAZOLIDINONES

#### 2.1.12.1   LINEZOLID

**FDA Category: C**
***Risk Summary:*** The reproduction studies in animals have shown evidence of fetal toxicity, however, no teratogenicity was observed. The pregnancy experience in humans is not available. It should be used when there is no safer alternative.

**Further Reading:**
• *Drug Information*. Zyvox. Pharmacia & Upjohn.

#### 2.1.12.2   TEDIZOLID PHOSPHATE

**FDA Category: C**
***Risk Summary:*** The reproduction studies in animals have shown evidence of fetal toxicity, however, no teratogenicity was observed. The pregnancy experience in humans is not available. It should be used when there is no safer alternative.

**Further Reading:**
• Cada, D. J., Ingram, K., & Baker, D. E., (2014). Tedizolid phosphate. *Hospital Pharmacy*, *49*(10), 961–971. doi: 10.1310/hpj4910-961.

### 2.1.13   AMINOGLYCOSIDES

#### 2.1.13.1   GENTAMYCIN

**FDA Category: D**
***Risk Summary:*** Human pregnancy experience suggests low risk. However, it should only be used parenterally in serious infections caused by difficult gram-negative pathogens, and when first-choice antibiotics fail.

**Further Reading:**
• Czeizel, A. E., Rockenbauer, M., Olsen, J., & Sorensen, H. T., (2000). A teratological study of aminoglycoside antibiotic treatment during pregnancy. *Scand J. Infect. Dis.*, *32*, 309–313.

- *Drug Information*. Garamycin. Schering.
- Hulton, S. A., & Kaplan, B. S., (1995). Renal dysplasia associated with in utero exposure to gentamicin and corticosteroids. *Am. J. Med Genet*, *58*, 91–93.
- Smaoui, H., Mallie, J. P., Schaeverbeke, M., Robert, A., & Schaeverbeke, J., (1993). Gentamicin administered during gestation alters glomerular basement membrane development. *Antimicrob Agents Chemother*, *37*, 1510–1517.

## 2.1.13.2   AMIKACIN

**FDA Category: D**
***Risk Summary:*** Human pregnancy experience suggests low risk. However, it should only be used parenterally in serious infections caused by difficult gram-negative pathogens, and when first-choice antibiotics fail.

**Further Reading:**
- Bernard, B., Abate, M., Thielen, P., Attar, H., Ballard, C., & Wehrle, P., (1977). Maternal–fetal pharmacological activity of amikacin. *J. Infect. Dis., 135*, 925–931.
- *Drug Information*. Amikacin. Elkins-Sinn.
- Mallie, J. P., Coulon, G., Billerey, C., Faucourt, A., & Morin, J. P., (1988). In utero aminoglycosides-induced nephrotoxicity in rat neonates. *Kidney Inter, 33*, 36–44.

## 2.1.13.3   KANAMYCIN

**FDA Category: D**
***Risk Summary:*** Human pregnancy experience suggests Eighth cranial nerve damage following in utero exposure to kanamycin. It should only be used parenterally in serious infections caused by difficult gram-negative pathogens, and when first-choice antibiotics fail.

**Further Reading:**
- Jones, H. C., (1973). Intrauterine ototoxicity. A case report and review of literature. *J. Natl. Med. Assoc., 65*, 201–203.
- Nishimura, H., & Tanimura, T., (1976). *Clinical Aspects of the Teratogenicity of Drugs* (p. 131). New York, NY: American Elsevier.

## 2.1.13.4   STREPTOMYCIN

**FDA Category: D**

***Risk Summary:*** Human pregnancy experience suggests fetal ototoxicity and deafness in newborns. It should only be used parenterally in serious infections caused by difficult gram-negative pathogens, and when first-choice antibiotics fail.

**Further Reading:**
- Czeizel, A. E., Rockenbauer, M., Olsen, J., & Sorensen, H. T., (2000). A teratological study of aminoglycoside antibiotic treatment during pregnancy. *Scand J. Infect. Dis., 32*, 309–313.
- Donald, P. R., & Sellars, S. L., (1981). Streptomycin ototoxicity in the unborn child. *S. Afr. Med. J., 60*, 316–318.

## 2.1.13.5   PAROMOMYCIN

**FDA Category: N**

***Risk Summary:*** The pregnancy experience in humans is limited. However, Paromomycin is poorly absorbed, with nearly 100% of an orally given dose excreted unchanged in the feces, minute if any of the drugs will reach the fetus.

**Further Reading:**
- D'Alauro, F., Lee, R. V., Pao-In, K., & Khairallah, M., (1985). Intestinal parasites and pregnancy. *Obstet. Gynecol., 66*, 639–643.
- Kreutner, A. K., Del Bene, V. E., & Amstey, M. S., (1981). Giardiasis in pregnancy. *Am. J. Obstet. Gynecol., 140*, 895–901.

## 2.1.13.6   NEOMYCIN

**FDA Category: D**

***Risk Summary:*** Human pregnancy experience suggests Eighth cranial nerve damage following in utero exposure to Neomycin. It should only be used parenterally in serious infections caused by difficult gram-negative pathogens, and when first-choice antibiotics fail.

**Further Reading:**
- Czeizel, A. E., Rockenbauer, M., Olsen, J., & Sorensen, H. T., (2000). A teratological study of aminoglycoside antibiotic treatment during pregnancy. *Scand J. Infect. Dis., 32*, 309–313.
- Heinonen, O. P., Slone, D., & Shapiro, S., (1977). *Birth Defects and Drugs in Pregnancy* (pp. 297–301). Littleton, MA: Publishing Sciences Group.

## 2.1.14  SULFONAMIDES

**FDA Category (1ˢᵗ & 2ⁿᵈ Trimesters): C**

**FDA Category (3ʳᵈ Trimester): D**

*Risk Summary:* Taken all together, sulfonamides do not seem to pose a major teratogenic risk. One study has uncovered links with birth defects, but a causative link cannot be determined with this kind of study and they may have been caused by other factors, mainly if trimethoprim was used along with the sulfonamide. Verification is needed. Due to the possible toxicity to the newborn, sulfonamides must be avoided in the 3rd Trimester.

**Further Reading:**
- Crider, K. S., Cleves, M. A., Reefhuis, J., Berry, R. J., Hobbs, C. A., & Hu, D. J., (2009). Antibacterial medication use during pregnancy and risk of birth defects. *Arch. Pediatr. Adolesc. Med., 163*, 978–985.
- Dunn, P. M., (1964). The possible relationship between the maternal administration of sulphamethoxypyridazine and hyperbilirubinemia in the newborn. *J. Obstet. Gynaecol Br Commonw, 71*, 128–131.
- Ito, S., Blajchman, A., Stephenson, M., Eliopoulos, C., & Koren, G., Prospective follow-up of adverse reactions in breast-fed infants exposed to maternal medication. *Am. J. Obstet. Gynecol., 168*, 1393–1399.
- Lucey, J. F., & Driscoll, T. J. Jr., (1959). Hazard to newborn infants of administration of long-acting sulfonamides to pregnant women. *Pediatrics, 24*, 498–499.

## 2.1.14.1  TRIMETHOPRIM AND TRIMETHOPRIM/SULFAMETHOXAZOLE

**FDA Category: D**

*Risk Summary:* The pregnancy experience in humans and the reproduction studies in animals have shown that Trimethoprim is teratogenic. However, there is an opinion of giving Folate, concomitantly with Trimethoprim, to mitigate the expected harmful effects.

**Further Reading:**
- Czeizel, A. E., Rockenbauer, M., Sorensen, H. T., & Olsen, J., (2001). The teratogenic risk of trimethoprim-sulfonamides: A population-based case-control study. *Reprod Toxicol, 15,* 637–646.
- *Drug Information.* Septra. Monarch Pharmaceuticals.
- Hernandez-Diaz, S., Werler, M. M., Walker, A. M., & Mitchell, A. A., (2000). Folic acid antagonists during pregnancy and the risk of birth defects. *N. Engl. J. Med., 343,* 1608–1614.

### 2.1.15   *NITROFURANTOIN*

**FDA Category (1st & 2nd Trimesters): B**

**FDA Category (3rd Trimester): C\***

*Risk Summary:* Nitrofurantoin has been found, generally, safe during the 1st and 2nd trimesters; however, the pregnancy experience in humans suggests the risk of hemolytic anemia in newborns that are exposed in-utero to nitrofurantoin in the late days of the 3rd Trimester.

**Further Reading:**
- Bruel, H., Guillemant, V., Saladin-Thiron, C., Chabrolle, J. P., Lahary, A., Poinsot, J., (2000). Hemolytic anemia in a newborn after maternal treatment with nitrofurantoin at the end of pregnancy. *Arch Pediatr, 7,* 745–747.
- Crider, K. S., Cleves, M. A., Reefhuis, J., Berry, R. J., Hobbs, C. A., & Hu, D. J., (2009). Antibacterial medication use during pregnancy and risk of birth defects. *Arch Pediatr. Adolesc. Med., 163,* 978–985.
- *Drug Information,* (2001). Macrodantin. Procter & Gamble Pharmaceuticals.
- Powell, R. D., DeGowin, R. L., & Alving, A. S., (1963). Nitrofurantoin-induced hemolysis. *J. Lab Clin. Med., 62,* 1002–1003.

\*It is the author's opinion regarding the most accurate, possible, classification of Nitrofurantoin during the 3rd Trimester—it is not an official FDA classification.

## 2.1.16 QUINOLONES

### 2.1.16.1 NALIDIXIC ACID

**FDA Category: C**
*Risk Summary:* The reproduction studies in animals have shown teratogenic and embryocidal effects for Nalidixic Acid. The pregnancy experience in humans is limited; however, one significant case-control study shed a light on the association between the intake of Nalidixic Acid in the 3rd Trimester and the increased prevalence of pyloric stenosis in the newborns.

**Further Reading:**
- Belton, E. M., & Jones, R. V., (1965). Hemolytic anemia due to nalidixic acid. *Lancet, 2,* 691.
- Czeizel, A. E., Sorensen, H. T., Rockenbauer, M., & Olsen, J., (2001). A population-based case-control teratologic study of nalidixic acid. *Int. J. Gynaecol Obstet, 73,* 221–228.
- *Drug Information.* NegGram. Sanofi Winthrop Pharmaceuticals.

### 2.1.16.2 NORFLOXACIN

**FDA Category: C**
*Risk Summary:* The pregnancy experience in humans suggests low risk; however, the authors of one study recommended avoid giving Norfloxacin during pregnancy because safer alternatives are generally available. However, fluoroquinolones are commonly avoided in the perinatal period because of fears from fetal cartilage damage.

**Further Reading:**
- *Drug Information.* Noroxin. Merck & Company.
- Norrby, S. R., & Lietman, P. S., (1993). Safety and tolerability of fluoroquinolones. *Drugs, 45*(Suppl 3), 59–64.
- Pastuszak, A., Andreou, R., Schick, B., Sage, S., Cook, L., Donnenfeld, A., & Koren, G., (1995). New postmarketing surveillance data supports a lack of association between quinolone use in pregnancy and fetal and neonatal complications. *Reprod Toxicol, 9,* 584.
- Schaefer, C., Amoura-Elefant, E., Vial, T., Ornoy, A., Garbis, H., Robert, E., Rodriguez-Pinilla, E., Pexieder, T., Prapas, N., & Merlob, P., (1996). Pregnancy outcome after prenatal quinolone exposure. Evaluation of a case registry of the European Network of Teratology

Information Services (ENTIS). *Eur. J. Obstet. Gynecol Reprod. Biol.,* *69*, 83–89.

## 2.1.16.3   *CIPROFLOXACIN*

**FDA Category: C**

*Risk Summary:* The pregnancy experience in humans suggests low risk; however, the authors of one study recommended avoid giving Ciprofloxacin during pregnancy because safer alternatives are generally available. However, fluoroquinolones are commonly avoided in the perinatal period because of fears from fetal cartilage damage.

**Further Reading:**
  - *Drug Information*. Cipro. Miles Pharmaceutical.
  - Norrby, S. R., & Lietman, P. S., (1993). Safety and tolerability of fluoroquinolones. *Drugs, 45*(Suppl 3), 59–64.
  - Schaefer, C., Amoura-Elefant, E., Vial, T., Ornoy, A., Garbis, H., Robert, E., Rodriguez-Pinilla, E., Pexieder, T., Prapas, N., & Merlob, P., (1996). Pregnancy outcome after prenatal quinolone exposure. Evaluation of a case registry of the European Network of Teratology Information Services (ENTIS). *Eur, J, Obstet. Gynecol Reprod Biol., 69*, 83–89.

## 2.1.16.4   *OFLOXACIN*

**FDA Category: C**

*Risk Summary:* The pregnancy experience in humans suggests low risk; however, the authors of one study recommended avoid giving Ofloxacin during pregnancy because safer alternatives are generally available. However, fluoroquinolones are commonly avoided in the perinatal period because of fears from fetal cartilage damage.

**Further Reading:**
  - *Drug Information*. Floxin. Ortho-McNeil Pharmaceutica.
  - Norrby, S. R., & Lietman, P. S., (1993). Safety and tolerability of fluoroquinolones. *Drugs, 45*(Suppl 3), 59–64.
  - Schaefer, C., Amoura-Elefant, E., Vial, T., Ornoy, A., Garbis, H., Robert, E., Rodriguez-Pinilla, E., Pexieder, T., Prapas, N., & Merlob, P., (1996). Pregnancy outcome after prenatal quinolone exposure. Evaluation of a case registry of the European Network of Teratology

Information Services (ENTIS). *Eur. J. Obstet. Gynecol Reprod Biol.,* *69*, 83–89.

## 2.1.16.5  LOMEFLOXACIN

**FDA Category: C**
*Risk Summary:* The pregnancy experience in humans suggests low risk; however, the authors of one study recommended avoid giving Lomefloxacin during pregnancy because safer alternatives are generally available. However, fluoroquinolones are commonly avoided in the perinatal period because of fears from fetal cartilage damage.

**Further Reading:**
- *Drug Information.* Maxaquin. G.D. Searle.
- Norrby, S. R., & Lietman, P. S., (1993). Safety and tolerability of fluoroquinolones. *Drugs, 45*(Suppl 3), 59–64.
- Schaefer, C., Amoura-Elefant, E., Vial, T., Ornoy, A., Garbis, H., Robert, E., Rodriguez-Pinilla, E., Pexieder, T., Prapas, N., & Merlob, P., (1996). Pregnancy outcome after prenatal quinolone exposure. Evaluation of a case registry of the European Network of Teratology Information Services (ENTIS). *Eur. J. Obstet. Gynecol Reprod Biol., 69*, 83–89.

## 2.1.16.6  LEVOFLOXACIN

**FDA Category: C**
*Risk Summary:* The pregnancy experience in humans suggests low risk; however, the authors of one study recommended avoid giving Levofloxacin during pregnancy because safer alternatives are generally available. However, fluoroquinolones are commonly avoided in the perinatal period because of fears from fetal cartilage damage.

**Further Reading:**
- *Drug Information.* Levaquin. Ortho-McNeil Pharmaceutical.
- Meaney-Delman, D., Rasmussen, S. A., Beigi, R. H., Zotti, M. E., Hutchings, Y., Bower, W. A., Treadwell, T. A., & Jamieson, D. J., (2013). Prophylaxis and treatment of anthrax in pregnant women. *Obstet. Gynecol., 122*, 885–900.

- Norrby, S. R., & Lietman, P. S., (1993). Safety and tolerability of fluoroquinolones. *Drugs, 45*(Suppl 3), 59–64.
- Schaefer, C., Amoura-Elefant, E., Vial, T., Ornoy, A., Garbis, H., Robert, E., Rodriguez-Pinilla, E., Pexieder, T., Prapas, N., & Merlob, P., (1996). Pregnancy outcome after prenatal quinolone exposure. Evaluation of a case registry of the European Network of Teratology Information Services (ENTIS). *Eur. J. Obstet. Gynecol Reprod Biol., 69*, 83–89.

## 2.1.16.7   MOXIFLOXACIN

**FDA Category: C**
***Risk Summary:*** The pregnancy experience in humans suggests low risk; however, the authors of one study recommended avoid giving Moxifloxacin during pregnancy because safer alternatives are generally available. However, fluoroquinolones are commonly avoided in the perinatal period because of fears from fetal cartilage damage.

**Further Reading:**
- *Drug Information*. Avelox. Schering Plough.
- Meaney-Delman, D., Rasmussen, S. A., Beigi, R. H., Zotti, M. E., Hutchings, Y., Bower, W. A., Treadwell, T. A., & Jamieson, D. J., (2013). Prophylaxis and treatment of anthrax in pregnant women. *Obstet. Gynecol., 122*, 885–900.
- Schaefer, C., Amoura-Elefant, E., Vial, T., Ornoy, A., Garbis, H., Robert, E., Rodriguez-Pinilla, E., Pexieder, T., Prapas, N., & Merlob, P., (1996). Pregnancy outcome after prenatal quinolone exposure. Evaluation of a case registry of the European Network of Teratology Information Services (ENTIS). *Eur. J. Obstet. Gynecol Reprod Biol., 69*, 83–89.

## 2.1.17   CHLORAMPHENICOL

**FDA Category: C**
***Risk Summary:*** One report suggested an association between near term administration of Chloramphenicol and the incidence of gray baby syndrome. Therefore, it is recommended to avoid Chloramphenicol at term.

## Further Reading:

- Oberheuser, F., (1971). Praktische Erfahrungen mit Medikamenten in der Schwangerschaft. *Therapie Woche, 31*, 2200. As reported in Manten A. Antibiotic drugs. In: Dukes, M. N. G., (ed.), *Meyler's Side Effects of Drugs* (Vol. VIII, p. 604). New York, NY: American Elsevier, 1975.
- Schwarz, R. H., & Crombleholme, W. R., (1979). Antibiotics in pregnancy. *South Med. J., 72*, 1315–1318.
- Weiss, C. V., Glazko, A. J., & Weston, J. K., (1960). Chloramphenicol in the newborn infant. A physiologic explanation of its toxicity when given in excessive doses. *N. Engl. J. Med., 262*, 787–794.

## 2.2    ANTI-MYCOBACTERIAL DRUGS

### *2.2.1    ISONIAZID*

**FDA Category: C**
***Risk Summary:*** The American Thoracic Society advises the use of the appropriate anti-mycobacterial agents for tuberculosis happening during pregnancy because keeping tuberculosis without treatment is much hazardous for the pregnant mother and the baby than giving the appropriate anti-mycobacterial drugs.

## Further Reading:

- American Thoracic Society (1986). Treatment of tuberculosis and tuberculosis infection in adults and children. *Am. Rev. Respir Dis., 134*, 355–363.
- *Drug Information*. Rifamate. Hoechst Marion Roussel.
- Keskin, N., & Yilmaz, S., (2008). Pregnancy and tuberculosis: To assess tuberculosis cases in pregnancy in a developing region retrospectively and two case reports. *Arch Gynecol Obstet, 278*, 451–455.
- Kingdom, J. C. P., & Kennedy, D. H., (1989). Tuberculous meningitis in pregnancy. *Br. J. Obstet. Gynaecol, 96*, 233–235.

### *2.2.2    RIFAMPIN*

**FDA Category: C**
***Risk Summary:*** The reproduction studies in animals have shown no evidence of fetal harm or impaired fertility. The pregnancy experience in humans is

adequate to exhibit that the embryo-fetal risk is nonexistent or very low. It is noteworthy to mention that one study has recommended a prophylactic vitamin K administration to pregnant women given Rifampin for treating tuberculosis.

**Further Reading:**
- American Thoracic Society (1986). Treatment of tuberculosis and tuberculosis infection in adults and children. *Am. Rev. Respir Dis., 134*, 355–363.
- *Drug Information*. Rifadin. Hoechst Marion Roussel.
- Keskin, N., & Yilmaz, S., (2008). Pregnancy and tuberculosis: To assess tuberculosis cases in pregnancy in a developing region retrospectively and two case reports. *Arch Gynecol Obstet, 278,* 451–455.
- Medchill, M. T., & Gillum, M., (1989). Diagnosis and management of tuberculosis during pregnancy. *Obstet. Gynecol Surv.*, *44,* 81–84.

### 2.2.3   PYRAZINAMIDE

**FDA Category: C**
*Risk Summary:* Although there is limited data from the human pregnancy experience, but the expected maternal benefit extremely outweighs the unknown or known embryo/fetal risk.

**Further Reading:**
- API Consensus Expert Committee (2006). API TB consensus guidelines 2006: Management of pulmonary tuberculosis, extra-pulmonary tuberculosis, and tuberculosis in special situations. *J. Assoc. Physicians India, 54,* 219–234.
- Jana, N., Vasishta, K., Saha, S. C., & Ghosh, K., (1999). Obstetrical outcomes among women with extrapulmonary tuberculosis. *N. Engl. J. Med., 341,* 645–649.
- Keskin, N., & Yilmaz, S., (2008). Pregnancy and tuberculosis: To assess tuberculosis cases in pregnancy in a developing region retrospectively and two case reports. *Arch Gynecol Obstet, 278,* 451–455.

### 2.2.4   ETHAMBUTOL

**FDA Category: B**
*Risk Summary:* The reproduction studies in animals have shown no evidence of fetal harm or impaired fertility. The pregnancy experience in humans is adequate to exhibit that the embryo-fetal risk is nonexistent or very low.

**Further Reading:**
- Bobrowitz, I. D., (1974). Ethambutol in pregnancy. *Chest, 66,* 20–24.
- Brock, P. G., & Roach, M., (1981). Antituberculous drugs in pregnancy. *Lancet, 1,* 43.
- Kingdom, J. C. P., & Kennedy, D. H., (1989). Tuberculous meningitis in pregnancy. *Br. J. Obstet. Gynaecol, 96,* 233–235.
- Lewit, T., Nebel, L., Terracina, S., & Karman, S., (1974). Ethambutol in pregnancy: Observations on embryogenesis. *Chest, 66,* 25–26.

### 2.2.5   RIFABUTIN

**FDA Category: B**
*Risk Summary:* Although Rifabutin has been assigned with the letter (B), according to the FDA categorization, but it should be used with caution because no human data is available and the reproduction studies in animals have shown low risk.

**Further Reading:**
- *Drug Information*. Mycobutin. Pharmacia & Upjohn.

### 2.2.6   RIFAPENTINE

**FDA Category: C**
*Risk Summary:* No human data is available and the reproduction studies in animals have shown a low risk of fetal harm and teratogenicity. It is better to be avoided in the 1st Trimester.

**Further Reading:**
- Briggs, G. G., & Freeman, R. K. (2015). Drugs in pregnancy and lactation: A reference guide to fetal and neonatal risk. Philadelphia, PA: Lippincott Williams & Wilkins.
- CDC (2003). Treatment of tuberculosis. *MMWR, 52*(RR11), 1–77.
- Center for Drug Evaluation and Research (1998). FDA. Approval package: Priftin (Rifapentine) 150 mg tablets. Hoechst Marion Roussel.
- *Drug Information*. Priftin. Aventis Pharmaceuticals.

## 2.2.7  *DAPSONE*

**FDA Category: C**

*Risk Summary:* Although there is limited data from the human pregnancy experience, but the expected maternal benefit extremely outweighs the unknown or known embryo/fetal risk.

**Further Reading:**
- Bhargava, P., Kuldeep, C. M., & Mathur, N. K., (1996). Antileprosy drugs, pregnancy and fetal outcome. *Int. J. Lepr Other Mycobact Dis., 64,* 457.
- *Drug Information.* Dapsone. Jacobus Pharmaceutical.
- Greenwood, A. M., Menendez, C., Todd, J., & Greenwood, B. M., (1994). The distribution of birth weights in Gambian women who received malaria chemoprophylaxis during their first pregnancy and in control women. *Trans R. Soc. Trop. Med. Hyg., 88,* 311–312.
- Sanders, S. W., Zone, J. J., Foltz, R. L., Tolman, K. G., & Rollins, D. E., (1982). Hemolytic anemia induced by dapsone transmitted through breast milk. *Ann Intern. Med., 96,* 465–466.

## 2.3  ANTIFUNGAL AGENTS

### 2.3.1  *AZOLES*

#### 2.3.1.1  *KETOCONAZOLE*

**FDA Category: C**

*Risk Summary:* The pregnancy experience in humans is limited. The reproduction studies in animals revealed that Ketoconazole is embryotoxic and teratogenic in rats at a dose 10 times the maximum recommended human.

**Further Reading:**
- Amado, J. A., Pesquera, C., Gonzalez, E. M., Otero, M., Freijanes, J., & Alvarez, A., (1990). Successful treatment with ketoconazole of Cushing's syndrome in pregnancy. *Postgrad Med. J., 66,* 221–223.
- *Drug Information.* Nizoral. Janssen Pharmaceutics.
- Lind, J., (1985). Limb malformations in the case of hydrops fetal is with ketoconazole use during pregnancy (abstract). *Arch Gynecol., 237*(Suppl), 398.

- Nishikawa, S., Hara, T., Miyazaki, H., & Ohguro, Y., (1984). Reproduction studies of KW-1414 in rats and rabbits. *Clin. Rep., 18,* 1433–1488. As cited in Shepard, T. H., Catalog of Teratogenic Agents. 6th ed. Baltimore, MD: The Johns Hopkins University Press, 1989:1075.

## 2.3.1.2  ITRACONAZOLE

**FDA Category: C**
*Risk Summary:* It is better to be avoided during the 1st Trimester because the pregnancy experience in humans has shown a low risk of teratogenicity associated with the use of Itraconazole.

**Further Reading:**
- De Santis, M., Gianantonio, E. D., Cesari, E., Ambrosini, G., Straface, G., & Clementi, M., (2009). First-trimester itraconazole exposure and pregnancy outcome; a prospective cohort study of women contacting teratology information services in Italy. *Drug Safety, 32,* 239–244.
- *Drug Information*. Sporanox. Janssen Pharmaceutica.
- Rosa, F., (1996). *Azole Fungicide Pregnancy Risks*. Presented at the Ninth International Conference of the Organization of Teratology Information Services, May 2–4, 1996, Salt Lake City, Utah.

## 2.3.1.3  FLUCONAZOLE

**FDA Category: D (Multiple doses)**
**FDA Category: C (150 single doses)**
*Risk Summary:* The use of Fluconazole should be avoided in pregnant women, especially during the 1st Trimester, because the pregnancy experience in humans has shown the risk of teratogenicity at doses ≥400 mg/day.

**Further Reading:**
- *Drug Information*. Diflucan. Pfizer, 2001.
- Lee, B. E., Feinberg, M., Abraham, J. J., & Murthy, A. R., (1992). Congenital malformations in an infant born to a woman treated with fluconazole. *Pediatr. Infect. Dis. J., 11,* 1062–1064.
- Molgaard-Nielsen, D., Pasternak, B., & Hviid, A., (2013). Use of oral fluconazole during pregnancy and the risk of birth defects. *N. Engl. J. Med., 369,* 830–839.

- Pursley, T. J., Blomquist, I. K., Abraham, J., Andersen, H. F., & Bartley, J. A., (1996). Fluconazole-induced congenital anomalies in three infants. *Clin. Infect. Dis., 22,* 336–340.

## 2.3.1.4  *VORICONAZOLE*

**FDA Category: C**
***Risk Summary:*** The use of Voriconazole is better to be avoided in pregnant women, especially during the 1st Trimester, because the pregnancy experience in humans is limited and the reproduction studies in animals have shown low risk.

**Further Reading:**
- *Drug Information.* Vfend. Pfizer.
- Moudgal, V. V., & Sobel, J. D., (2003). Antifungal drugs in pregnancy: A review. *Expert Opin. Drug Saf., 2,* 475–483.

## 2.3.1.5  *POSACONAZOLE*

**FDA Category: C**
***Risk Summary:*** The use of Posaconazole is better to be avoided in pregnant women, especially during the 1st Trimester, because the pregnancy experience in humans is limited and the reproduction studies in animals have shown low risk.

**Further Reading:**
- *Drug Information.* Noxafil. Schering.

## *2.3.2  POLYENES*

### 2.3.2.1  *AMPHOTERICIN B*

**FDA Category: B**
***Risk Summary:*** The reproduction studies in animals have shown no evidence of fetal harm or impaired fertility. The pregnancy experience in humans is adequate to exhibit that the embryo-fetal risk is nonexistent or very low.

**Further Reading:**
- Aitken, G. W. E., & Symonds, E. M., (1962). Cryptococcal meningitis in pregnancy treated with amphotericin. A case report. *Br. J. Obstet. Gynaecol. 69,* 677–679.
- *Drug Information.* Ambisome. Fujisawa Healthcare.
- Ismail, M. A., & Lerner, S. A., (1982). Disseminated blastomycosis in a pregnant woman. Review of amphotericin B usage during pregnancy. Am. Rev. Respir. Dis., *126,* 350–353.

### 2.3.2.2   NYSTATIN

**FDA Category: A (Vaginal Tablets)**

**FDA Category: C (Topical cream, ointment, and powder)**

*Risk Summary:* The reproduction studies in animals have shown no evidence of fetal harm or impaired fertility. The pregnancy experience in humans is adequate to exhibit that the embryo-fetal risk is nonexistent or very low.

**Further Reading:**
- David, J. E., Frudenfeld, J. H., & Goddard, J. L., (1974). Comparative evaluation of Monistat and Mycostatin in the treatment of vulvovaginal candidiasis. *Obstet. Gynecol., 44,* 403–406.
- Heinonen, O. P., Slone, D., & Shapiro, S., (1977). *Birth Defects and Drugs in Pregnancy.* Littleton, MA: Publishing Sciences Group.
- Rosa, F. W., Baum, C., & Shaw, M., (1987). Pregnancy outcomes after first-trimester vaginitis drug therapy. *Obstet. Gynecol., 69,* 751–755.

## 2.3.3   ECHINOCANDINS

### 2.3.3.1   CASPOFUNGIN

**FDA Category: C**

*Risk Summary:* It is better to be avoided during the 1st Trimester because the pregnancy experience in humans is limited, and the reproduction studies in animals have shown the risk of teratogenicity associated with the use of Caspofungin.

**Further Reading:**
- *Drug Information.* Cancidas. Merck.
- Moudgal, V. V., & Sobel, J. D., (2003). Antifungal drugs in pregnancy: A review. *Expert Opin. Drug Saf., 2,* 475–483.

## 2.3.3.2   *MICAFUNGIN*

**FDA Category: C**
*Risk Summary:* It is better to be avoided during the 1st Trimester because the pregnancy experience in humans is limited, and the reproduction studies in animals have shown the risk of teratogenicity associated with the use of Micafungin.

**Further Reading:**
 • *Drug Information*. Mycamine. Astellas Pharma US.

## 2.3.3.3   *ANIDULAFUNGIN*

**FDA Category: C**
*Risk Summary:* It is better to be avoided during the 1st Trimester because the pregnancy experience in humans is limited, and the reproduction studies in animals have shown the risk of teratogenicity associated with the use of Anidulafungin.

**Further Reading:**
 • *Drug Information*. Eraxis. Pfizer.

## 2.3.4   *ALLYLAMINE*

### 2.3.4.1   *TERBINAFINE*

**FDA Category: B**
*Risk Summary:* Although Terbinafine has been assigned with the letter (B), according to the FDA categorization, but it should be used with caution because no human data is available and the reproduction studies in animals have shown low risk.

**Further Reading:**
 • Briggs, G. G., & Freeman, R. K., (2015). Drugs in pregnancy and lactation: A reference guide to fetal and neonatal risk. Philadelphia, PA: Lippincott Williams & Wilkins.
 • *Drug Information*. Lamisil. Novartis Pharmaceuticals.

## 2.3.5  PYRIMIDINE ANALOG

### 2.3.5.1  FLUCYTOSINE

**FDA Category (1ˢᵗ Trimester): D***
**FDA Category (2ⁿᵈ & 3ʳᵈ Trimester): C**

*Risk Summary:* Flucytosine is contraindicated during the 1st Trimester because it is partially metabolized to 5-Fluorouracil, antineoplastic agent, which is known for its teratogenicity. Although Terbinafine has been assigned with the letter (B), according to the FDA categorization, but it should be used with caution because no human data is available and the reproduction studies in animals have shown low risk.

**Further Reading:**
- Diasio, R. B., Lakings, D. E., & Bennett, J. E., (1978). Evidence for conversion of 5-fluorocytosine to 5-fluorouracil in humans: Possible factor in 5-fluorocytosine clinical toxicity. *Antimicrob Agents Chemother, 14,* 903–908.
- *Drug Information.* Ancobon. ICN Pharmaceuticals.
- Schonebeck, J., & Segerbrand, E., (1973). Candida albicans septicemia during the first half of pregnancy successfully treated with 5-fluorocytosine. *Br. Med. J., 4,* 337–338.
- Stafford, C. R., Fisher, J. F., Fadel, H. E., Espinel-Ingroff, A. V., Shadomy, S., & Hamby, M., (1983). Cryptococcal meningitis in pregnancy. *Obstet. Gynecol., 62*(3 Suppl), 35s–37s.

*It is the author's opinion regarding the most accurate classification of Flucytosine during the 1ˢᵗ Trimester, and it is not an official FDA classification.

## 2.4  ANTIVIRAL AGENTS

### 2.4.1  ANTI-HERPES AGENTS

### 2.4.1.1  ACYCLOVIR

**FDA Category: B**
*Risk Summary:* The reproduction studies in animals have shown no evidence of fetal harm or impaired fertility. The pregnancy experience in humans is adequate to exhibit that the embryo-fetal risk is nonexistent or very low.

**Further Reading:**
- American College of Obstetricians and Gynecologists (2007). Management of herpes in pregnancy. *ACOG Practice Bulletin. No. 82.*
- *Drug Information.* Zovirax. Glaxo Wellcome.
- Moore, H. L., Szczech, G. M., Rodwell, D. E., Kapp, R. W. Jr., De Miranda, P., Tucker, W. E. Jr., (1983). Preclinical toxicology studies with acyclovir: Teratologic, reproductive, and neonatal tests. *Fund Appl Toxicol, 3,* 560–568.
- Stone, K. M., Reiff-Eldridge, R., White, A. D., Cordero, J. F., Brown, Z., Alexander, E. R., & Andrews, E. B., (2004). Pregnancy outcomes following systemic prenatal acyclovir exposure: Conclusions from the International Acyclovir Pregnancy Registry, 1984–1999. *Birth Defects Res. A Clin. Mol. Teratol., 70,* 201–207.

### 2.4.1.2   VALACYCLOVIR

**FDA Category: B**

***Risk Summary:*** The reproduction studies in animals have shown no evidence of fetal harm or impaired fertility. The pregnancy experience in humans is adequate to exhibit that the embryo-fetal risk is nonexistent or very low.

**Further Reading:**
- *Drug Information.* Valtrex. Glaxo Wellcome.
- Mills, J. L., & Carter, T. C., (2010). Acyclovir exposure and birth defects—an important advance, but more are needed. *JAMA, 304,* 905–906.
- Sheffield, J. S., Hill, J. B., Hollier, L. M., Laibl, V. R., Roberts, S. W., Sanchez, P. J., & Wendel, G. D. Jr., (2006). Valacyclovir prophylaxis to prevent recurrent herpes at delivery. *Obstet. Gynecol., 108,* 141–147.

### 2.4.1.3   GANCICLOVIR

**FDA Category: C**

***Risk Summary:*** Due to the carcinogenic and mutagenic effects of Ganciclovir in animals and the potential for fetal toxicity, some experts recommend that ganciclovir should only be used during pregnancy for immunocompromised patients with major CMV infections, such as retinitis or for life-threatening disease.

**Further Reading:**
- *Drug Information.* Cytovene. Roche Laboratories.
- Pescovitz, M. D., (1999). Absence of teratogenicity of oral ganciclovir used during early pregnancy in a liver transplant recipient. *Transplantation, 67,* 758–759.
- Puliyanda, D. P., Silverman, N. S., Lehman, D., Vo, A., Bunnapradist, S., Radha, R. K., Toyoda, M., & Jordan, S. C., (2005). Successful use of oral ganciclovir for the treatment of intrauterine cytomegalovirus (CMV) infection in a renal allograft recipient. *Transpl. Infect. Dis., 7,* 71–74.

## 2.4.1.4  VALGANCICLOVIR

**FDA Category: C**
*Risk Summary:* Due to the carcinogenic and mutagenic effects of Valganciclovir in animals and the potential for fetal toxicity, some experts recommend that Valganciclovir should only be used during pregnancy for immunocompromised patients with major CMV infections, such as retinitis or for life-threatening disease.

**Further Reading:**
- *Drug Information.* Valcyte. Roche Pharmaceuticals.

## 2.4.1.5  PENCICLOVIR (TOPICAL)

**FDA Category: B**
*Risk Summary:* The reproduction studies in animals have shown no evidence of fetal harm or impaired fertility. The pregnancy experience in humans is limited.

**Further Reading:**
- *Drug Information.* Denavir. New American Therapeutics.
- Pasternak, B., & Hviid, A., (2010). Use of acyclovir, valacyclovir, and famciclovir in the first trimester of pregnancy and the risk of birth defects. *JAMA, 304,* 859–866.

## 2.4.1.6   FAMCICLOVIR

**FDA Category: B**
*Risk Summary:* Although Famciclovir has been assigned with the letter (B), according to the FDA categorization, but it should be used with caution because no human data is available and the reproduction studies in animals have shown low risk.

**Further Reading:**
- *Drug Information.* Famvir. Novartis Pharmaceuticals.
- Mubareka, S., Leung, V., Aoki, F. Y., & Vinh, D. C., (2010). Famciclovir: A focus on efficacy and safety. *Expert Opin. Drug Saf., 9,* 643–658.

## 2.4.1.7   CIDOFOVIR

**FDA Category: C**
*Risk Summary:* Although there is limited data from the human pregnancy experience, but the possible maternal benefit extremely outweighs the unknown or known embryo/fetal risk.

**Further Reading:**
- Brown, Z. A., & Watts, D. H., (1990). Antiviral therapy in pregnancy. *Clin. Obstet. Gynecol., 33,* 276–289.
- *Drug Information.* Vistide. Gilead Sciences.
- Van de Perre, P., (1995). Postnatal transmission of human immunodeficiency virus type 1: The breastfeeding dilemma. *Am. J. Obstet. Gynecol., 173,* 483–487.

## 2.4.1.8   FOSCARNET

**FDA Category: C**
*Risk Summary:* Although there is limited data from the human pregnancy experience, but the possible maternal benefit extremely outweighs the unknown or known embryo/fetal risk.

**Further Reading:**
- Alvarez-McLeod, A., Havlik, J., & Drew, K. E., (1999). Foscarnet treatment of genital infection due to acyclovir-resistant herpes simplex virus type 2 in a pregnant patient with AIDS: a case report. *Clin. Infect. Dis., 29,* 937–938.
- *Drug Information.* Foscavir. AstraZeneca.
- Watts, D. H., (1992). Antiviral agents. *Obstet. Gynecol Clin North Am., 19,* 563–585.

### 2.4.1.9   FOMIVIRSEN

**FDA Category: C**
***Risk Summary:*** Although there is limited data from the human pregnancy experience, but the possible maternal benefit extremely outweighs the unknown or known embryo/fetal risk.

**Further Reading:**
- Avalos, L. A., Chen, H., Yang, C., Andrade, S. E., Cooper, W. O., Cheetham, C. T., & Li, D., (2014). The Prevalence and trends of antiviral medication use during pregnancy in the US: A population-based study of 664, 297 deliveries in 2001–2007. *Maternal and Child Health Journal, 18*(1), 64–72. doi: 10.1007/s10995-013-1234-9.

### 2.4.2   ANTI-HIV NRTI AGENTS

### 2.4.2.1   ZIDOVUDINE

**FDA Category: C**
***Risk Summary:*** Although there is limited data from the human pregnancy experience, but the possible maternal benefit extremely outweighs the unknown or known embryo/fetal risk.

**Further Reading:**
- *Drug Information.* Retrovir. Glaxo Wellcome.
- Nosbisch, C., Ha, J. C., Sackett, G. P., Conrad, S. H., Ruppenthal, G. C., & Unadkat, J. D., (1994). Fetal and infant toxicity of zidovudine in Macaca nemestrina (abstract). *Teratology, 49,* 415.

- Stojanov, S., Wintergerst, U., Belohradsky, B. H., & Rolinski, B., (2000). Mitochondrial and peroxisomal dysfunction following perinatal exposure to antiretroviral drugs. *AIDS, 14,* 1669.
- Toltzis, P., Marx, C. M., Kleinman, N., Levine, E. M., & Schmidt, E. V., (1991). Zidovudine-associated embryonic toxicity in mice. *J. Infect. Dis.,* 1212–1218.

## 2.4.2.2 STAVUDINE

**FDA Category: C**
*Risk Summary:* Although there is limited data from the human pregnancy experience, but the possible maternal benefit extremely outweighs the unknown or known embryo/fetal risk.

**Further Reading:**
- *Drug Information.* Zerit. Bristol-Myers Squibb.
- Richardson, M. P., Osrin, D., Donaghy, S., Brown, N. A., Hay, & Sharland, M., (2000). Spinal malformations in the fetuses of HIV infected women receiving combination antiretroviral therapy and co-trimoxazole. *Eur. J. Obstet. Gynecol Reprod Biol., 93,* 215–217.

## 2.4.2.3 LAMIVUDINE

**FDA Category: C**
*Risk Summary:* Although there is limited data from the human pregnancy experience, but the possible maternal benefit extremely outweighs the unknown or known embryo/fetal risk.

**Further Reading:**
- *Drug Information.* Epivir. Glaxo Wellcome.
- McGowan, J. P., Crane, M., Wiznia, A. A., & Blum, S., (1999). Combination antiretroviral therapy in human immunodeficiency virus-infected pregnant women. *Obstet. Gynecol., 94,* 641–646.
- Lorenzi, P., Spicher, V. M., Laubereau, B., Hirschel, B., Kind, C., Rudin, C., Irion, O., & Kaiser, L., (1998). Antiretroviral therapies in pregnancy: maternal, fetal and neonatal effects. Swiss HIV cohort study, the swiss collaborative HIV and pregnancy study, and the swiss neonatal HIV Study. *AIDS, 12,* F241–247.

## 2.4.2.4 *DIDANOSINE*

**FDA Category: B**
***Risk Summary:*** Although there is limited data from the human pregnancy experience, but the possible maternal benefit extremely outweighs the unknown or known embryo/fetal risk.

**Further Reading:**
- *Drug Information.* Videx. Bristol-Myers Squibb.
- Esterman, A. L., Rosenberg, C., Brown, T., & Dancis, J., (1995). The effect of zidovudine and 2'3'-dideoxyinosine on human trophoblast in culture. *Pharmacol Toxicol, 76,* 89–92.
- Minkoff, H., (2003). Human immunodeficiency virus infection in pregnancy. *Obstet. Gynecol., 101,* 797–810.

## 2.4.2.5 *ABACAVIR*

**FDA Category: C**
***Risk Summary:*** Although there is limited data from the human pregnancy experience, but the possible maternal benefit extremely outweighs the unknown or known embryo/fetal risk.

**Further Reading:**
- *Drug Information.* Ziagen. Glaxo Wellcome.
- Carpenter, C. C. J., Fischi, M. A., Hammer, S. M., Hirsch, M. S., Jacobsen, D. M., Katzenstein, D. A., & Montaner, J. S. G., Richman, D. D., Saag, M. S., Schooley, R. T., Thompson, M. A., Vella, S., Yeni, P. G., & Volberding, P. A., (1996). Antiretroviral therapy for HIV infection in 1996. *JAMA, 276,* 146–154.

## 2.4.2.6 *TENOFOVIR DISOPROXIL*

**FDA Category: B**
***Risk Summary:*** Although there is limited data from the human pregnancy experience, but the possible maternal benefit extremely outweighs the unknown or known embryo/fetal risk.

**Further Reading:**
- *Drug Information.* Viread. Gilead Sciences.

- Tarantal, A. F., Castillo, A., Ekert, J. E., Bischofberger, N., & Martin, R. B., (2002). Fetal and maternal outcome after administration of tenofovir to gravid rhesus monkeys (Macaca mulatta). *J. Acquir Immune Defic. Syndrome, 29,* 207–220.

## 2.4.2.7   EMTRICITABINE

**FDA Category: B**
*Risk Summary:* There is limited data from the human pregnancy experience, and the animal data suggest low risk; however, the possible maternal benefit extremely outweighs the unknown or known embryo/fetal risk.

**Further Reading:**
- *Drug Information*. Emtriva. Gilead Sciences.
- Furco, A., Gosrani, B., Nicholas, S., Williams, A., Braithwaite, W., Pozniak, A., Taylor, G., Asboe, D., Lyall, H., Shaw, A., & Kapembwa, M., (2009). Successful use of darunavir, etravirine, enfuvirtide and tenofovir/emtricitabine in a pregnant woman with multiclass HIV resistance. *AIDS, 23,* 434–435.
- Szczech, G. M., Wang, L. H., Walsh, J. P., & Rousseau, F. S., (2003). Reproductive toxicology profile of emtricitabine in mice and rabbits. *Reprod Toxicol, 17,* 95–108.

## 2.4.3   ANTI-HBV AGENTS

## 2.4.3.1   ADEFOVIR

**FDA Category: C**
*Risk Summary:* There is limited data from the human pregnancy experience, and the animal data suggest low risk; however, the possible maternal benefit extremely outweighs the unknown or known embryo/fetal risk.

**Further Reading:**
- Carpenter, C. C. J., Fischi, M. A., Hammer, S. M., Hirsch, M. S., Jacobsen, D. M., Katzenstein, D. A., Montaner, J. S. G., Richman, D. D., Saag, M. S., Schooley, R. T., Thompson, M. A., Vella, S., Yeni, P. G., & Volberding, P. A., (1996). Antiretroviral therapy for HIV infection in 1996. *JAMA, 276,* 146–154.

- *Drug Information*. Hepsera. Gilead Sciences.


## 2.4.3.2   ENTECAVIR

**FDA Category: C**
***Risk Summary:*** There is limited data from the human pregnancy experience, and the animal data suggest low risk; however, the possible maternal benefit extremely outweighs the unknown or known embryo/fetal risk.

**Further Reading:**
- *Drug Information*. Baraclude. Bristol-Meyers Squibb.


## 2.4.4   ANTI-HCV AGENTS

### 2.4.4.1   RIBAVIRIN

**FDA Category: X**
***Risk Summary:*** It is contraindicated during pregnancy. Ribavirin should be discontinued, at least six months, before the planned conception.

**Further Reading:**
- *Drug Information*. Copegus. Roche Laboratories.
- Rezvani, M., & Koren, G., (2006). Pregnancy outcome after exposure to injectable ribavirin during embryogenesis. *Reprod Toxicol*, *21*, 113–115.
- Polifka, J. E., & Friedman, J. M., (2003). Developmental toxicity of ribavirin/IFα combination therapy: Is the label more dangerous than the drugs? *Birth Defects Res. A Clin. Mol. Teratol.*, *67*, 8–12.


## 2.4.4.2   INTERFERON ALFA-2A, INTERFERON ALFA-2B, AND PEGINTERFERON ALFA-2B

**FDA Category: C**
***Risk Summary:*** The reproduction studies in animals have shown no evidence of fetal harm or impaired fertility. The pregnancy experience in humans is limited.

**Further Reading:**
- Beauverd, Y., Radia, D., Cargo, C., Knapper, S., Drummond, M., Pillai, A., & Robinson, S., (2016). Pegylated interferon-alpha-2a for essential thrombocythemia during pregnancy: Outcome and safety. A case series. *Haematologica, 101*(5). doi: 10.3324/haematol.2015.139691.
- *Drug Information. Intron. A.* Schering.
- *Drug Information. Roferon-A.* Roche Laboratories.
- Kuroiwa, M., Gondo, H., Ashida, K., Kamimura, T., Miyamoto, T., Niho, Y., Tsukimori, K., Nakano, H., & Ohga, S., (1998). Interferon-alpha therapy for chronic myelogenous leukemia during pregnancy. *Am. J. Hematol, 59,* 101–102.
- Trotter, J. F., & Zygmunt, A. J., (2001). Conception and pregnancy during interferon-alpha therapy for chronic hepatitis C. *J. Clin. Gastroenterol, 32,* 76–78.

### 2.4.4.3   SOFOSBUVIR

**FDA Category: B**
***Risk Summary:*** The reproduction studies in animals have shown no evidence of fetal harm or impaired fertility. The pregnancy experience in humans is adequate to exhibit that the embryo-fetal risk is nonexistent or very low. However, Sofosbuvir is contraindicated during pregnancy if taken in combination with Ribavirin and peginterferon alfa.

**Further Reading:**
- Food and Drug Administration. *U.S. Food and Drug Administration.* Sovaldi highlights of prescribing information.
- Food and Drug Administration. *U.S. National Library of Medicine.* National Center for Biotechnology Information. Compound Summary for CID 45375808 Sofosbuvir.

### 2.4.4.4   LEDIPASVIR

**FDA Category: B**
***Risk Summary:*** The reproduction studies in animals have shown no evidence of fetal harm or impaired fertility. The pregnancy experience in humans is adequate to exhibit that the embryo-fetal risk is nonexistent or very low.

However, Ledipasvir is contraindicated during pregnancy if taken in combination with Ribavirin and peginterferon alfa.

**Further Reading:**
- European Medicines Agency – Science Medicine Health. Harvoni summary of product characteristics
- Food and Drug Administration. U.S. National Library of Medicine. National Center for Biotechnology Information. Compound Summary for CID 72734365 Sofosbuvir/Ledispasvir.

## 2.4.4.5  TELAPREVIR

**FDA Category: B**
*Risk Summary:* The reproduction studies in animals have shown no evidence of fetal harm or impaired fertility. The pregnancy experience in humans is adequate to exhibit that the embryo-fetal risk is nonexistent or very low. However, Telaprevir is contraindicated during pregnancy if taken in combination with Ribavirin and peginterferon alfa.

**Further Reading:**
- *Drug Information.* Incivek. Vertex Pharmaceuticals.

## 2.4.5  ANTI-INFLUENZA AGENTS

### 2.4.5.1  AMANTADINE AND RIMANTADINE

**FDA Category: C**
*Risk Summary:* It is better to be avoided during the 1st Trimester because the pregnancy experience in humans is limited, and the reproduction studies in animals have shown the risk of teratogenicity associated with the use of Amantadine. It is believed that Rimantadine has a lower risk of harmful effects than Amantadine

**Further Reading:**
- *Drug Information.* Flumadine. Forest Pharmaceuticals.
- *Drug Information.* Symmetrel. Endo Pharmaceuticals.
- Greer, L. G., Sheffield, J. S., Rogers, V. L., Roberts, S. W., McIntire, D. D., & Wendel, G. D. Jr., (2010). Maternal and neonatal outcomes

after antepartum treatment of influenza with antiviral medications. *Obstet. Gynecol., 115,* 711–716.
- Pandit, P. B., Chitayat, D., Jefferies, A. L., Landes, A., Qamar, I. U., & Koren, G., (1994). Tibial hemimelia and tetralogy of Fallot associated with first-trimester exposure to amantadine. *Reprod Toxicol, 8,* 89–92.
- Rosa, F., (1994). Amantadine pregnancy experience. *Reprod Toxicol, 8,* 531.

## 2.4.5.2   OSELTAMIVIR

**FDA Category: C**
***Risk Summary:*** Although there is limited data from the human pregnancy experience, but the possible maternal benefit extremely outweighs the unknown or known embryo/fetal risk.

**Further Reading:**
- Centers for Disease Control and Prevention (CDC), (2009). Novel influenza A (H1N1) virus infections in three pregnant women— United States, April–May 2009. *MMWR Morb. Mortal Wkly Rep., 58*(18), 497–500.
- *Drug Information.* Tamiflu. Roche Laboratories.
- Greer, L. G., Sheffield, J. S., Rogers, V. L., Roberts, S. W., McIntire, D. D., & Wendel, G. D. Jr., (2010). Maternal and neonatal outcomes after antepartum treatment of influenza with antiviral medications. *Obstet. Gynecol., 115,* 711–716.

## 2.4.5.3   ZANAMIVIR

**FDA Category: C**
***Risk Summary:*** Although there is limited data from the human pregnancy experience, but the possible maternal benefit extremely outweighs the unknown or known embryo/fetal risk.

**Further Reading:**
- *Drug Information.* Relenza. GlaxoSmithKline.

- Kiatboonsri, S., Kiatboonsri, C., & Theerawit, P., (2010). Fatal respiratory events caused by zanamivir nebulization. *Clin. Infect. Dis., 50,* 620.


## 2.4.6   OTHER ANTIVIRAL AGENTS

### 2.4.6.1   PALIVIZUMAB

**FDA Category: C**
***Risk Summary:*** It is only used for the treatment of respiratory syncytial virus in children. Therefore, no human or animal data is available regarding its safety profile in pregnancy.

**Further Reading:**
- *Drug Information.* Synagis. MedImmune.


### 2.4.6.2   LOPINAVIR/RITONAVIR

**FDA Category: C**
***Risk Summary:*** Although there is limited data from the human pregnancy experience, but the possible maternal benefit extremely outweighs the unknown or known embryo/fetal risk.

**Further Reading:**
- *Drug Information.* Kaletra. Abbott Laboratories.
- Fassett, M., Kramer, F., & Stek, A., (2000). Treatment with protease inhibitors in pregnancy is not associated with an increased incidence of gestational diabetes (abstract). *Am. J. Obstet. Gynecol., 182,* S97.
- Minkoff, H., & Augenbraun, M., (1997). Antiretroviral therapy for pregnant women. *Am. J. Obstet. Gynecol., 176,* 478–489.


### 2.4.6.3   TIPRANAVIR

**FDA Category: C**
***Risk Summary:*** Although there is limited data from the human pregnancy experience, but the possible maternal benefit extremely outweighs the unknown or known embryo/fetal risk.

**Further Reading:**
- *Drug Information*. Aptivus. Boehringer Ingelheim Pharmaceuticals.
- Minkoff, H., (2003). Human immunodeficiency virus infection in pregnancy. *Obstet. Gynecol., 101,* 797–810.
- Wensing, A. M. J., Boucher, C. A. B., van Kasteren, M., van Dijken, P. J., Geelen, S. P., & Juttmann, J. R., (2006). Prevention of mother-to-child transmission of multi-drug-resistant HIV-1 using maternal therapy with both enfuvirtide and tipranavir. *AIDS, 20,* 1465–1467.

## 2.4.6.4   ENFUVIRTIDE

**FDA Category: B**
*Risk Summary:* Although there is limited data from the human pregnancy experience, but the possible maternal benefit extremely outweighs the unknown or known embryo/fetal risk.

**Further Reading:**
- Brennan-Benson, P., Pakianathan, M., Rice, P., Bonora, S., Chakraborty, R., Sharland, M., & Hay, P., (2006). Enfuvirtide prevents vertical transmission of multidrug-resistant HIV-1 in pregnancy but does not cross the placenta. *AIDS, 20,* 297–299.
- *Drug Information*. Fuzeon. Roche Pharmaceuticals.
- Furco, A., Gosrani, B., Nicholas, S., Williams, A., Braithwaite, W., Pozniak, A., Taylor, G., Asboe, D., Lyall, H., Shaw, A., & Kapembwa, M., (2009). Successful use of darunavir, etravirine, enfuvirtide and tenofovir/emtricitabine in a pregnant woman with multiclass HIV resistance. *AIDS, 23,* 434–435.

## 2.4.6.5   DELAVIRDINE

**FDA Category: C**
*Risk Summary:* Although there is limited data from the human pregnancy experience, but the possible maternal benefit extremely outweighs the unknown or known embryo/fetal risk.

**Further Reading:**
- Carpenter, C. C. J., Fischi, M. A., Hammer, S. M., Hirsch, M. S., Jacobsen, D. M., Katzenstein, D. A., Montaner, J. S. G., Richman, D.

D., Saag, M. S., Schooley, R. T., Thompson, M. A., Vella, S., Yeni, P. G., & Volberding, P. A., (1996). Antiretroviral therapy for HIV infection in 1996. *JAMA, 276,* 146–154.
- *Drug Information.* Rescriptor. Pfizer.

### 2.4.6.6  NEVIRAPINE

**FDA Category: B**
***Risk Summary:*** Although there is limited data from the human pregnancy experience, but the possible maternal benefit extremely outweighs the unknown or known embryo/fetal risk.

**Further Reading:**
- *Drug Information.* Viramune. Roxane Laboratories.
- Musoke, P., Guay, L. A., Bagenda, D., Mirochnick, M., Nakabiito, C., Fleming, T., Elliott, T., Horton, S., Dransfield, K., Pav, J. W., Murarka, A., Allen, M., Fowler, M. G., Mofenson, L., Hom, D., Mmiro, F., & Jackson, J. B., (1999). A phase I/II study of the safety and pharmacokinetics of nevirapine in HIV-1-infected pregnant Ugandan women and their neonates (HIVNET 006). *AIDS, 13,* 479–486.
- Taylor, G. P., Lyall EGH, Back, D., Ward, C., & Tudor-Williams, G., (2000). Pharmacological implications of lengthened in-utero exposure to nevirapine. *Lancet, 355,* 2134–2135.

## 2.5  ANTI-PROTOZOAL

### 2.5.1  ANTI-MALARIAL DRUGS

#### 2.5.1.1  CHLOROQUINE

**FDA Category: N**
***Risk Summary:*** Although there is limited data from the human pregnancy experience, but the possible maternal benefit extremely outweighs the unknown or known embryo/fetal risk.

**Further Reading:**
- *Drug Information.* Aralen. Sanofi Pharmaceuticals.

- Strang, A., Lachman, E., Pitsoe, S. B., Marszalek, A., & Philpott, R. H., (1984). Malaria in pregnancy with fatal complications: a case report. *Br. J. Obstet. Gynaecol, 91,* 399–403.
- Udalova, L. D., (1967). The effect of chloroquine on the embryonal development of rats. *Pharmacol Toxicol* (Russian), *2,* 226–228. As cited in Shepard, T. H., Catalog of Teratogenic Agents. (6<sup>th</sup> edn.) Baltimore, MD: Johns Hopkins University Press, 1989, 140–141.

## 2.5.1.2   HYDROXYCHLOROQUINE

**FDA Category: C**
***Risk Summary:*** The reproduction studies in animals have shown no evidence of fetal harm or impaired fertility. The pregnancy experience in humans is limited.

**Further Reading:**
- CDC (1990). Recommendations for the prevention of malaria among travelers. *MMWR, 39,* 1–10.
- *Drug Information. Plaquenil.* Sanofi Winthrop Pharmaceuticals.
- Parke, A., & West, B., (1996). Hydroxychloroquine in pregnant patients with systemic lupus erythematosus. *J. Rheumatol., 23,* 1715–1718.
- Suhonen, R., (1983). Hydroxychloroquine administration in pregnancy. *Arch Dermatol., 119,* 185–186.

## 2.5.1.3   MEFLOQUINE

**FDA Category: C**
***Risk Summary:*** The reproduction studies in animals have shown no evidence of fetal harm or impaired fertility. The pregnancy experience in humans is adequate to exhibit that the embryo-fetal risk is nonexistent or very low.

**Further Reading:**
- Centers for Disease Control (1990). Recommendations for the prevention of malaria among travelers. *MMWR, 39,* 1–10.
- Collignon, P., Hehir, J., & Mitchell, D., (1989). Successful treatment of falciparum malaria in pregnancy with mefloquine. *Lancet, 1,* 967.
- *Drug Information. Lariam.* Roche Laboratories.

## 2.5.1.4   *QUININE*

**FDA Category: C**
*Risk Summary:* The use of Quinine should be avoided in pregnant women because the pregnancy experience in humans has shown the risk of teratogenicity associated with the use of this drug.

**Further Reading:**
- *Drug Information. Quinamm.* Merrell Dow.
- Heinonen, O. P., Slone, D., & Shapiro, S., (1977). *Birth Defects and Drugs in Pregnancy.* Littleton, MA: Publishing Sciences Group, 1977:299, 302, 333.
- Robinson, G. C., Brummitt, J. R., & Miller, J. R., (1963). Hearing loss in infants and preschool children. II. Etiological considerations. *Pediatrics, 32,* 115–124.

## 2.5.1.5   *PRIMAQUINE*

**FDA Category: N**
*Risk Summary:* Since the fetuses are considered relatively G6PD deficient, Primaquine should not be used during pregnancy because it is known to generate acute hemolysis in those who are G6PD deficient.

**Further Reading:**
- *Drug Information. Primaquine Phosphate.* Sanofi-Aventis U.S.
- Nosten, F., McGready, R., d'Alessandro, U., Bonell, A., Verhoeff, F., Menendez, C., Mutabingwa, T., & Brabin, B., (2006). Antimalarial drugs in pregnancy: A review. *Curr Drug Saf., 1,* 1–15.
- Trenholme, G. M., & Parson, P. E., (1978). Therapy and prophylaxis of malaria. *JAMA, 240,* 2293–2295.

## 2.5.1.6   *PIPERAQUINE*

**FDA Category: C**
*Risk Summary:* The reproduction studies in animals have shown no evidence of fetal harm or impaired fertility. The pregnancy experience in humans is limited.

**Further Reading:**
- Clark, R. L., (2017). *"Animal Embryotoxicity Studies of Key Non-Artemisinin Antimalarials and Use in Women in the First Trimester"* (vol. 109(14), pp. 1075–1126). Birth Defects Research.
- Poespoprodjo, J. R., Fobia, W., Kenangalem, E., Lampah, D. A., Sugiarto, P., Tjitra, E., Anstey, N. M., & Price, R. N., (2014). Dihydroartemisinin-piperaquine treatment of multidrug-resistant falciparum and vivax malaria in pregnancy. *PLoS One, 9,* e84976.

### 2.5.1.7   AMODIAQUINE

**FDA Category: C**
***Risk Summary:*** The reproduction studies in animals have shown no evidence of fetal harm or impaired fertility. The pregnancy experience in humans is limited.

**Further Reading:**
- Clark, R. L., (2017). *"Animal Embryotoxicity Studies of Key Non-Artemisinin Antimalarials and Use in Women in the First Trimester"* (vol. 109(14), pp. 1075–1126). Birth Defects Research.
- Thomas, F., Erhart, A., & D'Alessandro, U., (2004). Can amodiaquine be used safely during pregnancy? *Lancet Infect Dis., 4,* 235–239.

### 2.5.1.8   PROGUANIL

**FDA Category: C**
***Risk Summary:*** Although there is limited data from the human pregnancy experience, but the possible maternal benefit extremely outweighs the unknown or known embryo/fetal risk.

**Further Reading:**
- Olsen, V. V., (1983). Why not proguanil in malaria prophylaxis? *Lancet, 1,* 649.
- Pasternak, B., & Hviid, A., (2011). Atovaquone-proguanil use in early pregnancy and the risk of birth defects. *Arch Intern. Med., 171,* 259–260.

## 2.5.1.9  *ARTEMETHER/LUMEFANTRINE*

**FDA Category: C**
*Risk Summary:* There is limited data from the human pregnancy experience in the 1st Trimester. But the adequate human experience of their use during the 2nd and 3rd Trimesters has shown a good safety profile.

**Further Reading:**
- Manyando, C., Mkandawire, R., Puma, L., et al., (2010). Safety of artemether-lumefantrine in pregnant women with malaria: Results of a prospective cohort study in Zambia. *Malar. J., 9,* 249.
- Mosha, D., Mazuguni, F., Mrema, S., et al., (2014). Safety of arte-mether-lumefantrine exposure in the first trimester of pregnancy: An observational cohort. *Malar. J., 13,* 197.
- Tarning, J., Kloprogge, F., Dhorda, M., et al., (2013). Pharmacokinetic properties of artemether, dihydroartemisinin, lumefantrine, and quinine in pregnant women with uncomplicated plasmodium falciparum malaria in Uganda. *Antimicrob Agents Chemother, 57,* 5096–5103.

## 2.5.2   *OTHER ANTI-PROTOZOAL*

## 2.5.2.1   *METRONIDAZOLE*

**FDA Category: B**
*Risk Summary:* Although Metronidazole has been assigned with the letter (B), according to the FDA categorization, but it should be used with caution especially during the 1st Trimester because the pregnancy experience in the human suggests low risk.

**Further Reading:**
- Berbel-Tornero, O., Lopez-Andreu, J. A., & Ferris-Tortajada, J., (1999). Prenatal exposure to metronidazole and risk of childhood cancer. A retrospective cohort study of children younger than 5 years. *Cancer, 85,* 2494–2495.
- Carvajal, A., Sanchez, A., & Hurtarte, G., (1995). Metronidazole during pregnancy. *Int. J. Gynecol Obstet, 48,* 323–324.
- *Drug Information.* Flagyl. G.D. Searle.

## 2.5.2.2    *TINIDAZOLE*

**FDA Category: C**
*Risk Summary:* The pregnancy experience in humans is limited, and the reproduction studies in animals have shown moderate risk. Therefore, it is advisable to use it only if Metronidazole has failed in eradicating the infection.

**Further Reading:**
- CDC (2006). Sexually transmitted diseases treatment guidelines, 2006. *MMWR, 55*(RR11), 1–94.
- Czeizel, A. E., Kazy, Z., & Vargha, P., (2003). Oral tinidazole treatment during pregnancy and teratogenesis. *Int. J. Gynecol Obstet, 83,* 305–306.
- *Drug Information.* Tindamaz. Presutti Laboratories.

## 2.5.2.3    *IODOQUINOL*

**FDA Category: N**
*Risk Summary:* It should be used only when the maternal benefit outweighs the fetal risk because there is very limited human pregnancy data, and the animal studies are not relevant.

**Further Reading:**
- *Drug Information.* Yodoxin. Glenwood.
- Heinonen, O. P., Slone, D., & Shapiro, S., (1977). *Birth Defects and Drugs in Pregnancy.* Littleton, MA: Publishing Sciences Group.
- Vedder, J. S., & Griem, S., (1956). Acrodermatitis enteropathica (Danbolt–Closs) in five siblings: Efficacy of diiodoquin in its management. *J. Pediatr., 48,* 212–219.

## 2.5.2.4    *PENTAMIDINE*

**FDA Category: C**
*Risk Summary:* Although there is limited data from the human pregnancy experience, but the possible maternal benefit extremely outweighs the unknown or known embryo/fetal risk.

**Further Reading:**
- Drake, S., Lampasona, V., Nicks, H. L., & Schwarzmann, S. W., (1985). Pentamidine isethionate in the treatment of Pneumocystis carinii pneumonia. *Clin. Pharm., 4*, 507–516.
- *Drug Information.* Pentam. Lyphomed, Inc.
- Harstad, T. W., Little, B. B., Bawdon, R. E., Knoll, K., Roe, D., & Gilstrap, L. C. III., (1990). Embryofetal effects of pentamidine isethionate administered to pregnant Sprague-Dawley rats. *Am. J. Obstet. Gynecol., 163*, 912–916.

## 2.5.2.5   SODIUM STIBOGLUCONATE

**FDA Category: N**
***Risk Summary:*** Because of the potential risk to the fetus, it is advisable to use it only when safer alternatives are not available or have failed.

**Further Reading:**
- Long, Sarah, S., et al., (2018). *Principles and Practice of Pediatric Infectious Diseases.* Elsevier.

## 2.5.2.6   NITAZOXANIDE

**FDA Category: B**
***Risk Summary:*** No human data is available and the reproduction studies in animals have shown low risk.

**Further Reading:**
- *Drug Information.* Alinia. Romark Pharmaceuticals.
- Murphy, J. R., & Friedman, J. C., (1985). Pre-clinical toxicology of nitazoxanide—A new antiparasitic compound. *J. Appl. Toxicol, 5*, 49–52.
- Romero Cabello, R., Guerrero, L. R., Munoz Garcia, M. D. R., & Geyne, C. A., (1997). Nitazoxanide for the treatment of intestinal protozoan and helminthic infections in Mexico. *Trans. R. Soc. Trop. Med. Hyg., 91*, 701–703.

## 2.6   ANTHELMINTIC

### *2.6.1   ALBENDAZOLE*

**FDA Category: C**

***Risk Summary:*** The reproduction studies in animals have shown no evidence of fetal harm or impaired fertility. The pregnancy experience in humans is adequate to exhibit that the embryo-fetal risk is nonexistent or very low.

**Further Reading:**
- Cowden, J., & Hotez, P., (2000). Mebendazole and albendazole treatment of geohelminth infections in children and pregnant women. *Pediatr. Infect. Dis. J., 19,* 659–660.
- *Drug Information.* Albenza. SmithKline Beecham Pharmaceuticals.
- Yilmaz, N., Kiymaz, N., Etlik, O., & Yazici, T., (2006). Primary hydatid cyst of the brain during pregnancy—case report. *Neurol Med Chir* (Tokyo), *46,* 415–417.

### *2.6.2   MEBENDAZOLE*

**FDA Category: C**

***Risk Summary:*** It should be used with caution because the human pregnancy experience has shown a low risk.

**Further Reading:**
- D'Alauro, F., Lee, R. V., Pao-In, K., & Khairallah, M., (1985). Intestinal parasites and pregnancy. *Obstet. Gynecol., 66,* 639–643.
- Diav-Citrin, O., Shechtman, S., Arnon, J., Lubart, I., & Ornoy, A., (2003). Pregnancy outcome after gestational exposure to mebendazole: A prospective controlled cohort study. *Am. J. Obstet. Gynecol., 188,* 282–285.
- *Drug Information. Vermox.* McNeil Consumer.

### *2.6.3   IVERMECTIN*

**FDA Category: C**

***Risk Summary:*** It should be used with caution because the human pregnancy experience has shown a low risk.

**Further Reading:**
- Chippaux, J. P., Gardon-Wendel, N., Gardon, J., & Ernould, J. C., (1993). Absence of any adverse effect of inadvertent ivermectin treatment during pregnancy. *Tran. R. Soc. Trop. Med. Hyg., 87,* 318.
- *Drug Information.* Stromectol. Merck.
- Pacque, M., Munoz, B., Poetschke, G., Foose, J., Greene, B. M., & Taylor, H. R., (1990). Pregnancy outcome after inadvertent ivermectin treatment during community-based distribution. *Lancet, 336,* 1486–1489.

## 2.6.4   PIPERAZINE

**FDA Category: N**
***Risk Summary:*** It should be used only when the maternal benefit outweighs the fetal risk because there is very limited human pregnancy data, and the animal studies are not relevant.

**Further Reading:**
- Heinonen, O. P., Slone, D., & Shapiro, S., (1977). *Birth Defects and Drugs in Pregnancy* (p. 299). Littleton, MA: Publishing Sciences Group.
- Leach, F. N., (1990). Management of threadworm infestation during pregnancy. *Arch Dis. Child, 65,* 399–400.

## 2.6.5   PYRANTEL PAMOATE

**FDA Category: C**
***Risk Summary:*** It should be used with caution because the human pregnancy experience has shown a low risk.

**Further Reading:**
- Owaki, Y., Sakai, T., & Momiyama, H., (1971). Teratological studies on pyrantel pamoate in rabbits. *Oyo Yakuri, 5,* 33–39. As cited in: Shepard, T. H., Catalog of Teratogenic Agents. (6th edn., p. 536). Baltimore, MD: The Johns Hopkins University Press, 1989.
- Owaki, Y., Sakai, T., & Momiyama, H., (1971). Teratological studies on pyrantel pamoate in rats. *Oyo Yakuri, 5,* 41–50. As cited

in: Shepard, T. H., Catalog of Teratogenic Agents. (6ᵗʰ edn., p. 536). Baltimore, MD: The Johns Hopkins University Press, 1989.

## 2.7   SCABICIDE

### 2.7.1   BENZYL ALCOHOL

**FDA Category: B**
*Risk Summary:* The reproduction studies in animals have shown no evidence of fetal harm or impaired fertility. The pregnancy experience in humans is limited.

**Further Reading:**
- Craig, D. B., & Habib, G. G., (1977). Flaccid paraparesis following obstetrical epidural anesthesia: Possible role of benzyl alcohol. *Anesth Analg., 56,* 219–221.
- *Drug Information.* Ulesfia. Shionogi Pharma.

### 2.7.2   CROTAMITON

**FDA Category: C**
*Risk Summary:* It should be used with caution because the pregnancy experience in humans is limited and the reproduction studies in animals have shown low risk.

**Further Reading:**
- Schaefer, Christof, Paul, P., & Richard, K. M., (2015). *Drugs During Pregnancy and Lactation Treatment Options and Risk Assessment.* Amsterdam: Elsevier.

### 2.7.3   PERMETHRIN

**FDA Category: B**
*Risk Summary:* The reproduction studies in animals have shown no evidence of fetal harm or impaired fertility. The pregnancy experience in humans is adequate to exhibit that the embryo-fetal risk is nonexistent or very low.

**Further Reading:**
- Clinical Effectiveness Group (Association of Genitourinary Medicine and the Medical Society for the Study of Venereal Diseases) (1999). National guideline for the management of scabies. *Sex Transm Inf.*, *75*(Suppl), S76–77.
- *Drug Information*. Elimite. Allergan.

## 2.7.4   *LINDANE*

**FDA Category: C**
***Risk Summary:*** It should be used with caution because the pregnancy experience in humans is limited and the reproduction studies in animals have shown low risk.

**Further Reading:**
- *Drug Information*. Lindane Lotion USP 1%. Alpharma.
- Palmer, A. K., Cozens, D. D., Spicer, E. J. F., & Worden, A. N., (1978). Effects of lindane upon reproduction function in a 3-generation study of rats. *Toxicology, 10,* 45–54.

## KEYWORDS

- **albendazole**
- **benzyl alcohol**
- **ivermectin**
- **mebendazole**
- **piperazine**
- **pyrantel pamoate**

# CHAPTER 3

# Cardiovascular Drugs

## 3.1 ANTIDYSRHYTHMIC DRUGS

### 3.1.1 ANTIDYSRHYTHMICS CLASS IA

#### 3.1.1.1 QUINIDINE

**FDA Category: C**

*Risk Summary:* The reproduction studies in animals have shown no evidence of fetal harm or impaired fertility. The pregnancy experience in humans is adequate to exhibit that the embryo-fetal risk is nonexistent or very low.

**Further Reading:**

- Guntheroth, W. G., Cyr, D. R., Mack, L. A., Benedetti, T., Lenke, R. R., & Petty, C. N., (1985). Hydrops from reciprocating atrioventricular tachycardia in a 27-week fetus requiring quinidine for conversion. *Obstet. Gynecol., 66*(Suppl), 29S–33S.
- Kambam, J. R., Franks, J. J., & Smith, B. E., (1987). Inhibitory effect of quinidine on plasma pseudocholinesterase activity in pregnant women. *Am. J. Obstet. Gynecol., 157*, 897–899.
- Tamari, I., Eldar, M., Rabinowitz, B., & Neufeld, H. N., (1982). Medical treatment of cardiovascular disorders during pregnancy. *Am. Heart J., 104*, 1357–1363.

## 3.1.1.2   PROCAINAMIDE

**FDA Category: C**
*Risk Summary:* It should be used only when the maternal benefit outweighs the fetal risk because there is very limited human pregnancy data, and the animal studies are not relevant.

**Further Reading:**
- Hallak, M., Neerhof, M. G., Perry, R., Nazir, M., & Huhta, J. C., (1991). Fetal supraventricular tachycardia and hydrops fetalis: Combined intensive, direct, and transplacental therapy. *Obstet. Gynecol., 78,* 523–525.
- Rotmensch, H. H., Elkayam, U., & Frishman, W., (1983). Antiarrhythmic drug therapy during pregnancy. *Ann. Intern. Med., 98,* 487–497.
- Weiner, C. P., & Thompson, M. I. B., (1988). Direct treatment of fetal supraventricular tachycardia after failed transplacental therapy. *Am. J. Obstet. Gynecol., 158,* 570–573.

## 3.1.1.3   DISOPYRAMIDE

**FDA Category: C**
*Risk Summary:* It should be used with caution, especially during the 3rd Trimester, because Disopyramide has been found to an Oxytocic effect.

**Further Reading:**
- *Drug Information.* Norpace. G. D. Searle and Company.
- Rotmensch, H. H., Rotmensch, S., & Elkayam, U., (1987). Management of cardiac arrhythmias during pregnancy: Current concepts. *Drugs, 33,* 623–633.
- Tadmor, O. P., Keren, A., Rosenak, D., Gal, M., Shaia, M., Hornstein, E., Yaffe, H., Graff, E., Stern, S., & Diamant, Y. Z., (1990). The effect of disopyramide on uterine contractions during pregnancy. *Am. J. Obstet. Gynecol., 162,* 482–486.

## 3.1.1.4   MORICIZINE

**FDA Category: B**
*Risk Summary:* Although Moricizine has been assigned with the letter (B), according to the FDA categorization, but it should be used with caution

because no human data is available and the reproduction studies in animals have shown low risk.

**Further Reading:**
- *Drug Information. Ethmozine.* Roberts Pharmaceutical.


### 3.1.2 ANTIDYSRHYTHMICS CLASS IB

#### 3.1.2.1 LIDOCAINE

**FDA Category: B**
**Risk Summary:** The reproduction studies in animals have shown no evidence of fetal harm or impaired fertility. The pregnancy experience in humans is adequate to exhibit that the embryo-fetal risk is nonexistent or very low.

**Further Reading:**
- Abboud, T. K., Williams, V., Miller, F., Henriksen, E. H., Doan, T., Van Dorsen, J. P., & Earl, S., (1981). Comparative fetal, maternal, and neonatal responses following epidural analgesia with bupivacaine, chloroprocaine, and lidocaine. *Anesthesiology, 55*(Suppl), A315.
- Cordina, R., & Mark, A. M., (2010). "Maternal cardiac arrhythmias during pregnancy and lactation." *Obstetric Medicine, 3*(1), 8–16.
- *Drug Information. Xylocaine.* AstraZeneca.


#### 3.1.2.2 PHENYTOIN

**FDA Category: D**
**Risk Summary:** The use of Phenytoin during pregnancy has been associated with teratogenic effects in the newborns. If its use was mandatory, it is recommended to give Folic Acid 5 mg/day at the beginning or even before the start of pregnancy.

**Further Reading:**
- D'Souza, S. W., Robertson, I. G., Donnai, D., & Mawer, G., (1990). Fetal phenytoin exposure, hypoplastic nails, and jitteriness. *Arch Dis. Child, 65*, 320–324.
- Hiilesmaa, V. K., Teramo, K., Granstrom, M. L., & Bardy, A. H., (1983). Serum folate concentrations during pregnancy in women

with epilepsy: Relation to antiepileptic drug concentrations, number of seizures, and fetal outcome. *Br. Med. J., 287*, 577–579.

- Lewin, P. K., (1973). Phenytoin associated congenital defects with Y-chromosome variant. *Lancet, 1*, 559.
- Sabry, M. A., & Farag, T. I., (1996). Hand anomalies in fetal-hydantoin syndrome: From nail/phalangeal hypoplasia to unilateral acheiria. *Am. J. Med. Genet., 62*, 410–412.
- Truog, W. E., Feusner, J. H., & Baker, D. L., (1980). Association of hemorrhagic disease and the syndrome of persistent fetal circulation with the fetal hydantoin syndrome. *J. Pediatr, 96*, 112–114.

### 3.1.2.3   MEXILETINE

**FDA Category: C**
***Risk Summary:*** It should be used with caution because the pregnancy experience in humans is limited and the reproduction studies in animals have shown low risk.

**Further Reading:**
- Brodsky, M., Doria, R., Allen, B., Sato, D., Thomas, G., & Sada, M., (1992). New-onset ventricular tachycardia during pregnancy. *Am Heart J., 123*, 933–941.
- *Drug Information*. Mexiletine. Watson Laboratories.
- Gregg, A. R., & Tomich, P. G., (1988). Mexiletine use in pregnancy. *J. Perinatol Winter, 8*, 33–35.
- Lownes, H. E., & Ives, T. J., (1987). Mexiletine use in pregnancy and lactation. *Am. J. Obstet. Gynecol., 157*, 446, 447.

### 3.1.3   ANTIDYSRHYTHMICS CLASS IC

### 3.1.3.1   FLECAINIDE

**FDA Category: C**
***Risk Summary:*** The pregnancy experience in humans is limited, and the reproduction studies in animals have shown moderate risk.

**Further Reading:**
- Connaughton, M., & Jenkins, B. S., (1994). Successful use of flecainide to treat new-onset maternal ventricular tachycardia in pregnancy. *Br. Heart J., 72,* 297.
- *Drug Information,* Tambocor. 3M Pharmaceuticals.
- Kofinas, A. D., Simon, N. V., Sagel, H., Lyttle, E., Smith, N., & King, K., (1991). Treatment of fetal supraventricular tachycardia with flecainide acetate after digoxin failure. *Am. J. Obstet. Gynecol., 165,* 630–631.
- Wren, C., & Hunter, S., (1988). Maternal administration of flecainide to terminate and suppress fetal tachycardia. *Br. Med. J., 296,* 249.

## 3.1.3.2   PROPAFENONE

**FDA Category: C**
*Risk Summary:* The pregnancy experience in humans is limited, and the reproduction studies in animals have shown moderate risk.

**Further Reading:**
- Brunozzi, L. T., Meniconi, L., Chiocchi, P., Liberati, R., Zuanetti, G., & Latini, R., (1988). Propafenone in the treatment of chronic ventricular arrhythmias in a pregnant patient. *Br. J. Clin. Pharmacol., 26,* 489–490.
- Capucci, A., & Boriani, G., (1995). Propafenone in the treatment of cardiac arrhythmias. A risk-benefit appraisal. *Drug Saf., 12,* 55–72.
- *Drug Information.* Rythmol. Knoll Pharmaceuticals.

## 3.1.4   ANTIDYSRHYTHMICS CLASS II

### 3.1.4.1   PROPRANOLOL

**FDA Category: C**
*Risk Summary:* Propranolol is not a teratogen; however, its use during the 2nd and 3rd Trimesters is discouraged because its administration, during this period, has been linked with the incidence of reduced placental weight and intrauterine growth restriction (IUGR).

**Further Reading:**
- Barnes, A. B., (1970). Chronic propranolol administration during pregnancy: A case report. *J. Reprod Med., 5*, 79–80.
- Fiddler, G. I., (1974). Propranolol and pregnancy. *Lancet, 2*, 722–723.
- Pruyn, S. C., Phelan, J. P., & Buchanan, G. C., (1979). Long-term propranolol therapy in pregnancy: Maternal and fetal outcome. *Am. J. Obstet. Gynecol., 135*, 485–489.

## 3.1.4.2   METOPROLOL

**FDA Category: C**
***Risk Summary:*** Metoprolol is not a teratogen; however, its use during the 2nd and 3rd Trimesters is discouraged because its administration, during this period, has been linked with the incidence of reduced placental weight and IUGR.

**Further Reading:**
- *Drug Information.* Lopressor. CibaGeneva Pharmaceuticals.
- Lindeberg, S., Sandstrom, B., Lundborg, P., & Regardh, C. G., (1984). Disposition of the adrenergic blocker metoprolol in the late-pregnant woman, the amniotic fluid, the cord blood, and the neonate. *Acta Obstet. Gynecol. Scand., 118*(Suppl), 61–64.
- Lundborg, P., Agren, G., Ervik, M., Lindeberg, S., & Sandstrom, B., (1981). Disposition of metoprolol in the newborn. *Br. J. Clin. Pharmacol., 12*, 598–600.
- Sandstrom, B., (1978). Antihypertensive treatment with the adrenergic beta-receptor blocker metoprolol during pregnancy. *Gynecol. Invest., 9*, 195–204.

## 3.1.4.3   NADOLOL

**FDA Category: C**
***Risk Summary:*** Nadolol is not a teratogen; however, its use during the 2nd and 3rd Trimesters is discouraged because its administration, during this period, has been linked with the incidence of reduced placental weight and IUGR.

**Further Reading:**

- *Drug Information*. Corgard. Bristol Laboratories.
- Fox, R. E., Marx, C., & Stark, A. R., (1985). Neonatal effects of maternal nadolol therapy. *Am, J. Obstet. Gynecol., 152*, 1045–1046.
- Saegusa, T., Suzuki, T., & Narama, I., (1983). Reproduction studies of nadolol a new β-adrenergic blocking agent. *Yakuri to Chiryo, 11*, 5119–5138. As cited in: Shepard, T. H., & Lemire, R. J., Catalog of Teratogenic Agents. (12th edn., p. 304). Baltimore, MD: The Johns Hopkins University Press, 2007.

### 3.1.4.4   ATENOLOL

**FDA Category: D**

***Risk Summary:*** Atenolol is not a teratogen; however, its use during the 2nd and 3rd Trimesters is discouraged because its administration, during this period, has been linked with the incidence of reduced placental weight, and IUGR.

**Further Reading:**

- *Drug Information. Tenormin.* Zeneca Pharmaceuticals.
- Ghanem, F. A., & Movahed, A., (2008). Use of antihypertensive drugs during pregnancy and lactation. *Cardiovascular Drug Reviews, 26*(1), 38–49.
- Lardoux, H., Gerard, J., Blazquez, G., Chouty, F., & Flouvat, B., (1983). Hypertension in pregnancy: Evaluation of two beta-blockers atenolol and labetalol. *Eur. Heart J., 4*(Suppl G), 35–40.
- Lip, G. Y., Beevers, M., Churchill, D., Shaffer, L. M., & Beevers, D., (1997). Effect of atenolol on birth weight. *The American Journal of Cardiology, 79*(10), 1436–1438.
- Satge, D., Sasco, A. J., Col, J. Y., Lemonnier, P. G., Hemet, J., & Robert, E., (1997). Antenatal exposure to atenolol and retroperitoneal fibromatosis. *Reprod Toxicol., 11*, 539–541.
- Woods, D. L., & Morrell, D. F., (1982). Atenolol: Side effects in a newborn infant. *Br. Med. J., 285*, 691–692.

### 3.1.4.5   PINDOLOL

**FDA Category: C**

***Risk Summary:*** Pindolol is not a teratogen; however, its use during the 2nd and 3rd Trimesters is discouraged because its administration, during this

period, has been linked with the incidence of reduced placental weight and IUGR.

**Further Reading:**
- *Drug Information*. Visken. Sandoz Pharmaceuticals.
- Ghanem, F. A., & Movahed, A., (2008). Use of Antihypertensive Drugs during Pregnancy and Lactation. *Cardiovascular Drug Reviews*, *26*(1), 38–49.
- Montan, S., Ingemarsson, I., Marsal, K., & Sjoberg, N. O., (1992). A randomized controlled trial of atenolol and pindolol in human pregnancy: Effects on fetal hemodynamics. *Br. Med. J., 304*, 946–949.
- Tuimala, R., & Hartikainen-Sorri, A. L., (1988). Randomized comparison of atenolol and pindolol for treatment of hypertension in pregnancy. *Curr. Ther. Res., 44*, 579–584.

## 3.1.4.6  TIMOLOL

**FDA Category: C**
***Risk Summary:*** Timolol is not a teratogen; however, its use during the 2nd and 3rd Trimesters is discouraged because its administration, during this period, has been linked with the incidence of reduced placental weight and IUGR.

**Further Reading:**
- Devoe, L. D., O'Dell, B. E., Castillo, R. A., Hadi, H. A., & Searle, N., (1986). Metastatic pheochromocytoma in pregnancy and fetal biophysical assessment after maternal administration of alpha-adrenergic, beta-adrenergic, and dopamine antagonists. *Obstet. Gynecol., 68*, 15S–18S.
- *Drug Information*. Blocadren. Merck.
- Ghanem, F. A., & Movahed, A., (2008). Use of Antihypertensive Drugs during Pregnancy and Lactation. *Cardiovascular Drug Reviews*, *26*(1), 38–49.
- Wagenvoort, A. M., Van Vugt, J. M. G., Sobotka, M., & Van Geijn, H. P., (1998). Topical timolol therapy in pregnancy: Is it safe for the fetus? *Teratology, 58*, 258–262.

## 3.1.4.7  ESMOLOL

**FDA Category: C**
*Risk Summary:* Although there is limited data from the human pregnancy experience, but the possible maternal benefit extremely outweighs the unknown or known embryo/fetal risk.

**Further Reading:**
- Ducey, J. P., & Knape, K. G., (1992). Maternal esmolol administration resulting in fetal distress and cesarean section in a term pregnancy. *Anesthesiology, 77*, 829–832.
- Gilson, G. J., Knieriem, K. J., Smith, J. F., Izquierdo, L., Chatterjee, M. S., & Curet, L. B., (1992). Short-acting beta-adrenergic blockade and the fetus. A case report. *J. Reprod Med., 37*, 277–279.
- Losasso, T. J., Muzzi, D. A., & Cucchiara, R. F., (1991). Response of fetal heart rate to maternal administration of esmolol. *Anesthesiology, 74*, 782–784.

## 3.1.4.8  ACEBUTOLOL

**FDA Category: B**
*Risk Summary:* Although Acebutolol has been assigned with the letter (B), according to the FDA categorization, but it should be used with caution because the human data is limited, and the reproduction studies in animals have shown low risk. Nevertheless, Acebutolol has Intrinsic Sympathomimetic activity, and it is expected that Acebutolol has lower fetal risks than other β-Blockers (see Atenolol and Nadolol) that lack this property.

**Further Reading:**
- *Drug Information.* Lopressor. CibaGeneva Pharmaceuticals.
- Ghanem, F. A., & Movahed, A., (2008). Use of antihypertensive drugs during pregnancy and lactation. *Cardiovascular Drug Reviews, 26*(1), 38–49.
- Kaaja, R., Hiilesmaa, V., Holma, K., & Jarvenpaa, A. L., (1992). Maternal antihypertensive therapy with beta-blockers associated with poor outcome in very low birth weight infants. *Int. J. Gynecol. Obstet., 38*, 195–199.

### 3.1.4.9   SOTALOL

**FDA Category: B**
***Risk Summary:*** Although Sotalol has been assigned with the letter (B), according to the FDA categorization, but it should be used with caution because the human data is limited, and the reproduction studies in animals have shown low risk.

**Further Reading:**
- *Drug Information*. Betapace. Berlex Laboratories.
- Oudijk, M. A., Michon, M. M., Kleinman, C. S., Kapusta, L., Stoutenbeek, P., Visser, G. H. A, & Meijboom, E. J., (2000). Sotalol in the treatment of fetal dysrhythmias. *Circulation, 101,* 2721–2726.
- Wagner, X., Jouglard, J., Moulin, M., Miller, A. M., Petitjean, J., & Pisapia, A., (1990). Coadministration of flecainide acetate and sotalol during pregnancy: Lack of teratogenic effects, passage across the placenta, and excretion in human breast milk. *Am. Heart J., 119,* 700–702.

## 3.1.5   ANTIDYSRHYTHMICS CLASS III

### 3.1.5.1   AMIODARONE

**FDA Category: D**
***Risk Summary:*** The use of Amiodarone should be avoided in pregnant women because the pregnancy experience in humans has shown the risk of congenital goiter/hyperthyroidism and hypothyroidism after in-utero exposure.

**Further Reading:**
- *Drug Information*. Cordarone. Wyeth-Ayerst Laboratories.
- Magee, L. A., Downar, E., Sermer, M., Boulton, B. C., Allen, L. C., & Koren, G., (1995). Pregnancy outcome after gestational exposure to amiodarone in Canada. *Am. J. Obstet. Gynecol., 172,* 1307–1311.
- Pitcher, D., Leather, H. M., Storey, G. A. C., & Holt, D. W., (1983). Amiodarone in pregnancy. *Lancet, 1,* 597–598.
- Plomp, T. A., Vulsma, T., & de Vijlder, J. J. M., (1992). Use of amiodarone during pregnancy. *Eur. J. Obstet. Gynecol. Reprod. Biol., 43,* 201–207.

## 3.1.5.2 BRETYLIUM

**FDA Category: C**
***Risk Summary:*** The reproduction studies in animals have shown no evidence of fetal harm or impaired fertility. The pregnancy experience in humans is very limited.

**Further Reading:**
- West, G. B., (1962). Drugs and Rat Pregnancy. *Journal of Pharmacy and Pharmacology*, *14*(1), 828–830.

## 3.1.6 ANTIDYSRHYTHMICS CLASS IV

### 3.1.6.1 IBUTILIDE

**FDA Category: C**
***Risk Summary:*** The pregnancy experience in humans is limited, and the reproduction studies in animals have shown moderate risk. Nevertheless, the use of Ibutilide rational because it is usually used for correcting a life-threatening arrhythmia in the mother that would be, by itself, more harmful to the baby if untreated.

**Further Reading:**
- Burkart, T. A., Kron, J., Miles, W. M., Conti, J. B., & Gonzalez, M. D., (2007). Successful termination of atrial flutter by ibutilide during pregnancy. *Pacing Clin. Electrophysiol., 30*, 283–286.
- *Drug Information.* Corvert, Pharmacia & Upjohn.
- Kockova, R., Kocka, V., Kiernan, T., & Fahy, G. J., (2007). Ibutilide-induced cardioversion of atrial fibrillation during pregnancy. *J. Cardiovasc. Electrophysiol., 18*, 545–547.
- Marks, T. A., & Terry, R. D., (1996). Developmental toxicity of ibutilide fumarate in rats after oral administration. *Teratology, 54*, 157–164.

### 3.1.6.2 DOFETILIDE

**FDA Category: C**
***Risk Summary:*** It is better to look for an alternative drug, if possible, because the pregnancy experience in humans is limited, and the reproduction studies in animals have shown the risk of teratogenicity and fetal toxicity.

**Further Reading:**
- *Drug Information*. Tikosyn. Pfizer.
- Webster, W. S., Brown-Woodman, P. D. C, Snow, M. D., & Danielsson, B. R. G., (1996). Teratogenic potential of almokalant, dofetilide, and d-sotalol: Drugs with potassium channel blocking activity. *Teratology, 53*, 168–175.

### 3.1.6.3   VERAPAMIL

**FDA Category: C**
***Risk Summary:*** Although Verapamil has been assigned with the letter "C" by the FDA, but many experts believe Verapamil use is mostly safe because the reproduction studies in animals have shown no evidence of fetal harm or impaired fertility. Furthermore, the pregnancy experience in humans is adequate to exhibit that the embryo-fetal risk is nonexistent or very low.

**Further Reading:**
- *Drug Information*. Calan. G.D. G.D. Searle.
- Gummerus, M., (1977). Treatment of premature labor and antagonization of the side effects of tocolytic therapy with verapamil. *Z Geburtshilfe Perinatol., 181*, 334–340.
- Klein, V., & Repke, J. T., (1984). Supraventricular tachycardia in pregnancy: Cardioversion with verapamil. *Obstet, Gynecol., 63*, 16S–18S.
- Lilja, H., Karlsson, K., Lindecrantz, K., & Sabel, K. G., (1984). Treatment of intrauterine supraventricular tachycardia with digoxin and verapamil. *J. Perinat. Med., 12*, 151–154.

### 3.1.6.4   DILTIAZEM

**FDA Category: C**
***Risk Summary:*** It should be used with extreme caution because the human pregnancy experience has shown low risk, and the animal reproduction studies have found a high risk to the fetus.

**Further Reading:**
- *Drug Information*. Cardizem. Hoechst Marion Roussel.

- El-Sayed, Y., & Holbrook, R. H, Jr., (1996). Diltiazem (D) for the maintenance tocolysis of preterm labor (PTL): A prospective randomized trial (abstract). *Am. J. Obstet. Gynecol., 174*, 468.
- Lubbe, W. F., (1987). Use of diltiazem during pregnancy. *NZ Med. J., 100*, 121.

## 3.1.6.5  BEPRIDIL

**FDA Category: C**
*Risk Summary:* Bepridil has not been studied during pregnancy.

**Further Reading:**
- Drugs@FDA: FDA Approved Drug Products. (n.d.). Retrieved from https://www.accessdata.fda.gov/scripts/cder/daf/index.cfm?event= overview.process&ApplNo=019002 (accessed on 30 January 2020).

## 3.1.7  MISCELLANEOUS ANTIDYSARRHYTHMIC AGENTS

### 3.1.7.1  DIGOXIN

**FDA Category: C**
*Risk Summary:* The reproduction studies in animals have shown no evidence of fetal harm or impaired fertility. The pregnancy experience in humans is adequate to exhibit that the embryo-fetal risk is nonexistent or very low.

**Further Reading:**
- Lingman, G., Ohrlander, S., & Ohlin, P., (1980). Intrauterine digoxin treatment of fetal paroxysmal tachycardia: a case report. *Br. J. Obstet. Gynaecol., 87*, 340–342.
- Shepard, T. H., (1980). *Catalog of Teratogenic Agents*. Baltimore, M. D., (3rd edn., pp. 116,117). Johns Hopkins University Press.
- Simpson, P. C., Trudinger, B. J., Walker, A., & Baird, P. J., (1983). The intrauterine treatment of fetal cardiac failure in a twin pregnancy with an acardiac, acephalic monster. *Am. J. Obstet. Gynecol., 147*, 842–844.

## 3.1.7.2   *ADENOSINE*

**FDA Category: C**
***Risk Summary:*** Although there is limited data from the human pregnancy experience, but the possible maternal benefit extremely outweighs the unknown or known embryo/fetal risk.

**Further Reading:**
*   Dangel, J. H., Roszkowski, T., Bieganowska, K., Kubicka, K., & Ganowicz, J., (2000). Adenosine triphosphate for cardioversion of supraventricular tachycardia in two hydropic fetuses. *Fetal Diagn Ther., 15*, 326–330.
*   Elkayam, U., & Goodwin, T. M. Jr., (1995). Adenosine therapy for supraventricular tachycardia during pregnancy. *Am. J. Cardiol., 75*, 521–523.

## 3.2   ANTI-ANGINAL DRUGS

### 3.2.1   *ATENOLOL*

**FDA Category: D**
***Risk Summary:*** Atenolol is not a teratogen; however, its use during the 2nd and 3rd Trimesters is discouraged because its administration, during this period, has been linked with the incidence of reduced placental weight, and IUGR. |

**Further Reading:**
*   *Drug Information*. Tenormin. Zeneca Pharmaceuticals.
*   Ghanem, F. A., & Movahed, A., (2008). Use of antihypertensive drugs during pregnancy and lactation. *Cardiovascular Drug Reviews, 26*(1), 38–49.
*   Lardoux, H., Gerard, J., Blazquez, G., Chouty, F., & Flouvat, B., (1983). Hypertension in pregnancy: Evaluation of two beta-blockers atenolol and labetalol. *Eur. Heart J., 4*(Suppl G), 35–40.
*   Lip, G. Y., Beevers, M., Churchill, D., Shaffer, L. M., & Beevers, D., (1997). Effect of atenolol on birth weight. *The American Journal of Cardiology, 79*(10), 1436–1438.

- Satge, D., Sasco, A. J., Col, J. Y., Lemonnier, P. G., Hemet, J., & Robert, E., (1997). Antenatal exposure to atenolol and retroperitoneal fibromatosis. *Reprod Toxicol., 11*, 539–541.
- Woods, D. L., & Morrell, D. F., (1982). Atenolol: Side effects in a newborn infant. *Br Med. J., 285*, 691–692.

## 3.2.2 METOPROLOL

**FDA Category: C**
***Risk Summary:*** Metoprolol is not a teratogen; however, its use during the 2nd and 3rd Trimesters is discouraged because its administration, during this period, has been linked with the incidence of reduced placental weight and IUGR.

**Further Reading:**
- *Drug Information*. Lopressor. CibaGeneva Pharmaceuticals.
- Lindeberg, S., Sandstrom, B., Lundborg, P., & Regardh, C. G., (1984). Disposition of the adrenergic blocker metoprolol in the late-pregnant woman, the amniotic fluid, the cord blood, and the neonate. *Acta Obstet. Gynecol. Scand, 118*(Suppl):61–64.
- Lundborg, P., Agren, G., Ervik, M., Lindeberg, S., & Sandstrom, B., (1981). Disposition of metoprolol in the newborn. *Br. J. Clin. Pharmacol., 12*, 598–600.
- Sandstrom, B., (1978). Antihypertensive treatment with the adrenergic beta-receptor blocker metoprolol during pregnancy. *Gynecol. Invest., 9*, 195–204.

## 3.2.3 NADOLOL

**FDA Category: C**
***Risk Summary:*** Nadolol is not a teratogen; however, its use during the 2nd and 3rd Trimesters is discouraged because its administration, during this period, has been linked with the incidence of reduced placental weight and IUGR.

**Further Reading:**
- *Drug Information*. Corgard. Bristol Laboratories.

- Fox, R. E., Marx, C., & Stark, A. R., (1985). Neonatal effects of maternal nadolol therapy. *Am. J. Obstet. Gynecol., 152*, 1045–1046.
- Saegusa, T., Suzuki, T., & Narama, I., (1983). Reproduction studies of nadolol a new β-adrenergic blocking agent. *Yakuri to Chiryo, 11*, 5119–5138. As cited in: Shepard, T. H., & Lemire, R. J., (2007). *Catalog of Teratogenic Agents* (12th edn., p. 304). Baltimore, MD: The Johns Hopkins University Press.

### 3.2.4	PROPRANOLOL

**FDA Category: C**

*Risk Summary:* Propranolol is not a teratogen; however, its use during the 2nd and 3rd Trimesters is discouraged because its administration, during this period, has been linked with the incidence of reduced placental weight and IUGR.

**Further Reading:**

- Barnes, A. B., (1970). Chronic propranolol administration during pregnancy: A case report. *J. Reprod Med., 5*, 79–80.
- Fiddler, G. I., (1974). Propranolol and pregnancy. *Lancet, 2*, 722–723.
- Pruyn, S. C., Phelan, J. P., & Buchanan, G. C., (1979). Long-term propranolol therapy in pregnancy: Maternal and fetal outcome. *Am. J. Obstet. Gynecol., 135*, 485–489.

### 3.2.5	DILTIAZEM

**FDA Category: C**

*Risk Summary:* It should be used with extreme caution because the human pregnancy experience has shown low risk, and the animal reproduction studies have found a high risk to the fetus.

**Further Reading:**

- *Drug Information*. Cardizem. Hoechst Marion Roussel.
- El-Sayed, Y., & Holbrook, R. H. Jr., (1996). Diltiazem (D) for the maintenance tocolysis of preterm labor (PTL): A prospective random-ized trial (abstract). *Am. J. Obstet. Gynecol., 174*, 468.
- Lubbe, W. F., (1987). Use of diltiazem during pregnancy. *NZ Med. J., 100*, 121.

## 3.2.6   VERAPAMIL

**FDA Category: C**
*Risk Summary:* Although Verapamil has been assigned with the letter "C" by the FDA, but many experts believe Verapamil use is mostly safe because the reproduction studies in animals have shown no evidence of fetal harm or impaired fertility. Furthermore, the pregnancy experience in humans is adequate to exhibit that the embryo-fetal risk is nonexistent or very low.

**Further Reading:**
- *Drug Information*. Calan. G.D. G.D. Searle.
- Gummerus, M., (1977). Treatment of premature labor and antagonization of the side effects of tocolytic therapy with verapamil. *Z Geburtshilfe Perinatol., 181*, 334–340.
- Klein, V., & Repke, J. T., (1984). Supraventricular tachycardia in pregnancy: Cardioversion with verapamil. *Obstet. Gynecol., 63*, 16S–18S.
- Lilja, H., Karlsson, K., Lindecrantz, K., & Sabel, K. G., (1984). Treatment of intrauterine supraventricular tachycardia with digoxin and verapamil. *J. Perinat. Med., 12*, 151–154.

## 3.2.7   ISOSORBIDE DINITRATE

**FDA Category: C**
*Risk Summary:* It should be used with caution because the pregnancy experience in humans is limited and the reproduction studies in animals have shown low risk. Interestingly, isosorbide dinitrate may be beneficial in inverting the effects of increased vascular resistance to flow in the utero-placental circulation, and the generalized vasoconstriction associated with preeclampsia.

**Further Reading:**
- Amit, A., Thaler, I., Paz, Y., & Itskovity-Eldor, J., (1998). The effect of a nitric oxide donor on Doppler flow velocity waveforms in the uterine artery during the first trimester of pregnancy. *Ultrasound Obstet. Gynecol., 11*, 94–98.
- *Drug Information*. Isordil. Wyeth-Ayerst Laboratories.
- Thaler, I., Amit, A., & Itskovitz, J., (1995). The effect of isosorbide dinitrate, a nitric oxide donor, on human uterine and placental

vascular resistance in patients with preeclampsia (abstract). *Am. J. Obstet. Gynecol.,172*, 387.
- Thaler, I., Amit, A., Jakobi, P., & Itskovitz-Eldor, J., (1996). The effect of isosorbide dinitrate on uterine artery and umbilical artery flow velocity waveforms at mid-pregnancy. *Obstet. Gynecol., 88*, 838–843.

## 3.2.8  ISOSORBIDE MONONITRATE

**FDA Category: C**
***Risk Summary:*** It should be used with caution because the pregnancy experience in humans is limited and the reproduction studies in animals have shown low risk.

**Further Reading:**
- Bollapragada, S. S., MacKenzie, F., Norrie, J. D., Eddama, O., Petrou, S., Reid, M., & Norman, J. E., (2009). Randomized placebo-controlled trial of outpatient (at home) cervical ripening with isosorbide mononitrate (IMN) prior to induction of labor-clinical trial with analyses of efficacy and acceptability. The IMOP study. *BJOG, 116*, 1185–1195.
- *Drug Information. Ismo.* Wyeth-Ayerst Laboratories.

## 3.2.9  NITROGLYCERIN

**FDA Category: C**
***Risk Summary:*** It should be used with caution because the human pregnancy experience has shown a low risk.

**Further Reading:**
- Bootstaylor, B., Roman, C., Heymann, M. A., & Parer, J. T., (1994). Fetal cardiorespiratory effects of nitroglycerin in the near-term pregnant sheep (abstract). *Am. J. Obstet. Gynecol., 170*, 281.
- Hood, D. D., Dewan, D. M., James, F. M. III., Bogard, T. D., & Floyd, H. M., (1983). The use of nitroglycerin in preventing the hypertensive response to tracheal intubation in severe preeclamptics. *Anesthesiology, 59*, A423.

- Oketani, Y., Mitsuzono, T., Ichikawa, K., Itono, Y., Gojo, T., Gofuku, M., & Konoha, N., (1981). Toxicological studies on nitroglycerin (NK-843). 6. Teratological studies in rabbits. *Oyo Yakuri, 22,* 633–638. As cited in: Schardein, J. L., *Chemically Induced Birth Defects.* (2nd edn., p. 91). New York, NY: Marcel Dekker, 1993.

## 3.3 ANTI-HYPERTENSIVES

### *3.3.1 B-BLOCKERS*

#### *3.3.1.1 ATENOLOL*

**FDA Category: D**
***Risk Summary:*** Atenolol is not a teratogen; however, its use during the 2nd and 3rd Trimesters is discouraged because its administration, during this period, has been linked with the incidence of reduced placental weight, and IUGR.

**Further Reading:**
- *Drug Information.* Tenormin. Zeneca Pharmaceuticals.
- Ghanem, F. A., & Movahed, A., (2008). Use of antihypertensive drugs during pregnancy and lactation. *Cardiovascular Drug Reviews, 26*(1), 38–49.
- Lardoux, H., Gerard, J., Blazquez, G., Chouty, F., & Flouvat, B., (1983). Hypertension in pregnancy: Evaluation of two beta-blockers atenolol and labetalol. *Eur. Heart J., 4*(Suppl G), 35–40.
- Lip, G. Y., Beevers, M., Churchill, D., Shaffer, L. M., & Beevers, D., (1997). Effect of atenolol on birth weight. *The American Journal of Cardiology, 79*(10), 1436–1438.
- Satge, D., Sasco, A. J., Col, J. Y., Lemonnier, P. G., Hemet, J., & Robert, E., (1997). Antenatal exposure to atenolol and retroperitoneal fibromatosis. *Reprod Toxicol., 11,* 539–541.
- Woods, D. L., & Morrell, D. F., (1982). Atenolol: Side effects in a newborn infant. *Br. Med. J., 285,* 691–692.

## 3.3.1.2   ACEBUTOLOL

**FDA Category: B**
*Risk Summary:* Although Acebutolol has been assigned with the letter (B), according to the FDA categorization, but it should be used with caution because the human data is limited, and the reproduction studies in animals have shown low risk. Nevertheless, Acebutolol has Intrinsic Sympathomimetic activity, and it is expected that Acebutolol has lower fetal risks than other β-Blockers (see Atenolol and Nadolol) that lack this property.

**Further Reading:**
- *Drug Information.* Lopressor. CibaGeneva Pharmaceuticals.
- Ghanem, F. A., & Movahed, A., (2008). Use of Antihypertensive Drugs during Pregnancy and Lactation. *Cardiovascular Drug Reviews, 26*(1), 38–49.
- Kaaja, R., Hiilesmaa, V., Holma, K., & Jarvenpaa, A. L., (1992). Maternal antihypertensive therapy with beta-blockers associated with poor outcome in very low birth weight infants. *Int. J. Gynecol. Obstet., 38*, 195–199.

## 3.3.1.3   ESMOLOL

**FDA Category: C**
*Risk Summary:* Although there is limited data from the human pregnancy experience, but the possible maternal benefit extremely outweighs the unknown or known embryo/fetal risk.

**Further Reading:**
- Ducey, J. P., & Knape, K. G., (1992). Maternal esmolol administration resulting in fetal distress and cesarean section in a term pregnancy. *Anesthesiology, 77*, 829–832.
- Gilson, G. J., Knieriem, K. J., Smith, J. F., Izquierdo, L., Chatterjee, M. S., & Curet, L. B., (1992). Short-acting beta-adrenergic blockade and the fetus. A case report. *J. Reprod Med., 37*, 277–279.
- Losasso, T. J., Muzzi, D. A., & Cucchiara, R. F., (1991). Response of fetal heart rate to maternal administration of esmolol. *Anesthesiology, 74*, 782–784.

## 3.3.1.4   *METOPROLOL*

**FDA Category: C**
***Risk Summary:*** Metoprolol is not a teratogen; however, its use during the 2nd and 3rd Trimesters is discouraged because its administration, during this period, has been linked with the incidence of reduced placental weight and IUGR.

**Further Reading:**
- *Drug Information.* Lopressor. CibaGeneva Pharmaceuticals.
- Lindeberg, S., Sandstrom, B., Lundborg, P., & Regardh, C. G.,(1984). Disposition of the adrenergic blocker metoprolol in the late-pregnant woman, the amniotic fluid, the cord blood, and the neonate. *Acta Obstet. Gynecol. Scand., 118*(Suppl), 61–64.
- Lundborg, P., Agren, G., Ervik, M., Lindeberg, S., & Sandstrom, B.,(1981). Disposition of metoprolol in the newborn. *Br. J. Clin. Pharmacol., 12*, 598–600.
- Sandstrom, B., (1978). Antihypertensive treatment with the adrenergic beta-receptor blocker metoprolol during pregnancy. *Gynecol. Invest., 9*, 195–204.

## 3.3.1.5   *NADOLOL*

**FDA Category: C**
***Risk Summary:*** Nadolol is not a teratogen; however, its use during the 2nd and 3rd Trimesters is discouraged because its administration, during this period, has been linked with the incidence of reduced placental weight and IUGR.

**Further Reading:**
- *Drug Information.* Corgard. Bristol Laboratories.
- Fox, R. E., Marx, C., & Stark, A. R., (1985). Neonatal effects of maternal nadolol therapy. *Am. J. Obstet. Gynecol.,152*, 1045–1046.
- Saegusa, T., Suzuki, T., & Narama, I., (1983). Reproduction studies of nadolol a new β-adrenergic blocking agent. *Yakuri to Chiryo, 11*, 5119–5138. As cited in: Shepard, T. H., & Lemire, R. J., *Catalog of Teratogenic Agents.* (12th edn., p. 304). Baltimore, MD: The Johns Hopkins University Press, 2007.

### 3.3.1.6   PROPRANOLOL

**FDA Category: C**
***Risk Summary:*** Propranolol is not a teratogen; however, its use during the 2nd and 3rd Trimesters is discouraged because its administration, during this period, has been linked with the incidence of reduced placental weight and IUGR.

**Further Reading:**
- Barnes, A. B., (1970). Chronic propranolol administration during pregnancy: A case report. *J, Reprod. Med., 5,* 79–80.
- Fiddler, G. I., (1974). Propranolol and pregnancy. *Lancet, 2,* 722–723.
- Pruyn, S. C., Phelan, J. P., & Buchanan, G. C., (1979). Long-term propranolol therapy in pregnancy: Maternal and fetal outcome. *Am. J. Obstet. Gynecol., 135,* 485–489.

### 3.3.1.7   PINDOLOL

**FDA Category: C**
***Risk Summary:*** Pindolol is not a teratogen; however, its use during the 2nd and 3rd Trimesters is discouraged because its administration, during this period, has been linked with the incidence of reduced placental weight and IUGR.

**Further Reading:**
- *Drug Information*. Visken. Sandoz Pharmaceuticals.
- Ghanem, F. A., & Movahed, A., (2008). Use of antihypertensive drugs during pregnancy and lactation. *Cardiovascular Drug Reviews, 26*(1), 38–49.
- Montan, S., Ingemarsson, I., Marsal, K., & Sjoberg, N. O., (1992). A randomized controlled trial of atenolol and pindolol in human pregnancy: Effects on fetal hemodynamics. *Br Med. J., 304,* 946–949.
- Tuimala, R., & Hartikainen-Sorri, A. L., (1988). Randomized comparison of atenolol and pindolol for treatment of hypertension in pregnancy. *Curr. Ther. Res., 44,* 579–584.

### 3.3.1.8  TIMOLOL

**FDA Category: C**
*Risk Summary:* Timolol is not a teratogen; however, its use during the 2nd and 3rd Trimesters is discouraged because its administration, during this period, has been linked with the incidence of reduced placental weight and IUGR.

**Further Reading:**
- Devoe, L. D., O'Dell, B. E., Castillo, R. A., Hadi, H. A., & Searle, N., (1986). Metastatic pheochromocytoma in pregnancy and fetal biophysical assessment after maternal administration of alpha-adrenergic, beta-adrenergic, and dopamine antagonists. *Obstet. Gynecol.*, *68*, 15S–18S.
- *Drug Information*. Blocadren. Merck.
- Ghanem, F. A., & Movahed, A., (2008). Use of antihypertensive drugs during pregnancy and lactation. *Cardiovascular Drug Reviews*, *26*(1), 38–49.
- Wagenvoort, A. M., Van Vugt, J. M. G., Sobotka, M., & Van Geijn, H. P., (1998). Topical timolol therapy in pregnancy: Is it safe for the fetus? *Teratology*, *58*, 258–262.

### 3.3.1.9  LABETALOL

**FDA Category: C**
*Risk Summary:* It should be used with caution because the human pregnancy experience has shown a low risk.

**Further Reading:**
- *Drug Information*. Normodyne. Schering.
- Nylund, L., Lunell, N. O., Lewander, R., Sarby, B., & Thornstrom, S., (1984). Labetalol for the treatment of hypertension in pregnancy. *Acta Obstet. Gynecol. Scand.*, *118*(Suppl):71–73.
- Plouin, P. F, Breart, G., Maillard, F., Papiernik, E., & Relier, J. P., (1988). Comparison of antihypertensive efficacy and perinatal safety of labetalol and methyldopa in the treatment of hypertension in pregnancy: A randomized controlled trial. *Br. J. Obstet. Gynaecol.*, *95*, 868–876.

## 3.3.1.10   CARVEDILOL

**FDA Category: C**
***Risk Summary:*** It should be used with caution because the human pregnancy experience is very limited. However, it is plausible to expect that Carvedilol has the same kind of problems associated with the use of β-Blockers during pregnancy.

**Further Reading:**
- *Drug Information*. Coreg. GlaxoSmithKline.

## 3.3.2   CALCIUM CHANNEL BLOCKERS

### 3.3.2.1   AMLODIPINE

**FDA Category: C**
***Risk Summary:*** The pregnancy experience in humans is limited, and the reproduction studies in animals have shown moderate risk.

**Further Reading:**
- *Drug Information*. Norvasc. Pfizer.
- Ghanem, F. A., & Movahed, A., (2008). Use of antihypertensive drugs during pregnancy and lactation. *Cardiovascular Drug Reviews*, *26*(1), 38–49.
- Nahapetian, A., & Oudiz, R. J., (2008). Serial hemodynamics and complications of pregnancy in severe pulmonary arterial hypertension. *Cardiology*, *109*, 237–240.

### 3.3.2.2   FELODIPINE

**FDA Category: C**
***Risk Summary:*** It should be used with caution because the pregnancy experience in humans is limited, and the reproduction studies in animals have shown the risk of teratogenicity associated with the use of Felodipine.

**Further Reading:**
- Casele, H. L., Windley, K. C., Prieto, J. A., Gratton, R., & Laifer, S. A., (1997). Felodipine use in pregnancy. Report of three cases. *J. Reprod. Med., 42*, 378–381.
- *Drug Information*. Plendil. Merck Sharp & Dohm.
- Magee, L. A., Schick, B., Donnenfeld, A. E., Sage, S. R., Conover, B., Cook, L., McElhatton, P. R., Schmidt, M. A., & Koren, G., (1996). The safety of calcium channel blockers in human pregnancy: A prospective, multicenter cohort study. *Am. J. Obstet. Gynecol., 174*, 823–828.

## 3.3.2.3   NIFEDIPINE

**FDA Category: C**
***Risk Summary:*** It should be used with caution because the human pregnancy experience has shown a low risk.

**Further Reading:**
- *Drug Information*. Procardia. Pfizer.
- Harake, B., Gilbert, R. D., Ashwal, S., & Power, G. G., (1987). Nifedipine: Effects on fetal and maternal hemodynamics in pregnant sheep. *Am. J. Obstet. Gynecol., 157*, 1003–1008.
- Snyder, S. W., & Cardwell, M. S., (1989). Neuromuscular blockade with magnesium sulfate and nifedipine. *Am. J. Obstet. Gynecol., 161*, 35, 36.

## 3.3.2.4   NIMODIPINE

**FDA Category: C**
***Risk Summary:*** It should be used with caution because the pregnancy experience in humans is limited, and the reproduction studies in animals have shown the risk of teratogenicity associated with the use of Nimodipine.

**Further Reading:**
- Belfort, M. A., Carpenter, R. J. Jr., Kirshon, B., Saade, G. R., & Moise, K. J. Jr., (1993). The use of nimodipine in a patient with eclampsia: Color flow doppler demonstration of retinal artery relaxation. *Am. J. Obstet. Gynecol., 169*, 204–206.

- Belfort, M. A., Saade, G. R., Moise, K. J. Jr., Cruz, A., Adam, K., Kramer, W., & Kirshon, B., (1994). Nimodipine in the management of preeclampsia: Maternal and fetal effects. *Am. J. Obstet. Gynecol., 171*, 417–424.
- Belfort, M. A., Saade, G. R., Yared, M., Grunewald, C., Herd, J. A., Varner, M. A., & Nisell, H., (1999). Change in estimated cerebral perfusion pressure after treatment with nimodipine or magnesium sulfate in patients with preeclampsia. *Am. J. Obstet. Gynecol., 181*, 402–407.
- *Drug Information*. Nimotop. Bayer.

### 3.3.2.5   NICARDIPINE

**FDA Category: C**
***Risk Summary:*** It should be used with caution because the pregnancy experience in humans is limited, and the reproduction studies in animals have shown the risk of embryotoxicity associated with the use of Nicardipine.

**Further Reading:**
- *Drug Information*. Cardene. Wyeth-Ayerst Pharmaceuticals.
- Jannet, D., Abankwa, A., Guyard, B., Carbonne, B., Marpeau, L., & Milliez, J., (1997). Nicardipine versus salbutamol in the treatment of premature labor. A prospective randomized study. *Eur. J. Obstet. Gynecol Reprod Med., 73*, 11–16.
- Parisi, V. M., Salinas, J., & Stockmar, E. J., (1989). Fetal vascular responses to maternal nicardipine administration in the hypertensive ewe. *Am. J. Obstet. Gynecol., 161*, 1035–1039.

### 3.3.2.6   DILTIAZEM

**FDA Category: C**
***Risk Summary:*** It should be used with extreme caution because the human pregnancy experience has shown low risk, and the animal reproduction studies have found a high risk to the fetus.

**Further Reading:**
- *Drug Information*. Cardizem. Hoechst Marion Roussel.

- El-Sayed, Y., & Holbrook, R. H. Jr., (1996). Diltiazem (D) for the maintenance tocolysis of preterm labor (PTL): A prospective randomized trial (abstract). *Am. J. Obstet. Gynecol., 174,* 468.
- Lubbe, W. F., (1987). Use of diltiazem during pregnancy. *NZ Med. J., 100,* 121.

## 3.3.2.7   VERAPAMIL

**FDA Category: C**
*Risk Summary:* Although Verapamil has been assigned with the letter "C" by the FDA, but many experts believe Verapamil use is mostly safe because the reproduction studies in animals have shown no evidence of fetal harm or impaired fertility. Furthermore, the pregnancy experience in humans is adequate to exhibit that the embryo-fetal risk is nonexistent or very low.

**Further Reading:**
- *Drug Information.* Calan. G.D. G.D. Searle.
- Gummerus, M., (1977). Treatment of premature labor and antagonization of the side effects of tocolytic therapy with verapamil. *Z Geburtshilfe Perinatol., 181,* 334–340.
- Klein, V., & Repke, J. T., (1984). Supraventricular tachycardia in pregnancy: Cardioversion with verapamil. *Obstet. Gynecol., 63,* 16S–18S.
- Lilja, H., Karlsson, K., Lindecrantz, K., & Sabel, K. G., (1984). Treatment of intrauterine supraventricular tachycardia with digoxin and verapamil. *J. Perinat. Med., 12,* 151–154.

## 3.3.3   ANGIOTENSIN-CONVERTING ENZYME INHIBITORS

### 3.3.3.1   CAPTOPRIL

**FDA Category (1st Trimester): C**
**FDA Category (2nd and 3rd Trimesters): D**
*Risk Summary:* Captopril is contraindicated during the 2nd and 3rd Trimesters because the pregnancy experience in humans showed a profound potentiality of teratogenicity and severe fetal toxicity associated with its use during this period.

**Further Reading:**
- Barr, M., (1990). Fetal effects of angiotensin-converting enzyme inhibitor (abstract). *Teratology, 41,* 536.
- Lumbers, E. R., Kingsford, N. M., Menzies, R. I., & Stevens, A. D., (1992). Acute effects of captopril, an angiotensin-converting enzyme inhibitor, on the pregnant ewe and fetus. *Am. J. Physiol., 262* (Regul Integrative Comp Physiol 31), R754–760.
- Millar, J. A., Wilson, P. D., & Morrison, N., (1983). Management of severe hypertension in pregnancy by a combined drug regimen including captopril: Case report. *NZ Med. J., 96,* 796–798.
- Smith, A. M., (1989). Are ACE inhibitors safe in pregnancy? *Lancet, 2,* 750–751.

## 3.3.3.2   ENALAPRIL

**FDA Category: D**
***Risk Summary:*** Enalapril is contraindicated during the 2nd and 3rd Trimesters because the pregnancy experience in humans showed a profound potentiality of teratogenicity and severe fetal toxicity associated with its use during this period.

**Further Reading:**
- Cunniff, C., Jones, K. L., Phillipson, J., Benirschke, K., Short, S., & Wujek, J., (1990). Oligohydramnios sequence and renal tubular malformation associated with maternal enalapril use. *Am. J. Obstet. Gynecol., 162,* 187–189.
- Kreft-Jais, C., Plouin, P. F, Tchobroutsky, C., & Boutroy, M. J., (1988). Angiotensin-converting enzyme inhibitors during pregnancy: A survey of 22 patients given captopril and nine given enalapril. *Br. J. Obstet. Gynaecol., 95,* 420–422.
- Smith, A. M., (1989). Are ACE inhibitors safe in pregnancy? *Lancet, 2,* 750–751.

## 3.3.3.3   LISINOPRIL

**FDA Category: D**
***Risk Summary:*** Lisinopril is contraindicated during the 2nd and 3rd Trimesters because the pregnancy experience in humans showed a profound

potentiality of teratogenicity and severe fetal toxicity associated with its use during this period.

**Further Reading:**
- Cooper, W. O., Hernandez-Diaz, S., Arbogast, P. G., Dudley, J. A., Dyer, S., Gideon, P. S., Hall, K., & Ray, W. A., (2006). Major congenital malformations after first-trimester exposure to ACE inhibitors. *N Engl. J. Med., 354*, 2443–2451.
- *Drug Information*. Prinivil. Merck.
- Tomlinson, A. J., Campbell, J., Walker, J. J., & Morgan, C., (2000). Malignant primary hypertension in pregnancy treated with lisinopril. *Ann Pharmacother., 34*, 180–182.

### 3.3.3.4 RAMIPRIL

**FDA Category: D**
***Risk Summary:*** Ramipril is contraindicated during the 2nd and 3rd Trimesters because the pregnancy experience in humans showed a profound potentiality of teratogenicity and severe fetal toxicity associated with its use during this period.

**Further Reading:**
- *Drug Information*. Altace. Monarch Pharmaceuticals.
- Friedman, J. M., (2006). ACE inhibitors and congenital anomalies. N. *Engl. J. Med.,354*, 2498–2500.
- Kolagasi, O., Sari, F., Akar, M., & Sari, R., (2009). Normal pregnancy and healthy child after continued exposure to gliclazide and ramipril during pregnancy. *Ann. Pharmacother, 43*, 147–149.
- Polifka, J. E., (2012). Is there an embryopathy associated with first-trimester exposure to angiotensin-converting enzyme inhibitors and angiotensin receptor antagonists? A critical review of the evidence. *Birth Defects Res* (Part A), *94*, 576–598.

### 3.3.4 ANGIOTENSIN II RECEPTOR BLOCKERS

### 3.3.4.1 VALSARTAN

**FDA Category: D**
***Risk Summary:*** Valsartan is contraindicated during the 2nd and 3rd Trimesters because the pregnancy experience in humans showed a profound

potentiality of teratogenicity and severe fetal toxicity associated with its use during this period.

**Further Reading:**

- Berkane, N., Carlier, P., Verstraete, L., Mathieu, E., Heim, N., & Uzan, S., (2004). Fetal toxicity of valsartan and possible reversible adverse side effects. *Birth Defects Res* (Part A), *70*, 547–549.
- *Drug Information*. Diovan. Novartis Pharmaceuticals.
- Vendemmia, M., Garcia-Meric, P., Rizzotti, A., Boubred, F., Lacroze, V., Liprandi, A., & Simeoni, U., (2005). Fetal and neonatal consequences of antenatal exposure to type 1 angiotensin II receptor antagonists. *J. Matern Fetal Neonatal Med., 19*, 137–140.

## 3.3.4.2   LOSARTAN

**FDA Category: D**

*Risk Summary:* Losartan is contraindicated during the 2nd and 3rd Trimesters because the pregnancy experience in humans showed a profound potentiality of teratogenicity and severe fetal toxicity associated with its use during this period.

**Further Reading:**

- Bass, J. K., & Faix, R. G., (2006). Gestational therapy with an angiotensin II receptor antagonist and transient renal failure in a premature infant. *Am. J. Perinatol., 23*, 313–318.
- *Drug Information*. Cozaar. Merck.
- Polifka, J. E., (2012). Is there an embryopathy associated with first-trimester exposure to angiotensin-converting enzyme inhibitors and angiotensin receptor antagonists? A critical review of the evidence. *Birth Defects Res.* (Part A), *94*, 576–598.
- Saji, H., Yamanaka, M., Hagiwara, A., & Ijiri, R., (2001). Losartan and fetal toxic effects. *Lancet, 357*, 363.

## 3.3.4.3   TELMISARTAN

**FDA Category: D**

*Risk Summary:* Telmisartan is contraindicated during the 2nd and 3rd Trimesters because the pregnancy experience in humans showed a profound

potentiality of teratogenicity and severe fetal toxicity associated with its use during this period.

**Further Reading:**
- *Drug Information*. Benicar. Sankyo Pharma.
- Polifka, J. E., (2012). Is there an embryopathy associated with first-trimester exposure to angiotensin-converting enzyme inhibitors and angiotensin receptor antagonists? A critical review of the evidence. *Birth Defects Res.* (Part A), *94*, 576–598.

### 3.3.4.4  CANDESARTAN CILEXETIL

**FDA Category: D**
***Risk Summary:*** Candesartan Cilexetil is contraindicated during the 2nd and 3rd Trimesters because the pregnancy experience in humans showed a profound potentiality of teratogenicity and severe fetal toxicity associated with its use during this period.

**Further Reading:**
- *Drug Information*. Atacand. AstraZeneca LP.
- Polifka, J. E., (2012). Is there an embryopathy associated with first-trimester exposure to angiotensin-converting enzyme inhibitors and angiotensin receptor antagonists? A critical review of the evidence. *Birth Defects Res.* (Part A), *94*, 576–598.
- Velazquez-Armenta, E. Y., Han, J. Y., Choi, J. S., Yang, K. M., & Nava-Ocampo, A. A., (2007). Angiotensin II receptor blockers in pregnancy: A case report and systematic review of the literature. *Hypertens Pregnancy*, *26*, 51–66.

### 3.3.4.5  OLMESARTAN

**FDA Category (1ˢᵗ Trimester): C**
**FDA Category (2ⁿᵈ and 3ʳᵈ Trimesters): D**
***Risk Summary:*** Olmesartan is contraindicated during the 2nd and 3rd Trimesters because the pregnancy experience in humans showed a profound potentiality of teratogenicity and severe fetal toxicity associated with its use during this period.

**Further Reading:**
- Accessdata.fda.gov. https://www.accessdata.fda.gov/drugsatfda_docs/label/2005/021286s010lbl.pdf (accessed on 30 January 2020).

### 3.3.4.6   IRBESARTAN

**FDA Category (1st Trimester): C**
**FDA Category (2nd and 3rd Trimesters): D**
*Risk Summary:* Irbesartan is contraindicated during the 2nd and 3rd Trimesters because the pregnancy experience in humans showed a profound potentiality of teratogenicity and severe fetal toxicity associated with its use during this period.

**Further Reading:**
- Boix, E., Zapater, P., Pico, A., & Moreno, O., (2005). Teratogenicity with angiotensin II receptor antagonists in pregnancy. *J. Endocrinol. Invest., 28*, 1029–1031.
- *Drug Information. Avapro*. Bristol-Myers Squibb.
- Velazquez-Armenta, E. Y., Han, J. Y., Choi, J. S., Yang, K. M., & Nava-Ocampo, A. A., (2007). Angiotensin II receptor blockers in pregnancy: A case report and systematic review of the literature. *Hypertens Pregnancy, 26*, 51–66.

### 3.3.5   ANGIOTENSIN A-1 BLOCKERS (PERIPHERALLY ACTING ADRENERGIC ANTAGONISTS)

### 3.3.5.1   PRAZOSIN

**FDA Category: C**
*Risk Summary:* It is better to be avoided during the 1st Trimester because the pregnancy experience in humans is limited and the reproduction studies in animals have shown low risk.

**Further Reading:**
- Bourget, P., Fernandez, H., Edouard, D., Lesne-Hulin, A., Ribou, F., Baton-Saint-Mleux, C., & Lelaidier, C., (1995). Disposition of a new rate-controlled formulation of prazosin in the treatment of hypertension during pregnancy: Transplacental passage of prazosin. *Eur. J. Drug Metab Pharmacokinet, 20*, 233–241.

- *Drug Information. Minipress*. Pfizer.
- Venuto, R., Burstein, P., & Schneider, R., (1984). Pheochromocy-toma: Antepartum diagnosis and management with tumor resection in the puerperium. *Am. J. Obstet. Gynecol., 150*, 431–432.

### 3.3.5.2   DOXAZOSIN

**FDA Category: C**
**Risk Summary:** It is better to be avoided during the 1st Trimester because the pregnancy experience in humans is limited and the reproduction studies in animals have shown low risk.

**Further Reading:**
- Accessdata.Fda.Gov. (2015). https://www.accessdata.fda.gov/drug-satfda_docs/label/2009/019668s021lbl.pdf (accessed on 12 February 2020).
- *Drug Information*. Cardura. Pfizer.
- Pirtskhalava, N., (2012). Pheochromocytoma and pregnancy: Complications and solutions (case report). *Georgian Med News* (pp. 208–209,76–82).

### 3.3.5.3   TERAZOSIN

**FDA Category: C**
**Risk Summary:** It is better to be avoided during the 1st Trimester because the pregnancy experience in humans is limited and the reproduction studies in animals have shown low risk.

**Further Reading:**
- *Drug Information. Hytrin*. Abbott Laboratories.

### 3.3.5.4   URAPIDIL

**FDA Category: C**
**Risk Summary:** Although there is limited data from the human pregnancy experience, but the possible maternal benefit extremely outweighs the unknown or known embryo/fetal risk.

**Further Reading:**
- Duley, L., Meher, S., & Jones, L., (2013). Drugs for treatment of very high blood pressure during pregnancy. *Cochrane Database of Systematic Reviews.*


### 3.3.6   ANGIOTENSIN A-2 BLOCKERS (CENTRALLY ACTING ADRENERGIC ANTAGONISTS)

#### 3.3.6.1   CLONIDINE

**FDA Category: C**
*Risk Summary:* It is better to be avoided during the 1st Trimester because the pregnancy experience in humans is limited and the reproduction studies in animals have shown risk.

**Further Reading:**
- *Drug Information.* Catapres. Boehringer Ingelheim Pharmaceuticals, 2000.
- Horvath, J. S., Phippard, A., Korda, A., Henderson-Smart, D. J., Child, A., & Tiller, D. J., (1985). Clonidine hydrochloride—A safe and effective antihypertensive agent in pregnancy. *Obstet. Gynecol., 66,* 634–638.


#### 3.3.6.2   RESERPINE

**FDA Category: C**
*Risk Summary:* It is better to be avoided during the 1st Trimester because the pregnancy experience in humans is limited and the reproduction studies in animals are not relevant.

**Further Reading:**
- Budnick, I. S., Leikin, S., & Hoeck, L. E., (1955). Effect in the newborn infant to reserpine administration antepartum. *Am. J. Dis. Child, 90,* 286–289.
- Czeizel, A., (1988). Reserpine is not a human teratogen. *J. Med. Genet.,* (p. 787).
- *Drug Information. Serpasil.* Ciba Pharmaceutical.

## 3.3.7   OTHER ANTIHYPERTENSIVE DRUGS

### 3.3.7.1   MINOXIDIL

**FDA Category: C**

*Risk Summary:* The pregnancy experience in humans is limited, and the reproduction studies in animals have shown moderate risk. Therefore, it is advisable to use it only if safer alternatives are not available.

**Further Reading:**
- *Drug Information*. Loniten. Pharmacia & Upjohn.
- Kaler, S. G., Patrinos, M. E., Lambert, G. H., Myers, T. F., Karlman, R., & Anderson, C. L., (1987). Hypertrichosis and congenital anomalies associated with maternal use of minoxidil. *Pediatrics, 79,* 434–436.
- Smorlesi, C., Caldarella, A., Caramelli, L., Di Lollo, S., & Moroni, F., (2003). Topically applied minoxidil may cause fetal malformation: A case report. *Birth Defects Res. A Clin. Mol. Teratol., 67,* 997–1001.

### 3.3.7.2   MAGNESIUM SULFATE

**FDA Category: D**

*Risk Summary:* Magnesium sulfate is contraindicated in pregnant women with cardiovascular and renal diseases, as in these situations the absorption of magnesium ions brings on a further burden.

**Further Reading:**
- *Drug Information. Magnesium Sulfate.* Abbott Pharmaceutical, Abbott Park, IL.
- Duley, L., Henderson-Smart, D. J., & Meher, S., (2006). Drugs for treatment of very high blood pressure during pregnancy. *Cochrane Database Syst Rev., 3.* CD001449.

### 3.3.7.3   ALISKIREN

**FDA Category: D**

*Risk Summary:* Aliskiren is contraindicated during the 2nd and 3rd Trimesters because the animal reproduction studies showed a profound potentiality of teratogenicity and severe fetal toxicity associated with its use during this period.

**Further Reading:**
- Azizi, M., Webb, R., Nussberger, J., & Hollenberg, N. K., (2006). Renin inhibition with aliskiren: Where are we now, and where are we going? *J. Hypertens*, *24*, 243–256.
- *Drug Information. Tekturna.* Novartis Pharmaceuticals.

## 3.3.7.4   SODIUM NITROPRUSSIDE

**FDA Category: C**
*Risk Summary:* The use of Sodium Nitroprusside is better to be avoided in pregnant women because of the risk of cyanide accumulation in the fetus.

**Further Reading:**
- Paull, J., (1975). Clinical report of the use of sodium nitroprusside in severe pre-eclampsia. *Anesth Intensive Care*, *3*, 72.
- Shoemaker, C. T., & Meyers, M., (1984). Sodium nitroprusside for control of severe hypertensive disease of pregnancy: A case report and discussion of potential toxicity. *Am. J. Obstet. Gynecol.*, *149*, 171–173.

## 3.3.7.5   PHENOXYBENZAMINE

**FDA Category: C**
*Risk Summary:* Although there is limited data from the human pregnancy experience, but the possible maternal benefit outweighs the unknown or known embryo/fetal risk.

**Further Reading:**
- Miller, C., Bernet, V., Elkas, J. C., Dainty, L., & Gherman, R. B., (2005). Conservative management of extra-adrenal pheochromocytoma during pregnancy. *Obstet. Gynecol.*, *105*, 1185–1188.
- Stenstrom, G., & Swolin, K., (1985). Pheochromocytoma in pregnancy. Experience of treatment with phenoxybenzamine in three patients. *Acta Obstet. Gynecol. Scand.*, *64*, 357–361.

## 3.3.7.6 HYDRALAZINE

**FDA Category: C**
*Risk Summary:* It should be used with caution during the 1st and 2nd Trimesters. However, it is better to avoid the use of Hydralazine during the 3rd Trimester because fetal toxicity has been associated with its use during the last Trimester.

**Further Reading:**
- Lodeiro, J. G., Feinstein, S. J., & Lodeiro, S. B., (1989). Fetal premature atrial contractions associated with hydralazine. *Am. J. Obstet. Gynecol., 160*, 105–107.
- Mabie, W. C., Gonzalez, A. R., Sibai, B. M., & Amon, E., (1987). A comparative trial of labetalol and hydralazine in the acute management of severe hypertension complicating pregnancy. *Obstet. Gynecol., 70*, 328–333.
- Widerlov, E., Karlman, I., & Storsater, J., (1980). Hydralazine-induced neonatal thrombocytopenia. *N Engl. J. Med., 303*, 1235.

## 3.4 DIURETICS

### 3.4.1 LOOP DIURETICS

#### 3.4.1.1 BUMETANIDE

**FDA Category: C**
*Risk Summary:* It should be used with caution because the pregnancy experience in humans is limited and the reproduction studies in animals have shown low risk. Nevertheless, diuretics are not preferred in the management of hypertension during pregnancy due to the expected risks of hypovolemia, and electrolyte disturbances.

**Further Reading:**
- *Drug Information.* Bumex. Roche Laboratories.
- McClain, R. M., & Dammers, K. D., (1981). Toxicologic evaluation of bumetanide, a potent diuretic agent. *J. Clin. Pharmacol., 21*, 543–554. As cited in: Shepard, T. H., Catalog of Teratogenic Agents. (6th edn., p. 92). Baltimore, MD: Johns Hopkins University Press, 1989.

- Wood, S. M., & Blainey, J. D., (1981). Hypertension and renal disease. In: Wood, S. M., & Beeley, L., (eds.) *Prescribing in Pregnancy. Clin. Obstet. Gynaecol., 8*, 439–453.

## 3.4.1.2   ETHACRYNIC ACID

**FDA Category: B**

*Risk Summary:* Although Ethacrynic acid has been assigned with the letter (B), according to the FDA categorization, but it should be used with caution because no human data is available and the reproduction studies in animals have shown low risk. Nevertheless, diuretics are not preferred in the management of hypertension during pregnancy due to the expected risks of hypovolemia, and electrolyte disturbances.

**Further Reading:**
- *Drug Information.* Edecrin. Merck.
- Felman, D., Theoleyre, J., & Dupoizat, H., (1967). Investigation of ethacrynic acid in the treatment of excessive gain in weight and pregnancy arterial hypertension. *Lyon Med., 217*, 1421–1428.
- Harrison, K. A., Ajabor, L. N., & Lawson, J. B., (1971). Ethacrynic acid and packed-blood-cell transfusion in the treatment of severe anemia in pregnancy. *Lancet, 1*, 11–14.

## 3.4.1.3   FUROSEMIDE

**FDA Category: C**

*Risk Summary:* It should be used with caution because the human pregnancy experience has shown a low risk. Nevertheless, diuretics are not preferred in the management of hypertension during pregnancy due to the expected risks of hypovolemia, and electrolyte disturbances.

**Further Reading:**
- *Drug Information.* Lasix. Hoechst–Roussel Pharmaceuticals.
- Suonio, S., Saarikoski, S., Tahvanainen, K., Paakkonen, A., & Olkkonen, H., (1985). Acute effects of dihydralazine mesylate, furosemide, and metoprolol on maternal hemodynamics in pregnancy-induced hypertension. *Am. J. Obstet. Gynecol., 155*, 122–125.

- Wladimiroff, J. W., (1975). Effect of furosemide on fetal urine production. *Br. J. Obstet. Gynaecol., 82*, 221–224.

### 3.4.1.4  TORSEMIDE

**FDA Category: B**
*Risk Summary:* The reproduction studies in animals have shown no evidence of fetal harm or impaired fertility. The pregnancy experience in humans is limited. Nevertheless, diuretics are not preferred in the management of hypertension during pregnancy due to the expected risks of hypovolemia, and electrolyte disturbances.

**Further Reading:**
- Accessdata.fda.gov.https://www.accessdata.fda.gov/drugsatfda_docs/label/2012/020136s014lbl.pdf. Published in 2018. (accessed on 30 January 2020).
- *Drug Information. Demadex.* Roche Pharmaceuticals.

### 3.4.2  POTASSIUM-SPARING DIURETICS

### 3.4.2.1  AMILORIDE

**FDA Category: B**
*Risk Summary:* It should be used with caution because the pregnancy experience in humans is limited and the reproduction studies in animals have shown low risk. Anyway, diuretics are not preferred in the management of hypertension during pregnancy due to the expected risks of hypovolemia, and electrolyte disturbances.

**Further Reading:**
- Deruelle, P., Dufour, P., Magnenant, E., Courouble, N., & Puech, F., (2004). Maternal Bartter's syndrome in pregnancy treated with amiloride. *Eur. J. Obstet. Gynecol. Reprod Biol., 115*, 106–107.
- *Drug Information. Midamor.* Merck.
- Krysiak, R., Samborek, M., & Stojko, R., (2012). Primary aldosteronism in pregnancy. *Acta Clin. Belg., 67*, 130–134.

### 3.4.2.2  *EPLERENONE*

**FDA Category: B**
*Risk Summary:* The reproduction studies in animals have shown no evidence of fetal harm or impaired fertility. The pregnancy experience in humans is adequate to exhibit that the embryo-fetal risk is nonexistent or very low. Nevertheless, diuretics are not preferred in the management of hypertension during pregnancy due to the expected risks of hypovolemia, and electrolyte disturbances.

**Further Reading:**
- Cabassi, A., Rocco, R., Berretta, R., et al., (2012). Eplerenone use in primary aldosteronism during pregnancy. *Hypertension, 59,* e18–19.
- Morton, A., Panitz, B., & Bush, A., (2011). Eplerenone for Gitelman syndrome in pregnancy. *Nephrology* (Carlton), *16,* 349.

### 3.4.2.3  *SPIRONOLACTONE*

**FDA Category: C**
*Risk Summary:* It should be used with caution because the pregnancy experience in humans is limited, and the reproduction studies in animals have shown the risk of teratogenicity associated with the use of Spironolactone. Nevertheless, diuretics are not preferred in the management of hypertension during pregnancy due to the expected risks of hypovolemia, and electrolyte disturbances.

**Further Reading:**
- *Drug Information. Aldactone.* G.D. Searle.
- Lindheimer, M. D., & Katz, A. I., (1973). Sodium and diuretics in pregnancy. *N Engl. J. Med., 288,* 891–894.
- Messina, M., Biffignandi, P., Ghiga, E., Jeantet, M. G., & Molinatti, G. M., (1979). Possible contraindication of spironolactone during pregnancy. *J. Endocrinol. Invest., 2,* 222.

### 3.4.2.4  *TRIAMTERENE*

**FDA Category: C**
*Risk Summary:* The use of Triamterene is better to be avoided in pregnant women because it has been found that Triamterene has weak folic acid

inhibitory effects. Nevertheless, diuretics are not preferred in the management of hypertension during pregnancy due to the expected risks of hypovolemia, and electrolyte disturbances.

**Further Reading:**
- *Drug Information. Dyrenium.* WellSpring Pharmaceuticals.
- Bozzo, P., & Einarson, A. (2009). Use of diuretics during pregnancy. *Canadian Family Physician, 55*(1), 44–45.
- Hernandez-Diaz, S., Werler, M. M., Walker, A. M., & Mitchell, A. A., (2000). Folic acid antagonists during pregnancy and the risk of birth defects. *N Engl. J. Med., 343*, 1608–1614.

### *3.4.3 THIAZIDE AND THIAZIDE-LIKE DIURETICS*

#### *3.4.3.1 BENDROFLUMETHIAZIDE*

**FDA Category: C**
*Risk Summary:* The reproduction studies in animals have shown no evidence of fetal harm or impaired fertility. The pregnancy experience in humans is limited. Nevertheless, diuretics are not preferred in the management of hypertension during pregnancy due to the expected risks of hypovolemia, and electrolyte disturbances.

**Further Reading:**
- Cuadros, A., & Tatum, H. J., (1964). The prophylactic and therapeutic use of bendroflumethiazide in pregnancy. *Am. J. Obstet. Gynecol., 89*, 891–897.

#### *3.4.3.2 BENZTHIAZIDE*

**FDA Category: C**
*Risk Summary:* The reproduction studies in animals have shown no evidence of fetal harm or impaired fertility. The pregnancy experience in humans is limited. Nevertheless, diuretics are not preferred in the management of hypertension during pregnancy due to the expected risks of hypovolemia, and electrolyte disturbances.

**Further Reading:**
- Briggs, G. G., & Freeman, R. K., (2015). *Drugs in Pregnancy and Lactation: A Reference Guide to Fetal and Neonatal Risk.* Philadelphia, PA: Lippincott Williams & Wilkins.

## 3.4.3.3   CHLOROTHIAZIDE

**FDA Category: C**
***Risk Summary:*** The reproduction studies in animals have shown no evidence of fetal harm or impaired fertility. The pregnancy experience in humans is limited. Nevertheless, diuretics are not preferred in the management of hypertension during pregnancy due to the expected risks of hypovolemia, and electrolyte disturbances.

**Further Reading:**
- *Drug Information*. Diuril. Merck.
- Flowers, C. E., Grizzle, J. E., Easterling, W. E., & Bonner, O. B., (1962). Chlorothiazide as a prophylaxis against toxemia of pregnancy. *Am. J. Obstet. Gynecol., 84,* 919–929.
- Menzies, D. N., (1964). Controlled trial of chlorothiazide in treatment of early pre-eclampsia. *Br Med. J., 1,* 739–742.
- Werthmann, M. W. Jr., & Krees, S. V., (1972). Excretion of chlorothiazide in human breast milk. *J. Pediatr., 81,* 781–783.

## 3.4.3.4   HYDROCHLOROTHIAZIDE

**FDA Category: B**
***Risk Summary:*** The reproduction studies in animals have shown no evidence of fetal harm or impaired fertility. The pregnancy experience in humans is limited. Nevertheless, diuretics are not preferred in the management of hypertension during pregnancy due to the expected risks of hypovolemia, and electrolyte disturbances.

**Further Reading:**
- Assoli, N. S., (1960). Renal effects of hydrochlorothiazide in normal and toxemic pregnancy. *Clin. Pharmacol. Ther., 1,* 48–52.
- Kraus, G. W., Marchese, J. R., & Yen, S. S. C., (1966). Prophylactic use of hydrochlorothiazide in pregnancy. *JAMA, 198,* 1150–1154.

## 3.4.3.5 HYDROFLUMETHIAZIDE

**FDA Category: C**

*Risk Summary:* The reproduction studies in animals have shown no evidence of fetal harm or impaired fertility. The pregnancy experience in humans is limited. Nevertheless, diuretics are not preferred in the management of hypertension during pregnancy due to the expected risks of hypovolemia, and electrolyte disturbances.

**Further Reading:**
- *Drug Information. Diucardin.* Wyeth-Ayerst Laboratories, Philadelphia, PA.
- Gray, M. J., (1968). Use and abuse of thiazides in pregnancy. *Clin. Obstet. Gynecol., 11*, 568–578.
- Tatum, H., & Waterman, E. A., (1961). The prophylactic and therapeutic use of the thiazides in pregnancy. *GP, 24*, 101–105.

## 3.4.3.6 CHLORTHALIDONE

**FDA Category: B**

*Risk Summary:* The reproduction studies in animals have shown no evidence of fetal harm or impaired fertility. The pregnancy experience in humans is limited. Nevertheless, diuretics are not preferred in the management of hypertension during pregnancy due to the expected risks of hypovolemia, and electrolyte disturbances.

**Further Reading:**
- *Drug Information. Thalitone.* Monarch Pharmaceuticals.
- Landesman, R., Aguero, O., Wilson, K., LaRussa, R., Campbell, W., & Penaloza, O., (1965). The prophylactic use of chlorthalidone, a sulfonamide diuretic, in pregnancy. *J Obstet. Gynaecol Br Commonw, 72*, 1004–1010.

## 3.4.3.7 CHLORTHALIDONE

**FDA Category: B**

*Risk Summary:* The reproduction studies in animals have shown no evidence of fetal harm or impaired fertility. The pregnancy experience in humans is limited. Nevertheless, diuretics are not preferred in the management of hypertension during pregnancy due to the expected risks of hypovolemia, and electrolyte disturbances.

**Further Reading:**
- *Drug Information. Thalitone.* Monarch Pharmaceuticals.
- Landesman, R., Aguero, O., Wilson, K., LaRussa, R., Campbell, W., Penaloza, O., (1965). The prophylactic use of chlorthalidone, a sulfon-amide diuretic, in pregnancy. *J. Obstet. Gynaecol. Br. Commonw, 72,* 1004–1010.


*3.4.3.8   METOLAZONE*

**FDA Category: B**
*Risk Summary:* The reproduction studies in animals have shown no evidence of fetal harm or impaired fertility. The pregnancy experience in humans is limited. Nevertheless, diuretics are not preferred in the management of hypertension during pregnancy due to the expected risks of hypovolemia, and electrolyte disturbances.

**Further Reading:**
- *Drug Information.* Mykrox. Medeva Pharmaceuticals.


## 3.4.4   OSMOTIC DIURETICS

*3.4.4.1   MANNITOL*

**FDA Category: C**
*Risk Summary:* The reproduction studies in animals have shown no evidence of fetal harm or impaired fertility. The pregnancy experience in humans is limited. Nevertheless, diuretics are not preferred in the management of hypertension during pregnancy due to the expected risks of hypovolemia, and electrolyte disturbances.

**Further Reading:**
- Craft, I. L., & Mus, B. D., (1971). Hypertonic solutions to induce abortions. *Br. Med. J., 2,* 49.

- *Drug Information. Osmitrol.* Baxter IV. Systems Division, Round Lake, IL.

## 3.4.5 CARBONIC ANHYDRASE INHIBITOR

### 3.4.5.1 ACETAZOLAMIDE

**FDA Category: C**
*Risk Summary:* The reproduction studies in animals have shown no evidence of fetal harm or impaired fertility. The pregnancy experience in humans is limited. Nevertheless, diuretics are not preferred in the management of hypertension during pregnancy due to the expected risks of hypovolemia, and electrolyte disturbances.

**Further Reading:**
- *Drug Information.* Acetazolamide. Teva Pharmaceuticals.
- Falardeau, J., Lobb, B. M., Golden, S., Maxfield, S. D., & Tanne, E., (2013). The use of acetazolamide during pregnancy in intracranial hypertension patients. *J. Neuroophthalmol., 33,* 9–12.
- Golan, S., Maslovitz, S., Kupferminc, M. J., & Kesler, A., (2013). Management and outcome of consecutive pregnancies complicated by idiopathic intracranial hypertension. *Isr. Med. Assoc. J., 15,* 160–163.

## 3.5 ANTI-DYSLIPIDEMIC DRUGS

### 3.5.1 HMG-COA INHIBITORS

### 3.5.1.1 ATORVASTATIN

**FDA Category: X**
*Risk Summary:* The use of Atorvastatin is contraindicated during pregnancy due to the fact that Cholesterol and products synthesized by cholesterol are essential during fetal development. Moreover, the discontinuation of Atorvastatin during pregnancy should have no influence on the long-term treatment of hyperlipidemia.

**Further Reading:**

- Dostal, L. A., Schardein, J. L., & Anderson, J. A., (1994). Developmental toxicity of the HMG-CoA reductase inhibitor, atorvastatin, in rats and rabbits. *Teratology, 50*, 387–394.
- *Drug Information. Lipitor.* Pfizer.
- Henck, J. W., Craft, W. R., Black, A., Colgin, J., & Anderson, J. A., (1998). Pre- and postnatal toxicity of the HMG-CoA reductase inhibitor atorvastatin in rats. *Toxicol. Sci., 41*, 88–99.
- Lipitor – Food and Drug Administration. Accessed August 18, 2018. https://www.accessdata.fda.gov/drugsatfda_docs/label/2009/020702s057lbl.pdf (accessed on 30 January 2020).
- McElhatton, P., (2005). Preliminary data on exposure to statins during pregnancy (abstract). *Reprod Toxicol., 20*, 471, 472.
- Taguchi, N., Rubin, E. T., Hosokawa, A., Choi, J., Ying, A. Y., Moretti, M., Koren, G., & Ito, S., (2008). Prenatal exposure to HMG-CoA reductase inhibitors: Effects on fetal and neonatal outcomes. *Reprod Toxicol., 26*, 175–177.

## 3.5.1.2   SIMVASTATIN

**FDA Category: X**

***Risk Summary:*** The use of simvastatin is contraindicated during pregnancy due to the fact that Cholesterol and products synthesized by cholesterol are essential during fetal development. Moreover, the discontinuation of Simvastatin during pregnancy should have no influence on the long-term treatment of hyperlipidemia.

**Further Reading:**

- *Drug Information. Zocor.* Merck
- Manson, J. M., Freyssinges, C., Ducrocq, M. B., & Stephenson, W. P., (1996). Postmarketing surveillance of lovastatin and simvastatin exposure during pregnancy. Reprod Toxicol., *10*, 439–446.
- McElhatton, P., (2005). Preliminary data on exposure to statins during pregnancy (abstract). *Reprod Toxicol., 20*, 471–472.
- Taguchi, N., Rubin, E. T., Hosokawa, A., Choi, J., Ying, A. Y., Moretti, M., Koren, G., & Ito, S., (2008). Prenatal exposure to HMG-CoA reductase inhibitors: Effects on fetal and neonatal outcomes. *Reprod Toxicol., 26*, 175–177.

- ZOCOR (simvastatin) Tablets – Accessdata.fda.gov. (accessed on 30 January 2020). https://www.accessdata.fda.gov/drugsatfda_docs/label/2018/019766s098lbl.pdf.

## 3.5.1.3 ROSUVASTATIN

**FDA Category: X**

***Risk Summary:*** The use of Rosuvastatin is contraindicated during pregnancy due to the fact that Cholesterol and products synthesized by cholesterol are essential during fetal development. Moreover, the discontinuation of Rosuvastatin during pregnancy should have no influence on the long-term treatment of hyperlipidemia.

**Further Reading:**
- "Crestor(rosuvastatinCalcium)Tablets–FoodandDrug."https://www.accessdata.fda.gov/drugsatfda_docs/label/2010/021366s016lbl.pdf (accessed on 30 January 2020).
- *Drug Information. Crestor.* AstraZeneca.
- Edison, R. J., & Muenke, M., (2004). Central nervous system and limb anomalies in case reports of first-trimester statin exposure. *New Engl. J. Med., 350,* 1579–1582.
- Edison, R. J., & Muenke, M., (2004). Mechanistic and epidemiologic considerations in the evaluation of adverse birth outcomes following gestational exposure to statins. *Am. J. Med. Genet., 131A,* 287–298.

## 3.5.1.4 PITAVASTATIN

**FDA Category: X**

***Risk Summary:*** The use of Pitavastatin is contraindicated during pregnancy due to the fact that Cholesterol and products synthesized by cholesterol are essential during fetal development. Moreover, the discontinuation of Pitavastatin during pregnancy should have no influence on the long-term treatment of hyperlipidemia.

**Further Reading:**
- *Drug Information. Livalo.* Kowa Pharmaceuticals America.

- "LIVALO Safely and Effectively. Se LIVALO. Initial U.S "https://www. accessdata.fda.gov/drugsatfda_docs/label/2009/022363s000lbl.pdf (accessed on 30 January 2020).

### 3.5.1.5    FLUVASTATIN

**FDA Category: X**
***Risk Summary:*** The use of Fluvastatin is contraindicated during pregnancy due to the fact that Cholesterol and products synthesized by cholesterol are essential during fetal development. Moreover, the discontinuation of Fluvastatin during pregnancy should have no influence on the long-term treatment of hyperlipidemia.

**Further Reading:**
- *Drug Information. Lescol.* Sandoz Pharmaceuticals.
- Prescribing Information – Food and Drug Administration. https:// www.accessdata.fda.gov/drugsatfda_docs/label/2000/20261S24lbl. pdf (accessed on 30 January 2020)
- Seguin, J., & Samuels, P., (1999). Fluvastatin exposure during pregnancy. *Obstet. Gynecol., 93*, 847.

### 3.5.2    FIBRATES

### 3.5.2.1    FENOFIBRATE

**FDA Category: C**
***Risk Summary:*** It should be used with caution because the pregnancy experience in humans is limited, and the reproduction studies in animals have shown the risk of embryocidal effect and teratogenicity.

**Further Reading:**
- *Drug Information. Lofibra.* GATE Pharmaceuticals.
- Sunman, H., Canpolat, U., Sahiner, L., & Aytemir, K., (2012). Use of fenofibrate during the first trimester of an unplanned pregnancy in a patient with hypertriglyceridemia. Ann. Pharmacother., *46*, e5. doi: 10.1345/aph.1Q626.

- Whitten, A. E., Lorenz, R. P., & Smith, J. M., (2011). Hyperlipid-emia-associated pancreatitis in pregnancy managed with fenofibrate. *Obstet. Gynecol., 117*, 517–519.

## 3.5.2.2   FENOFIBRATE

**FDA Category: C**
*Risk Summary:* It should be used with caution because the pregnancy experience in humans is limited, and the reproduction studies in animals have shown the risk of tumorigenic effects.

**Further Reading:**
- *Drug Information.* Gemfibrozil. Watson Laboratories.
- Saadi, H. F., Kurlander, D. J., Erkins, J. M., & Hoogwerf, B. J., (1999). Severe hypertriglyceridemia and acute pancreatitis during pregnancy: Treatment with gemfibrozil. *Endocr Pract., 5*, 33–36.
- Tsai, E, Brown, J. A., Veldee, M. Y., Anderson, G. J., Chait, A., & Brunzell, J. D., (2004). Potential of essential fatty acid deficiency with an extremely low-fat diet in lipoprotein lipase deficiency during pregnancy: A case report. *BMC Pregnancy Childbirth, 4*, 27.

## 3.5.3   BILE ACID SEQUESTRANTS

## 3.5.3.1   COLESTIPOL

**FDA Category: N**
*Risk Summary:* The reproduction studies in animals have shown no evidence of fetal harm or impaired fertility. The pregnancy experience in humans is limited. Colestipol should have no direct effect on the fetus because it is not absorbed systemically. However, it is well known that Colestipol reduces the absorption of fat-soluble vitamins (A, K, E, and D).

**Further Reading:**
- *Drug Information. Colestid.* Pharmacia & Upjohn.
- Rosa, F., (1994). *Anti-cholesterol Agent Pregnant Exposure Outcomes.* Presented at the 7th International Organization for Teratogen Information Services, Woods Hole, MA.

## 3.5.3.2   COLESEVELAM

**FDA Category: B**
*Risk Summary:* The reproduction studies in animals have shown no evidence of fetal harm or impaired fertility. The pregnancy experience in humans is limited. Colesevelam should have no direct effect on the fetus because it is not absorbed systemically. However, it is well known that Colesevelam reduces the absorption of fat-soluble vitamins (A, K, E, and D).

**Further Reading:**
*   *Drug Information. Welchol.* Sankyo Pharma.

## 3.5.3.3   CHOLESTYRAMINE

**FDA Category: C**
*Risk Summary:* The reproduction studies in animals have shown no evidence of fetal harm or impaired fertility. The pregnancy experience in humans is adequate to exhibit that the embryo-fetal risk is nonexistent or very low. However, it is well known that Cholestyramine reduces the absorption of fat-soluble vitamins (A, K, E, and D).

**Further Reading:**
*   Heikkinen, J., Maentausta, O., Ylostalo, P., & Janne, O., (1982). Serum bile acid levels in intrahepatic cholestasis of pregnancy during treatment with phenobarbital or cholestyramine. *Eur. J. Obstet. Gynecol. Reprod. Biol., 14*, 153–162.
*   Innis, S. M., (1983). Effect of cholestyramine administration during pregnancy in the rat. *Am. J. Obstet. Gynecol., 146*, 13–16.
*   Sadler, L. C., Lane, M., & North, R., (1995). Severe fetal intracranial hemorrhage during treatment with cholestyramine for intrahepatic cholestasis of pregnancy. *Br. J. Obstet. Gynaecol., 102*, 169–170.

## 3.5.4   MISCELLANEOUS AGENTS

## 3.5.4.1   EZETIMIBE

**FDA Category: C**
*Risk Summary:* It should be used with caution because the pregnancy experience in humans is limited and the reproduction studies in animals have

shown low risk. However, if treatment for hypercholesterolemia is needed to be given during pregnancy, Ezetimibe is considered a safer alternative to the Statins.

**Further Reading:**
- "ZETIA – Food and Drug Administration." https://www.accessdata. fda.gov/drugsatfda_docs/label/2008/021445s019lbl.pdf (accessed on 30 January 2020).

### 3.5.4.2 NIACIN

**FDA Category: B**

*Risk Summary:* The reproduction studies in animals have shown no evidence of fetal harm or impaired fertility. The pregnancy experience in humans is adequate to exhibit that the embryo-fetal risk is nonexistent or very low.

**Further Reading:**
- Baker, H., Frank, O., Thomson, A. D., Langer, A., Munves, E. D., De Angelis, B., & Kaminetzky, H. A., (1975). Vitamin profile of 174 mothers and newborns at parturition. *Am. J. Clin. Nutr., 28*, 59–65.
- "Dn2400v17-redlined-niaspan-2013-Jan-24." Accessed August 18, 2018. https://www.accessdata.fda.gov/drugsatfda_docs/ label/2013/020381s048lbl.pdf (accessed on 30 January 2020).

**KEYWORDS**

- **bile acid sequestrants**
- **cholestyramine**
- **fenofibrate**
- **fluvastatin**
- **intrauterine growth restriction**
- **miscellaneous agents**

# CHAPTER 4

# Hematologic Drugs

## 4.1 ANTICOAGULANTS

### 4.1.1 HEPARIN

**FDA Category: C**
*Risk Summary:* The reproduction studies in animals have shown no evidence of fetal harm or impaired fertility. The pregnancy experience in humans is adequate to exhibit that the embryo-fetal risk is nonexistent or very low.

**Further Reading:**
- De Swiet, M., Dorrington Ward, P., Fidler, J., Horsman, A., Katz, D., Letsky, E., Peacock, M., & Wise, P. H., (1983). Prolonged heparin therapy in pregnancy causes bone demineralization. *Br. J. Obstet. Gynaecol., 90,* 1129–1134.
- Griffiths, H. T., & Liu, D. T. Y., (1984). Severe heparin osteoporosis in pregnancy. *Postgrad Med. J., 60,* 424–425.
- Hall, J. G., Pauli, R. M., & Wilson, K. M., (1980). Maternal and fetal sequelae of anticoagulation during pregnancy. *Am. J. Med., 68,* 122–140.

### 4.1.2 APIXABAN

**FDA Category: B**
*Risk Summary:* It should be used with caution because the pregnancy experience in humans is limited and the reproduction studies in animals have shown low risk.

**Further Reading:**
- *Drug Information. Eliquis.* Bristol-Myers Squibb.

- Greer, I. A., (2012). Thrombosis in pregnancy: Updates in diagnosis and management. *Hematol. Am. Soc. Hematol. Educ. Program.*, 203–207. doi: 10.1182/asheducation-2012.1.203.
- Wang, L., He, K., Maxwell, B., Grossman, S. J., Tremaine, L. M., Humphreys, W. G., & Zhang, D., (2011). Tissue distribution and elimination of [14C] apixaban in rats. Drug Metab. Dispos., *39*, 256–264.

### 4.1.3 DALTEPARIN

**FDA Category: B**
***Risk Summary:*** The reproduction studies in animals have shown no evidence of fetal harm or impaired fertility. The pregnancy experience in humans is adequate to exhibit that the embryo-fetal risk is nonexistent or very low.

**Further Reading:**
- *Drug Information. Fragmin.* Pharmacia & Upjohn Company.
- Pettila, V., Kaaja, R., Leinonen, P., Ekblad, U., Kataja, M., & Ikkala, E., (1999). Thromboprophylaxis with low molecular weight heparin (dalteparin) in pregnancy. Thromb Res., *96*, 275–282.
- Rey, E., & Rivard, G. E., (2000). Prophylaxis and treatment of thromboembolic diseases during pregnancy with dalteparin. *Int. J. Gynecol. Obstet., 71*, 19–24.

### 4.1.4 DABIGATRAN ETEXILATE

**FDA Category: C**
***Risk Summary:*** The pregnancy experience in humans is limited, and the reproduction studies in animals have shown moderate risk. Therefore, it is advisable to avoid its use—if it is possible.

**Further Reading:**
- *Drug Information. Pradaxa.* Boehringer Ingelheim Pharmaceuticals.
- Huisman, M. V., (2010). Further issues with new oral anticoagulants. Curr. Pharm. Des., *16*, 3487–3489.

### 4.1.5 ENOXAPARIN

**FDA Category: B**
***Risk Summary:*** The reproduction studies in animals have shown no evidence of fetal harm or impaired fertility. The pregnancy experience in

humans is adequate to exhibit that the embryo-fetal risk is nonexistent or very low.

**Further Reading:**
- Casele, H. L., Laifer, S. A., Woelkers, D. A., & Venkataramanan, R., (1999). Changes in the pharmacokinetics of the low molecular-weight heparin enoxaparin sodium during pregnancy. *Am. J. Obstet. Gynecol.,181*, 1113–1117.
- *Drug Information. Lovenox*. Rhone-Poulenc Rorer.
- Magdelaine, A., Verdy, E., Coulet, F., Berkane, N., Girot, R., Uzan, S., & Soubrier, F., (2000). Deep vein thrombosis during enoxaparin prophylactic treatment in a young pregnant woman homozygous for factor V Leiden and heterozygous for the G127-A mutation in the thrombomodulin gene. *Blood Coagul Fibrinolysis, 11*, 761–765.

### *4.1.6 FONDAPARINUX*

**FDA Category: B**
*Risk Summary:* The reproduction studies in animals have shown no evidence of fetal harm or impaired fertility. The pregnancy experience in humans is limited.

**Further Reading:**
- Dempfle, C. E. H., (2004). Minor transplacental passage of fondaparinux in vivo. *N. Engl. J. Med., 350*, 1914, 1915.
- *Drug Information. Arixtra*. Sanofi-Synthelabo.
- Mazzolai, L., Hohlfeld, P., Spertini, F., Hayoz, D., Schapira, M., & Duchosal, M. A., (2006). Fondaparinux is a safe alternative in the case of heparin intolerance during pregnancy. *Blood, 108*, 1569, 1570.

### *4.1.7 REVIPARIN*

**FDA Category: C**
*Risk Summary:* The reproduction studies in animals have shown no evidence of fetal harm or impaired fertility. The pregnancy experience in humans is adequate to exhibit that the embryo-fetal risk is nonexistent or very low.

**Further Reading:**
- Laskin, C., Ginsberg, J., Farine, D., Crowther, M., Spitzer, K., Soloninka, C., Ryan, G., Seaward, G., & Ritchie, K., (1997). Low

molecular weight heparin and ASA therapy in women with autoanti-
bodies and unexplained recurrent fetal loss (U-RFL). Society of perinatal obstetricians abstracts. *Am. J. Obstet. Gynecol., 176*, S125.
- Reynold, J. E. F., & ed. Martindale, (1993). *The Extra Pharmaco-
poeia* (30th edn., p. 232). London, UK: The Pharmaceutical Press.


## 4.1.8   RIVAROXABAN

**FDA Category: C**
*Risk Summary:* The pregnancy experience in humans is limited, and the
reproduction studies in animals have shown moderate risk.

**Further Reading:**
- Cutts, B. A., Dasgupta, D., & Hunt, B. J., (2013). New directions in
the diagnosis and treatment of pulmonary embolism in pregnancy.
*Am. J. Obstet. Gynecol., 208*, 102–108.
- *Drug Information.* Xarelto. Janssen Pharmaceuticals.
- Greer, I. A., (2012). Thrombosis in pregnancy: Updates in diagnosis
and management. Hematology *Am. Soc. Hematol. Educ. Program*,
2012, 203–207. doi: 10.1182/asheducation-2012.1.203.


## 4.1.9   WARFARIN

**FDA Category: D (for women with mechanical heart valves)**
**FDA Category: X (all other indications)**
*Risk Summary:* It is generally contraindicated during pregnancy, especially
during the 1st Trimester, because of the high incidence of fetal warfarin
syndrome. However, it could be used only for women with mechanical heart
valves, who are at elevated risk of thromboembolism, and for whom the
advantages of this drug might surpass the risks.

**Further Reading:**
- Baillie, M., Allen, E. D., & Elkington, A. R., (1980). The congenital
warfarin syndrome: A case report. *Br. J. Ophthalmol., 64*, 633–635.
- Kaplan, L. C., Anderson, G. G., & Ring, B. A., (1982). Congenital
hydrocephalus and Dandy-Walker malformation associated with
warfarin use during pregnancy. *Birth Defects, 18*, 79–83.

- Lee, P. K., Wang, R. Y. C., Chow, J. S. F., Cheung, K. L., Wong, V. C. W., & Chan, T. K., (1986). Combined use of warfarin and adjusted subcutaneous (S.C) heparin during pregnancy in patients with an artificial heart valve. *J. Am. Coll. Cardiol., 8*, 221–224.
- Ruthnum, P., & Tolmie, J. L., (1987). Atypical malformations in an infant exposed to warfarin during the first trimester of pregnancy. *Teratology, 36*, 299–301.

## 4.2 ANTIPLATELET DRUGS

### 4.2.1 ASPIRIN

**FDA Category: N**
*Risk Summary:* The use of Aspirin at low doses (less than 150 mg/day) is generally considered safe during pregnancy; however, further studies are needed to assess precisely the risk to benefit ratio of such drugs.

**Further Reading:**
- Elder, M. G., DeSwiet, M., Robertson, A., Elder, M. A., Flloyd, E., & Hawkins, D. F., (1988). Low-dose aspirin in pregnancy. *Lancet, 1,* 410.
- Rudolph, A. M. (1981). Effects of aspirin and acetaminophen in pregnancy and in the newborn. *Arch Intern Med, 141*, 358–363.
- Spitz, B., Magness, R. R., Cox, S. M., Brown, C. E. L., Rosenfeld, C. R., & Gant, N. F., (1988). Low-dose aspirin. I. Effect on angiotensin II pressor responses and blood prostaglandin concentrations in pregnant women sensitive to angiotensin II. *Am. J. Obstet. Gynecol., 159*, 1035–1043.
- Wallenburg, H. C. S., & Rotmans, N., (1987). Prevention of recurrent idiopathic fetal growth retardation by low-dose aspirin and dipyridamole. *Am. J. Obstet. Gynecol., 157*, 1230–1235.

### 4.2.2 CLOPIDOGREL

**FDA Category: B**
*Risk Summary:* The reproduction studies in animals have shown no evidence of fetal harm or impaired fertility. The pregnancy experience in humans is limited.

**Further Reading:**
- Boztosun, B., Olcay, A., Avci, A., & Kirma, C., (2008). Treatment of acute myocardial infarction in pregnancy with coronary artery balloon angioplasty and stenting: Use of tirofiban and clopidogrel. *Int. J. Cardiol., 127,* 413–416.
- De Santis, M., De Luca, C., Mappa, I., Cesari, E., Mazza, A., Quattrocchi, T., & Caruso, A., (2011). Clopidogrel treatment during pregnancy: A case report and a review of the literature. *Intern. Med., 50,* 1769–1773.
- *Drug Information. Plavix,* Bristol-Myers Squibb.


### 4.2.3 CILOSTAZOL

**FDA Category: C**
*Risk Summary:* It should be used with caution because the pregnancy experience in humans is limited, and the reproduction studies in animals have shown the risk of teratogenicity associated with the use of Cilostazol.

**Further Reading:**
- *Drug Information.* Pletal. Otsuka America Pharma.


### 4.2.4 TICLOPIDINE

**FDA Category: B**
*Risk Summary:* It should be used with caution because the pregnancy experience in humans is limited and the reproduction studies in animals have shown low risk.

**Further Reading:**
- *Drug Information.* Ticlid. Roche Pharmaceuticals.
- Klinzing, P., Markert, U. R., Liesaus, K., & Peiker, G., (2001). Case report: Successful pregnancy and delivery after myocardial infarction and essential thrombocythemia treated with clopidogrel. *Clin. Exp. Obstet. Gynecol., 28,* 215–216.
- Sebastian, C., Scherlag, M., Kugelmass, A., & Schechter, E., (1998). Primary stent implantation for acute myocardial infarction during pregnancy: Use of abciximab, ticlopidine, and aspirin. *Cathet. Cardiovasc. Diagn., 45,* 275–279.

## 4.2.5 PRASUGREL

**FDA Category: B**
*Risk Summary:* It should be used with caution because the pregnancy experience in humans is limited and the reproduction studies in animals have shown low risk.

**Further Reading:**
- *Drug Information. Effient.* Eli Lilly.

## 4.2.6 TICAGRELOR

**FDA Category: C**
*Risk Summary:* It should be used with caution because the pregnancy experience in humans is limited, and the reproduction studies in animals have shown the risk of structural abnormalities associated with the use of Ticagrelor during organogenesis.

**Further Reading:**
- *Drug Information. Brilinta.* AstraZeneca.

## 4.2.7 ABCIXIMAB

**FDA Category: C**
*Risk Summary:* Although there is limited data from the human pregnancy experience, but the possible maternal benefit extremely outweighs the unknown or known embryo/fetal risk.

**Further Reading:**
- *Drug Information.* ReoPro. Eli Lilly.
- Sebastian, C., Scherlag, M., Kugelmass, A., & Schechter, E., (1998). Primary stent implantation for acute myocardial infarction during pregnancy: Use of abciximab, ticlopidine, and aspirin. *Cathet. Cardiovasc. Diagn., 45,* 275–279.
- Santiago-Diaz, P., Arrebola-Moreno, A. L., Ramirez-Hernandez, J. A., & Melgares-Moreno, R., (2009). Use of antiplatelet drugs during pregnancy. *Rev. Exp. Cardiol., 62,* 1197,1198.

### 4.2.8   EPTIFIBATIDE

**FDA Category: B**
*Risk Summary:* It should be used with caution because the pregnancy experience in humans is limited and the reproduction studies in animals have shown low risk.

**Further Reading:**
- Al-Aqeedi, R. F., & Al-Nabti, A. D., (2008). Drug-eluting stent implantation for acute myocardial infarction during pregnancy with the use of glycoprotein IIb/IIIa inhibitor. *J. Invasive Cardiol., 20*, E146–149.
- *Drug Information. Integrilin.* Schering.

### 4.2.9   TIROFIBAN

**FDA Category: B**
*Risk Summary:* Although there is limited data from the human pregnancy experience, but the possible maternal benefit extremely outweighs the unknown or known embryo/fetal risk.

**Further Reading:**
- Boztosun, B., Olcay, A., Avci, A., & Kirma, C., (2008). Treatment of acute myocardial infarction in pregnancy with coronary artery balloon angioplasty and stenting: Use of tirofiban and clopidogrel. *Int. J. Cardiol., 127*, 413–416.
- *Drug Information.* Aggrastat. Medicure International.

### 4.2.10   TIROFIBAN

**FDA Category: C**
*Risk Summary:* Although there is limited data from the human pregnancy experience, but the possible maternal benefit extremely outweighs the unknown or known embryo/fetal risk.

**Further Reading:**
- Alkindi, S., Dennison, D., & Pathare, A., (2005). Successful outcome with anagrelide in pregnancy. *Ann. Hematol., 84*, 758–759.

- Doubek, M., Brychtova, Y., Doubek, R., Janku, P., & Mayer, J., (2004). Anagrelide therapy in pregnancy: Report of a case of essential thrombocythemia. *Ann. Hematol., 83,* 726–727.
- *Drug Information. Agrylin.* Roberts Pharmaceutical.

## 4.2.11   DIPYRIDAMOLE

**FDA Category: B**
*Risk Summary:* The reproduction studies in animals have shown no evidence of fetal harm or impaired fertility. The pregnancy experience in humans is adequate to exhibit that the embryo-fetal risk is nonexistent or very low.

**Further Reading:**
- Beaufils, M., Uzan, S., Donsimoni, R., & Colau, J. C., (1986). Prospective controlled study of early antiplatelet therapy in prevention of preeclampsia. *Adv. Nephrol., 15,* 87–94.
- Biale, Y., Cantor, A., Lewenthal, H., & Gueron, M., (1980). The course of pregnancy in patients with artificial heart valves treated with dipyridamole. *Int. J. Gynaecol. Obstet.,* 1980 *18,* 128–32.
- *Drug Information.* Persantine. Boehringer Ingelheim Pharmaceuticals.

## 4.3   THROMBOLYTIC DRUGS

## 4.3.1   ALTEPLASE

**FDA Category: C**
*Risk Summary:* The reproduction studies in animals have shown no evidence of fetal harm or impaired fertility. The pregnancy experience in humans is adequate to exhibit that the embryo-fetal risk is nonexistent or very low.

**Further Reading:**
- *Drug Information.* Activase. Genentech.
- Flossdorf, T., Breulmann, M., Hopf, H. B., (1990). Successful treatment of massive pulmonary embolism with recombinant tissue-type plasminogen activator (rt-PA) in a pregnant woman with intact gravidity and preterm labor. *Intensive Care Med., 16,* 454–456.

- Song, J. Y., & Valentino, L., (2005). A pregnant patient with renal vein thrombosis successfully treated with low-dose thrombolytic therapy: A case report. *Am. J. Obstet. Gynecol., 192*, 2073–2075.

## 4.3.2 DROTRECOGIN ALFA (ACTIVATED)

**FDA Category: C**
*Risk Summary:* Although there is limited data from the human pregnancy experience, but the possible maternal benefit extremely outweighs the unknown or known embryo/fetal risk.

**Further Reading:**
- *Drug Information. Xigris.* Eli Lilly and Company.
- Eppert, H. D., Goddard, K. B., & King, C. L., (2011). Successful treatment with drotrecogin alfa (activated) in a pregnant women with severe sepsis. *Pharmacotherapy, 31*, 333. doi: 10.1592/phco.31.3.333.

## 4.3.3 RETEPLASE

**FDA Category: C**
*Risk Summary:* Although there is limited data from the human pregnancy experience, but the possible maternal benefit extremely outweighs the unknown or known embryo/fetal risk.

**Further Reading:**
- *Drug Information.* Retavase. Centocor.
- Yap, L. B., Alp, N. J., & Forfar, J. C., (2002). Thrombolysis for acute massive pulmonary embolism during pregnancy. *Int. J. Cardiol., 82*, 193–194.

## 4.3.4 TENECTEPLASE

**FDA Category: C**
*Risk Summary:* Although there is limited data from the human pregnancy experience, but the possible maternal benefit extremely outweighs the unknown or known embryo/fetal risk.

**Further Reading:**
- *Drug Information*. TNKase. Genentech.


## 4.3.5 UROKINASE

**FDA Category: B**
***Risk Summary:*** Although there is limited data from the human pregnancy experience, but the possible maternal benefit extremely outweighs the unknown or known embryo/fetal risk.

**Further Reading:**
- *Drug Information*. Abbokinase. Abbott Laboratories.
- Kramer, W. B., Belfort, M., Saade, G. R., Surani, S., & Moise, K. J. Jr., (1995). Successful urokinase treatment of massive pulmonary embolism in pregnancy. *Obstet. Gynecol.*, *86*, 660–662.
- Walker, J. E., Gow, L., Campbell, D. M., & Ogston, D., (1983). The inhibition by plasma of urokinase and tissue activator-induced fibrinolysis in pregnancy and the puerperium. Thromb Haemost, *49*, 21–23.


## 4.4 THROMBIN INHIBITORS

### 4.4.1 ANTITHROMBIN III (HUMAN)

**FDA Category: B**
***Risk Summary:*** The reproduction studies in animals have shown no evidence of fetal harm or impaired fertility. The pregnancy experience in humans is adequate to exhibit that the embryo-fetal risk is nonexistent or very low.

**Further Reading:**
- *Drug Information*. Thrombate III. Bayer Corporation, Pharmaceutical Division, Biological Products.
- Maki, M., Kobayashi, T., Terao, T., Ikenoue, T., Satoh, K., Nakabayashi, M., Sagara, Y., Kajiwara, Y., & Urata, M., (2000). Antithrombin therapy for severe preeclampsia. Results of a double-blind, randomized, placebo-controlled trial. *Thromb Haemost*, *84*, 583–590.

- Nakabayashi, M., Asami, M., & Nakatani, A., (1999). Efficacy of antithrombin replacement therapy in severe early-onset preeclampsia. *Semin Thromb Hemost, 25,* 463–466.

## 4.4.2 ARGATROBAN

**FDA Category: B**
***Risk Summary:*** It should be used with caution because the pregnancy experience in humans is limited and the reproduction studies in animals have shown low risk.

**Further Reading:**
- *Drug Information.* Argatroban. GlaxoSmithKline.
- Young, S. K., Al-Mondhiry, H. A., Vaida, S. J., Ambrose, A., & Botti, J. J., (2008). Successful use of argatroban during the third trimester of pregnancy: Case report and review of the literature. *Pharmacotherapy, 28,* 1531–1536.
- Tanimura, K., Ebina, Y., Sonoyama, A., Morita, H., Miyata, S., & Yamada, H., (2012). Argatroban therapy for heparin-induced thrombocytopenia during pregnancy in a woman with hereditary antithrombin deficiency. *J. Obstet. Gynaecol. Res., 38,* 749–752.

## 4.4.3 BIVALIRUDIN

**FDA Category: B**
***Risk Summary:*** It should be used with caution because the pregnancy experience in humans is limited and the reproduction studies in animals have shown low risk.

**Further Reading:**
- *Drug Information.* Angiomax. The Medicines Company.

## 4.4.4 DESIRUDIN

**FDA Category: C**
***Risk Summary:*** It should be used with caution because the pregnancy experience in humans is limited, and the reproduction studies in animals have shown the risk of teratogenicity associated with the use of Desirudin.

**Further Reading:**
- Accessdata.fda.gov. 2014 [cited 1 July 2019]. Available from: https://www.accessdata.fda.gov/drugsatfda_docs/label/2014/021271s006lbl.pdf (accessed on 30 January 2020).
- *Drug Information. Iprivask.* Aventis Pharmaceuticals.

### 4.4.5 LEPIRUDIN

**FDA Category: B**
*Risk Summary:* The reproduction studies in animals have shown no evidence of fetal harm or impaired fertility. The pregnancy experience in humans is limited.

**Further Reading:**
- Chapman, M. L., Martinez-Borges, A. R., & Mertz, H. L., (2008). Lepirudin for treatment of acute thrombosis during pregnancy. *Obstet. Gynecol., 112*, 432–433.
- *Drug Information.* Refludan. Aventis Pharmaceuticals.
- Furlan, A., Vianello, F., Clementi, M., & Prandoni, P., (2006). Heparin-induced thrombocytopenia occurring in the first trimester of pregnancy: Successful treatment with lepirudin. A case report. *Haematologica., 91*(8Suppl), ECR40.

## 4.5 HEMATOPOIETIC DRUGS

### 4.5.1 DARBEPOETIN ALFA

**FDA Category: C**
*Risk Summary:* Although there is limited data from the human pregnancy experience, but the possible maternal benefit extremely outweighs the unknown or known embryo/fetal risk.

**Further Reading:**
- *Drug Information.* Aranesp. Amgen.
- Ghosh, A., & Ayers, K. J., ( 2007). Darbepoetin alfa for treatment of anemia in a case of chronic renal failure during pregnancy—case report. *Clin. Exp. Obstet. Gynecol., 34*, 193,194.

- Sobito-Jarek, L., Popowska-Drojecka, J., Muszytowski, M., Wanic-Kossowska, M., Kobelski, M., & Czekalski, S., (2006). Anemia treatment with darbepoetin alpha in pregnant female with chronic renal failure: Report of two cases. *Adv. Med. Sci.*, *51*, 309–311.

### 4.5.2   ELTROMBOPAG

**FDA Category: C**
*Risk Summary:* Although there is limited data from the human pregnancy experience, but the possible maternal benefit extremely outweighs the unknown or known embryo/fetal risk.

**Further Reading:**
- Alkaabi, J., Alkindi, S., Riyami, N., Zia, F., Balla, L., & Balla, S., (2012). Successful treatment of severe thrombocytopenia with romiplostim in a pregnant patient with systemic lupus erythematosus. *Lupus*, *21*, 1571–1574.
- *Drug Information. Promacta.* GlaxoSmithKline.

### 4.5.3   EPOETIN ALFA

**FDA Category: C**
*Risk Summary:* Although there is limited data from the human pregnancy experience, but the possible maternal benefit extremely outweighs the unknown or known embryo/fetal risk.

**Further Reading:**
- *Drug Information.* Epogen. Amgen.
- Junca, J., Vela, D., Orts, M., Riutort, N., & Feliu, E., (1995). Treating the anemia of a pregnancy with heterozygous β thalassemia with recombinant human erythropoietin (r-HuEPO). *Eur. J. Haematol.*, *55*, 277–278.

### 4.5.4   FILGRASTIM

**FDA Category: C**
*Risk Summary:* Although there is limited data from the human pregnancy experience, but the possible maternal benefit extremely outweighs the unknown or known embryo/fetal risk.

## Further Reading:
- *Drug Information*. Neupogen. Amgen.
- Novales, J. S., Salva, A. M., Mondanlou, H. D., Kaplan, D. L., del Castillo, J., Andresen, J., & Medlock, E. S., (1993). Maternal administration of granulocyte colony-stimulating factor improves neonatal rat survival after a lethal group B streptococcal infection. *Blood., 81*, 923–927.

### 4.5.5  HEMIN

**FDA Category: C**
*Risk Summary:* It should be used only when the maternal benefit outweighs the fetal risk because there is very limited human pregnancy data, and animal studies are not relevant.

## Further Reading:
- *Drug Information. Panhematin*. Ovation Pharmaceuticals.
- Loftin, E. B. III., (1985). Hematin therapy in acute porphyria. *JAMA, 254*, 613.
- Wenger, S., Meisinger, V., Brücke, T., & Deecke, L., (1998). Acute porphyric neuropathy during pregnancy —effect of haematin therapy. *Eur. Neurol., 39*, 187–188.

### 4.5.6  PEGFILGRASTIM

**FDA Category: C**
*Risk Summary:* It should be used with caution because the pregnancy experience in humans is limited and the reproduction studies in animals have shown low risk.

## Further Reading:
- *Drug Information. Neulasta*. Amgen.

### 4.5.7  PEGINESATIDE

**FDA Category: C**
*Risk Summary:* It should be used with caution because the pregnancy experience in humans is limited, and the reproduction studies in animals have shown the risk of teratogenicity associated with the use of Peginesatide.

**Further Reading:**
- *Drug Information. Omontys.* Affymax.

## 4.5.8   SARGRAMOSTIM

**FDA Category: C**
*Risk Summary:* It should be used only when the maternal benefit outweighs the fetal risk because there is very limited human pregnancy data, and animal studies are not relevant.

**Further Reading:**
- *Drug Information.* Leukine. Berlex Laboratories.
- Perricone, R., De Carolis, C., Giacomelli, R., Guarino, M. D., De Sanctis, G., & Fontana, L., (2003). GM-CSF and pregnancy: Evidence of significantly reduced blood concentrations in unexplained recurrent abortion efficiently reverted by intravenous immunoglobulin treatment. *Am. J. Reprod. Immunol., 50,* 232–237.
- Sjöblom, C., Wikland, M., & Robertson, S. A., (). Granulocyte-macrophage colony-stimulating factor (GM-CSF) acts independently of the beta common subunit of the GM-CSF receptor to prevent inner cell mass apoptosis in human embryos. *Biol. Reprod., 67,* 1817–1823.

## 4.6   HEMOSTATIC DRUGS

### 4.6.1   AMINOCAPROIC ACID

**FDA Category: C**
*Risk Summary:* It should be used only when the maternal benefit outweighs the fetal risk because there is very limited human pregnancy data, and animal studies are not relevant.

**Further Reading:**
- *Drug Information.* Amicar. Immunex.

### 4.6.2   APROTININ

**FDA Category: B**
*Risk Summary:* Although Aprotinin has been assigned with the letter (B), according to the FDA categorization, but it should be used with caution

because no human data is available and the reproduction studies in animals have shown low risk.

**Further Reading:**
- *Drug Information. Trasylol.* Bayer.
- Sher, G., (1974). Trasylol in cases of accidental hemorrhage with coagulation disorder and associated uterine inertia. *S. Afr. Med. J., 48*, 1452–1455.

### 4.6.3 TRANEXAMIC ACID

**FDA Category: B**
***Risk Summary:*** Although Tranexamic Acid has been assigned with the letter (B), according to the FDA categorization, but it should be used with caution because no human data is available and the reproduction studies in animals have shown low risk.

**Further Reading:**
- Åstedt, B., & Nilsson, I. M. Recurrent abruptio placentae treated with the fibrinolytic inhibitor tranexamic acid.
- *Drug Information. Cyklokapron.* Pharmacia.
- Storm, O., & Weber, J., (1976). Prolonged treatment with tranexamic acid (Cyklokapron) during pregnancy. *Ugeskr Laeg., 138*, 1781–1782.

## 4.7 HEMORRHEOLOGIC DRUG

### 4.7.1 PENTOXIFYLLINE

**FDA Category: C**
***Risk Summary:*** The pregnancy experience in humans is limited, and the reproduction studies in animals have shown moderate risk.

**Further Reading:**
- *Drug Information. Trental.* Hoechst Roussel.
- Witter, F. R., & Smith, R. V., (1985). The excretion of pentoxifylline and its metabolites into human breast milk. *Am. J. Obstet. Gynecol., 151*, 1094–1097.

## 4.8  ANTI-HEPARIN

### *4.8.1  PROTAMINE*

**FDA Category: C**
*Risk Summary:* Although there is limited data from the human pregnancy experience, but the possible maternal benefit extremely outweighs the unknown or known embryo/fetal risk.

**Further Reading:**
- *Drug Information. Protamine sulfate.* Eli Lilly.

## 4.9  ANTI-HEMOPHILIC

### *4.9.1  FACTOR XIII CONCENTRATE (HUMAN)*

**FDA Category: C**
*Risk Summary:* The reproduction studies in animals have shown no evidence of fetal harm or impaired fertility. The pregnancy experience in humans is adequate to exhibit that the embryo-fetal risk is nonexistent or very low.

**Further Reading:**
- Asahina, T., Kobayashi, T., Takeuchi, K., & Kanayama, N., (2007). Congenital blood coagulation factor XIII deficiency and successful deliveries: A review of the literature. Obstet. Gynecol. Surv., *62,* 255–260.
- *Drug Information.* Corifact. CSL Behring.
- Rodeghiero, F., Castaman, G. C., Di Bona, E., Ruggeri, M., & Dini, E., (1987). Successful pregnancy in a woman with congenital factor XIII deficiency treats with substitutive therapy. Blut., *55,* 45–48.

## 4.10  BRADYKININ INHIBITOR

### *4.10.1  ICATIBANT*

**FDA Category: C**
*Risk Summary:* It should be used with caution because the pregnancy experience in humans is limited, and the reproduction studies in animals have shown the risk of developmental toxicity associated with the use of Icatibant.

**Further Reading:**
- *Drug Information*. Firazyr. Shire Orphan Therapies.
- Geng, B., & Riedl, M. A., (2013). HAE update: Special consideration in the female patient with hereditary angioedema. *Allergy Asthma Proc., 34*, 13–18.


## 4.11    KALLIKREIN INHIBITOR

### 4.11.1    ECALLANTIDE

**FDA Category: C**
***Risk Summary:*** It should be used with caution because the pregnancy experience in humans is limited and the reproduction studies in animals have shown low risk.

**Further Reading:**
- *Drug Information. Kalbitor*. Dyaz.


## KEYWORDS

- **anti-heparin**
- **aprotinin**
- **bradykinin inhibitor**
- **hemorheologic drug**
- **hemostatic drugs**
- **tranexamic acid**

# CHAPTER 5

# Drugs Affecting the Endocrine System

## 5.1 ANTIDIABETIC DRUGS

### 5.1.1 INSULINS

#### 5.1.1.1 REGULAR INSULIN

**FDA Category: B**
*Risk Summary:* The reproduction studies in animals have shown no evidence of fetal harm or impaired fertility. The pregnancy experience in humans is adequate to exhibit that the embryo-fetal risk is nonexistent or very low.

**Further Reading:**
- Buchanan, T. A., & Kjos, S. L., (2002). Diabetes in women. Early detection, prevention, and management. *Clin. Updates Women's Health Care.*, *1*(4/Fall), 47.
- Dignan, P. S. J., (1981). Teratogenic risk and counseling in diabetes. Clin Obstet. Gynecol 1981 *24*, 149–159.
- Kimmerle, R., Heinemann, L., Delecki, A., & Berger, M., (1992). Severe hypoglycemia incidence and predisposing factors in 85 pregnancies of type I diabetic women. *Diabetes Care, 15*, 1034–1037.

#### 5.1.1.2 INSULIN ASPART

**FDA Category: B**
*Risk Summary:* The reproduction studies in animals have shown no evidence of fetal harm or impaired fertility. The pregnancy experience in humans is limited.

**Further Reading:**
- *Drug Information*. Novolog. Novo Nordisk.
- Gonzalez, C., Santoro, S., Salzberg, S., Di Girolamo, G., & Alvarinas, J., (2005). Insulin analog therapy in pregnancies complicated by diabetes mellitus. *Expert Opin. Pharmacother*, *6*, 735–742.
- Pettitt, D. J., Ospina, P., Kolaczynski, J. W., & Jovanovic, L., (2003). Comparison of an insulin analog, insulin as part, and regular human insulin with no insulin in gestational diabetes mellitus. *Diabetes Care*, *26*, 183–186.

## 5.1.1.3   *INSULIN DETEMIR*

**FDA Category: B**
***Risk Summary:*** The reproduction studies in animals have shown no evidence of fetal harm or impaired fertility. The pregnancy experience in humans is limited.

**Further Reading:**
- *Drug Information*. Levemir. Novo Nordisk.
- Lambert, K., & Holt, R. I. G., (2013). The use of insulin analogs in pregnancy. *Diabetes Obes. Metab., 15*, 888–900.
- Lapolla, A., Di Cianni, G., Bruttomesso, D., Dalfra, M. G., Fresa, R., Mello, G., Napoli, A., Romanelli, T., Sciacca, L., Stefanelli, G., Torlone, E., & Mannino, G., (2009). Use of insulin detemir in pregnancy: A report on 10 type 1 diabetic women. *Diabet. Med., 26*, 1179, 1180.

## 5.1.1.4   *INSULIN GLARGINE*

**FDA Category: C**
***Risk Summary:*** The reproduction studies in animals have shown no evidence of fetal harm or impaired fertility. The pregnancy experience in humans is adequate to exhibit that the embryo-fetal risk is nonexistent or very low.

**Further Reading:**
- Devlin, J. T., Hothersall, L., & Wilkis, J. L., (2002). Use of insulin glargine during pregnancy in a type 1 diabetic woman. *Diabetes Care, 25*, 1095, 1096.

- *Drug Information*. Lantus. Sanofi-Aventis.
- Graves, D. E., White, J. C., & Kirk, J. K., (2006). The use of insulin glargine with gestational diabetes mellitus. *Diabetes Care, 29*, 471, 472.

## 5.1.1.5 INSULIN LISPRO

**FDA Category: B**

*Risk Summary:* The reproduction studies in animals have shown no evidence of fetal harm or impaired fertility. The pregnancy experience in humans is adequate to exhibit that the embryo-fetal risk is nonexistent or very low.

**Further Reading:**

- Cypryk, K., Sobczak, M., Pertyńska-Marczewska, M., Zawodniak-Szałapska, M., Szymczak, W., Wilczyński, J., & Lewiński, A. (2004). Pregnancy complications and perinatal outcome in diabetic women treated with Humalog (insulin lispro) or regular human insulin during pregnancy. *Medical Science Monitor, 10*(2), PI29–PI32.
- *Drug Information. Humalog*. Eli Lilly.
- Lewinski, A., (2004). Pregnancy complications and perinatal outcomes in diabetic women treated with Humalog (insulin lispro) or regular human insulin during pregnancy. *Med. Sci. Monit., 10*, P129–132.
- Scherbaum, W. A., Lankisch, M. R., Pawlowski, B., & Somville, T., (2002). Insulin lispro in pregnancy—a retrospective analysis of 33 cases and matched controls. *Exp. Clin. Endocrinol. Diabetes, 110*, 6–9.

## 5.1.2 SULFONYLUREAS

### 5.1.2.1 CHLORPROPAMIDE

**FDA Category: C**

*Risk Summary:* It should be used with caution during the 1st and 2nd Trimesters. However, it is better to avoid the use of Chlorpropamide during the 3rd Trimester because fetal toxicity has been associated with its use during the last Trimester.

**Further Reading:**
- American College of Obstetricians and Gynecologists (2005). Pregestational diabetes mellitus. ACOG Practice Bulletin. No. 60. March 2005. *Obstet. Gynecol., 105*, 675–685.
- Campbell, G. D., (1963). Chlorpropamide and fetal damage. *Br. Med. J., 1*, 59–60.
- Smoak, I. W., (1993). Embryopathic effects of the oral hypoglycemic agent chlorpropamide in cultured mouse embryos. *Am. J. Obstet. Gynecol., 169*, 409–414.

## 5.1.2.2   TOLBUTAMIDE

**FDA Category: C**
*Risk Summary:* It should be used with caution during the 1st and 2nd Trimesters. However, it is better to avoid the use of Tolbutamide during the 3rd Trimester because fetal toxicity has been associated with its use during the last Trimester.

**Further Reading:**
- American College of Obstetricians and Gynecologists (2005). Pregestational diabetes mellitus. ACOG Practice Bulletin. No. 60. March 2005. *Obstet. Gynecol., 105*, 675–685.
- Schiff, D., Aranda, J., & Stern, L., (1970). Neonatal thrombocytopenia and congenital malformation associated with the administration of tolbutamide to the mother. *J. Pediatr., 77*, 457–458.
- Smoak, I. W., (1992). Teratogenic effects of tolbutamide on early-somite mouse embryos in vitro. *Diabetes Res. Clin. Pract., 17*, 161–167.

## 5.1.2.3   TOLAZAMIDE

**FDA Category: C**
*Risk Summary:* It should be used with caution during the 1st and 2nd Trimesters. However, it is better to avoid the use of Tolazamide during the 3rd Trimester because fetal toxicity has been associated with its use during the last Trimester.

**Further Reading:**
- American College of Obstetricians and Gynecologists (2005). Pregestational diabetes mellitus. ACOG Practice Bulletin. No. 60. March 2005. *Obstet. Gynecol., 105*, 675–685.
- Piacquadio, K., Hollingsworth, D. R., & Murphy, H., (1991). Effects of in-utero exposure to oral hypoglycaemic drugs. *Lancet, 338*, 866–869.

## *5.1.2.4 GLIBENCLAMIDE*

**FDA Category: C**
***Risk Summary:*** It should be used with caution because the human pregnancy experience has shown a low risk.

**Further Reading:**
- Koren, G., (2001). Glyburide and fetal safety; transplacental pharmacokinetic considerations. *Reprod Toxicol., 15*, 227–229.
- Kremer, C. J., & Duff, P., (2004). Glyburide for the treatment of gestational diabetes. *Am. J. Obstet. Gynecol., 190*, 1438–1439.
- Langer, O., Conway, D. L., Berkus, M. D., Xenakis, E. M. J., & Gonzales, O., (2000). A comparison of glyburide and insulin in women with gestational diabetes mellitus. *N. Engl. J. Med., 343*, 1134–1138.

## *5.1.2.5 GLIPIZIDE*

**FDA Category: C**
***Risk Summary:*** It should be used with caution because the pregnancy experience in humans is limited and the reproduction studies in animals have shown low risk.

**Further Reading:**
- American College of Obstetricians and Gynecologists (2005). Pregestational diabetes mellitus. ACOG Practice Bulletin. No. 60. March 2005. *Obstet. Gynecol., 105*, 675–685.
- *Drug Information. Glucotrol.* Pfizer Inc.

## 5.1.3   THIAZOLIDINEDIONES

### 5.1.3.1   PIOGLITAZONE

**FDA Category: C**
*Risk Summary:* The pregnancy experience in humans is limited, and the reproduction studies in animals have shown moderate risk.

**Further Reading:**
- American College of Obstetricians and Gynecologists (2005). Pregestational diabetes mellitus. ACOG Practice Bulletin. No. 60. March 2005. *Obstet. Gynecol.,105*, 675–685.
- *Drug Information*. Actos. Takeda Pharmaceuticals America.

### 5.1.3.2   ROSIGLITAZONE

**FDA Category: C**
*Risk Summary:* The pregnancy experience in humans is limited, and the reproduction studies in animals have shown risk.

**Further Reading:**
- Belli, S. H., Graffigna, M. N., Oneto, A., Otero, P., Schurman, L., & Levalle, O. A., (2004). Effect of rosiglitazone on insulin resistance, growth factors, and reproductive disturbances in women with polycystic ovary syndrome. *Fertil Steril, 81*, 624–629.
- *Drug Information. Avandia.* SmithKline Beecham Pharmaceuticals.
- Yaris, F., Yaris, E., Kadioglu, M., Ulku, C., Kesim, M., & Kalyoncu, N. I., (2004). Normal pregnancy outcome following inadvertent exposure to rosiglitazone, gliclazide, and atorvastatin in a diabetic and hypertensive woman. *Reprod Toxicol., 18*, 619–621.

## 5.1.4   MEGLITINIDES

### 5.1.4.1   NATEGLINIDE

**FDA Category: C**
*Risk Summary:* The pregnancy experience in humans is limited, and the reproduction studies in animals have shown moderate risk.

**Further Reading:**
- *Drug Information. Starlix.* Novartis Pharmaceuticals.

## 5.1.4.2 REPAGLINIDE

**FDA Category: C**
*Risk Summary:* The pregnancy experience in humans is limited, and the reproduction studies in animals have shown moderate risk.

**Further Reading:**
- *Drug Information.* Prandin. Novo Nordisk.
- Mollar-Puchades, M. A., Martin-Cortes, A., Perez-Calvo, A., & Diaz-Garcia, C., (2007). Use of repaglinide on a pregnant woman during embryogenesis. *Diabetes Obes. Metab., 9*, 146, 147.
- Napoli, A., Ciampa, F., Colatrella, A., & Fallucca, F., (2006). Use of repaglinide during the first weeks of pregnancy in two type 2 diabetic women. *Diabetes Care, 29*, 2326–2327.

## 5.1.5   GLUCAGON-LIKE PEPTIDE 1 RECEPTOR AGONISTS

### 5.1.5.1   EXENATIDE

**FDA Category: C**
*Risk Summary:* The pregnancy experience in humans is limited, and the reproduction studies in animals have shown moderate risk.

**Further Reading:**
- *Drug Information. Byetta.* Amylin Pharmaceuticals.

### 5.1.5.2   LIRAGLUTIDE

**FDA Category: C**
*Risk Summary:* It should be used with caution because the pregnancy experience in humans is limited, and the reproduction studies in animals have shown the risk of developmental toxicity associated with the use of Liraglutide.

**Further Reading:**
• *Drug Information. Victoza.* Novo Nordisk.

## 5.1.6 DIPEPTIDYL PEPTIDASE-4 INHIBITORS

### 5.1.6.1 LINAGLIPTIN

**FDA Category: B**
*Risk Summary:* It should be used with caution because the pregnancy experience in humans is limited and the reproduction studies in animals have shown low risk.

**Further Reading:**
• American College of Obstetricians and Gynecologists (2005). Pregestational diabetes mellitus. ACOG Practice Bulletin No. 60, March 2005. *Obstet. Gynecol., 105*, 675–685.
• *Drug Information*, (2012). Tradjenta. Boehringer Ingelheim Pharmaceuticals and Eli Lilly.

### 5.1.6.2 SAXAGLIPTIN

**FDA Category: B**
*Risk Summary:* It should be used with caution because the pregnancy experience in humans is limited and the reproduction studies in animals have shown low risk.

**Further Reading:**
• American College of Obstetricians and Gynecologists (2005). Pregestational diabetes mellitus. ACOG Practice Bulletin. No. 60, March 2005. *Obstet. Gynecol., 105*, 675–685.
• *Drug Information. Onglyza.* AstraZeneca Pharmaceuticals.

### 5.1.6.3 SITAGLIPTIN

**FDA Category: B**
*Risk Summary:* It should be used with caution because the pregnancy experience in humans is limited and the reproduction studies in animals have shown low risk.

**Further Reading:**
- *Drug Information*. Januvia. Merck.
- Third Annual Report on exposure during pregnancy from the Merck Pregnancy Registry for Januvia (sitagliptin phosphate) and Janumet (sitagliptin phosphate/metformin hydrochloride) August 4, 2006, through August 3, 2009.

## 5.1.7  ALPHA-GLUCOSIDASE INHIBITORS

### 5.1.7.1  ACARBOSE

**FDA Category: B**
*Risk Summary:* It should be used with caution because the pregnancy experience in humans is limited and the reproduction studies in animals have shown low risk.

**Further Reading:**
- De Veciana, M., Trail, P. A., Evans, A. T., & Dulaney, K., (2002). A comparison of oral acarbose and insulin in women with gestational diabetes mellitus (abstract). *Obstet. Gynecol., 99*(Suppl), 5S.
- *Drug Information. Precose*. Bayer Corporation.
- Wilton, L. V., Pearce, G. L., Martin, R. M., Mackay, F. J., & Mann, R. D., (1998). The outcomes of pregnancy in women exposed to newly marketed drugs in general practice in England. *Br. J. Obstet. Gynaecol., 105*, 882–889.

### 5.1.7.2  MIGLITOL

**FDA Category: B**
*Risk Summary:* The reproduction studies in animals have shown no evidence of fetal harm or impaired fertility. The pregnancy experience in humans is limited.

**Further Reading:**
- Campbell, L. K., Baker, D. E., & Campbell, R. K., (2000). Miglitol: Assessment of its role in the treatment of patients with diabetes mellitus. Ann. Pharmacother., 2000 *34*, 1291–1301.
- *Drug Information. Glyset*. Pharmacia & Upjohn.

## *5.1.8   BIGUANIDES*

### *5.1.8.1   METFORMIN*

**FDA Category: B**
*Risk Summary:* It should be used with caution because the human pregnancy experience has shown a low risk.

**Further Reading:**
- Coetzee, R. J., & Jackson, W. P. U., (1979). Metformin in management of pregnant insulin-independent diabetics. *Diabetologia, 16,* 241–245.
- *Drug Information. Glucophage*. Bristol-Myers Squibb.
- Elliott, B., Schuessling, F., & Langer, O., (1997). The oral antihyperglycemic agent metformin does not affect glucose uptake and transport in the human diabetic placenta (abstract). *Am. J. Obstet. Gynecol., 176*, S182.

## *5.1.9   AMYLIN ANALOG*

### *5.1.9.1   PRAMLINTIDE*

**FDA Category: C**
*Risk Summary:* The pregnancy experience in humans is limited, and the reproduction studies in animals have shown moderate risk.

**Further Reading:**
- *Drug Information. Symlin*. Amylin Pharmaceuticals.

## 5.2   ADRENAL CORTICOSTEROID DRUGS

### *5.2.1   BECLOMETHASONE*

**FDA Category: C**
*Risk Summary:* The reproduction studies in animals have shown no evidence of fetal harm or impaired fertility. The pregnancy experience in humans is adequate to exhibit that the embryo-fetal risk is nonexistent or very low.

**Further Reading:**
- *Drug Information*. Beclovent. Glaxo Wellcome.
- Namazy, J., Schatz, M., Long, L., Lipkowitz, M., Lillie, M., Voss, M., Deitz, R. J., & Petitti, D., (2004). Use of inhaled steroids by pregnant asthmatic women does not reduce intrauterine growth. *J. Allergy Clin. Immunol., 113*, 427–432.
- Rahimi, R., Nikfar, S., & Abdollahi, M., (2006). Meta-analysis finds use of inhaled corticosteroids during pregnancy safe: A systematic meta-analysis review. Hum. Exp. Toxicol., *25*, 447–452.

### 5.2.2 BETAMETHASONE

**FDA Category: C**
*Risk Summary:* Although there is limited data from the human pregnancy experience, but the possible maternal benefit extremely outweighs the unknown or known embryo/fetal risk.

**Further Reading:**
- Gamsu, H. R., Mullinger, B. M., Donnai, P., & Dash, C. H., (1989). Antenatal administration of betamethasone to prevent respiratory distress syndrome in preterm infants: Report of a UK multicentre trial. *Br. J. Obstet. Gynaecol., 96*, 401–410.
- Helal, K. J., Gordon, M. C., Lightner, C. R., Barth, W. H. Jr., (2000). Adrenal suppression induced by betamethasone in women at risk for premature delivery. *Obstet. Gynecol., 96*, 287–290.
- Hoff, D. S., & Mammel, M. C., (1997). Suspected betamethasone-induced leukemoid reaction in a premature infant. *Pharmacotherapy, 17*, 1031–1034.
- Kuhn, R. J. P., Speirs, A. L., Pepperell, R. J., Eggers, T. R., Doyle, L. W., & Hutchison, A., (1982). Betamethasone, albuterol, and threatened premature delivery: Benefits and risks. *Obstet. Gynecol., 60*, 403–408.
- Yunis, K. A., Bitar, F. F., Hayek, P., Mroueh, S. M., & Mikati, M., (1999). Transient hypertrophic cardiomyopathy in the newborn following multiple doses of antenatal corticosteroids. *Am. J. Perinatol., 16*, 17–21.

## 5.2.3 BUDESONIDE

**FDA Category (Inhaled/Nasal): B**
**FDA Category (Oral): C**
1. *Risk Summary (Inhaled/Nasal):* The reproduction studies in animals have shown no evidence of fetal harm or impaired fertility. The pregnancy experience in humans is adequate to exhibit that the embryo-fetal risk is nonexistent or very low.
2. *Risk Summary (Oral):* It should be used with caution because the pregnancy experience in humans is limited, and the reproduction studies in animals have shown the risk of skeletal anomalies, fetal loss, and intrauterine growth restriction (IUGR) associated with the use of S.C. Budesonide.

**Further Reading:**
- *Drug Information. Pulmicort* Turbuhaler. AstraZeneca.
- *Drug Information. Rhinocort.* AstraZeneca.
- Kihlstrom, I., & Lundberg, C., (1987). Teratogenicity study of the new glucocorticosteroid budesonide in rabbits. *Arzneimittelforschung, 37,* 43–46.
- Norjavaara, E., Gerhardsson de Verdier, M., (2003). Normal pregnancy outcomes in a population-based study including 2968 pregnant women exposed to budesonide. *J. Allergy Clin. Immunol., 111,* 736–742.
- Rahimi, R., Nikfar, S., & Abdollahi, M., (2006). Meta-analysis finds use of inhaled corticosteroids during pregnancy safe: A systematic meta-analysis review. *Hum. Exp. Toxicol., 25,* 447–452.

## 5.2.4 DEXAMETHASONE

**FDA Category: C**
*Risk Summary:* Although there is limited data from the human pregnancy experience, but the possible maternal benefit extremely outweighs the small, absolute risk of oral clefts linked to its use during the 1st Trimester.

**Further Reading:**
- Anday, E. K., & Harris, M. C., (1982). Leukemoid reaction associated with antenatal dexamethasone administration. *J. Pediatr., 101,* 614–616.

- Kauppilla, A., (1977). ACTH levels in maternal, fetal and neonatal plasma after short term prenatal dexamethasone therapy. *Br. J. Obstet. Gynaecol., 84*, 128–134.
- Taeusch, H. W. Jr., Frigoletto, F., Kitzmiller, J., Avery, M. E., Hehre, A., Fromm, B., Lawson, E., & Neff, R. K., (1979). Risk of respiratory distress syndrome after prenatal dexamethasone treatment. *Pediatrics, 63*, 64–72.

## 5.2.5 HYDROCORTISONE

**FDA Category: C**
*Risk Summary:* The use of Hydrocortisone should be avoided in pregnant women because the pregnancy experience in humans has shown a slight risk of cleft lip, with/or without cleft palate, associated with the use of this drug. However, these adverse events should not withhold the administration of Hydrocortisone if medical condition of the pregnant mother needs it.

**Further Reading:**
- Gur, C., Diav-Citrin, O., Shechtman, S., Arnon, J., & Ornoy, A., (2004). Pregnancy outcome after first-trimester exposure to corticosteroids: A prospective controlled study. *Reprod Toxicol., 18*, 93–101.
- Harris, J. W. S., & Ross, I. P., (1956). Cortisone therapy in early pregnancy: Relation to cleft palate. *Lancet, 1*, 1045–1047.
- Kotas, R. V., Mims, L. C., & Hart, L. K., (1974). Reversible inhibition of lung cell number after glucocorticoid injection into fetal rabbits to enhance surfactant appearance. *Pediatrics, 53*, 358–361.
- Rodriguez-Pinilla, E., & Martinez-Frias, M. L., (1998). Corticosteroids during pregnancy and oral clefts: A case-control study. *Teratology, 58*, 2–5.
- Shepard, T. H., (1995). *Catalog of Teratogenic Agents.* (8th edn.) Baltimore, MD: The Johns Hopkins University Press.

## 5.2.6 PREDNISOLONE

**FDA Category: D**
*Risk Summary:* The use of c should be avoided in pregnant women because the pregnancy experience in humans has shown a slight risk of cleft lip, with/or without cleft palate, associated with the use of this drug. However,

these adverse events should not withhold the administration of Prednisolone if medical condition of the pregnant mother needs it.

**Further Reading:**

- Accessdata.fda.gov. (2018). [online] Available at: https://www. accessdata.fda.gov/drugsatfda_docs/label/2012/202020s000lbl.pdf (accessed on 31 January 2020).
- Carmichael, S. L., & Shaw, G. M., (). Maternal corticosteroid use and risk of selected congenital anomalies. *Am. J. Med. Genet.,* 1999 *86,* 242–244.
- Park-Wyllie, L., Mazzotta, P., Pastuszak, A., Moretti, M. E., Beique, L., Hunnisett, L., Friesen, M. H., Jacobson, S., Kasapinovic, S., Chang, D., Diav-Citrin, O., Chitayat, D., Nulman, I., Einarson, T. R., & Koren, G., (2000). Birth defects after maternal exposure to corticosteroids: Prospective cohort study and meta-analysis of epidemiological studies. *Teratology, 62,* 385–382.

### 5.2.7   PREDNISONE

**FDA Category: D**

**Risk Summary:** The use of Hydrocortisone should be avoided in pregnant women because the pregnancy experience in humans has shown a slight risk of cleft lip, with/or without cleft palate, associated with the use of this drug. However, these adverse events should not withhold the administration of hydrocortisone if the medical condition of the pregnant mother needs it.

**Further Reading:**

- Cote, C. J., Meuwissen, H. J., & Pickering, R. J., (1974). Effects on the neonate of prednisone and azathioprine administered to the mother during pregnancy. *J. Pediatr., 85,* 324–328.
- Jones, R. T., & Weinerman, E. R., (1979). MOPP (nitrogen mustard, vincristine, procarbazine, and prednisone) given during pregnancy. *Obstet. Gynecol., 54,* 477–478.
- Park-Wyllie, L., Mazzotta, P., Pastuszak, A., Moretti, M. E., Beique, L., Hunnisett, L., ... & Diav-Citrin, O. (2000). Birth defects after maternal exposure to corticosteroids: prospective cohort study and meta-analysis of epidemiological studies. *Teratology, 62*(6), 385–392.

## 5.2.8 *TRIAMCINOLONE*

**FDA Category (Local/Inhaled): B**

**FDA Category (Oral): C**

1. **Risk Summary (Local/Inhaled):** The reproduction studies in animals have shown no evidence of fetal harm or impaired fertility. The pregnancy experience in humans is adequate to exhibit that the embryo-fetal risk is nonexistent or very low.

2. **Risk Summary (Oral):** The use of Triamcinolone should be avoided in the 1st Trimester because the pregnancy experience in humans has shown a slight risk of cleft lip, with/or without cleft palate, associated with the use of this drug. However, these adverse events should not withhold the administration of Triamcinolone if the medical condition of the pregnant mother needs it.

**Further Reading:**

- *Drug Information*, (1994). *Azmacort*. Rhône-Poulenc Rorer Pharmaceuticals, Inc.
- Rahimi, R., Nikfar, S., & Abdollahi, M., (2006). Meta-analysis finds use of inhaled corticosteroids during pregnancy safe: A systematic meta-analysis review. *Hum. Exp. Toxicol.*, 25, 447–452.
- Tarara, R. P., Cordy, D. R., & Hendrickx, A. G., (1989). Central nervous system malformations induced by triamcinolone acetonide in nonhuman primates: Pathology. *Teratology*, 39, 75–84.
- Zhou, M., & Walker, B. E., (1993). Potentiation of triamcinolone-induced cleft palate in mice by maternal high dietary fat. *Teratology*, 48, 53–57.

## 5.3 ANDROGENIC DRUGS

### 5.3.1 *DANAZOL*

**FDA Category: X**

**Risk Summary:** Danazol is used in the treatment of various diseases, such as endometriosis, hereditary angioedema, and fibrocystic breast disease. However, Danazol is absolutely contraindicated during pregnancy. Therefore, women planning to become pregnant should stop taking Danazol first.

**Further Reading:**
- Brunskill, P. J., (1992). The effects of fetal exposure to danazol. *Br. J. Obstet. Gynaecol., 99*, 212–215.
- *Drug Information. Danocrine.* Sanofi Pharmaceuticals.
- Fayez, J. A., Collazo, L. M., & Vernon, C., (1988). Comparison of different modalities of treatment for minimal and mild endometriosis. *Am. J. Obstet. Gynecol., 159*, 927–932.
- Rosa, F. W., (1984). Virilization of the female fetus with maternal danazol exposure. *Am. J. Obstet. Gynecol., 149*, 99–100.

## 5.3.2   FLUOXYMESTERONE

**FDA Category: X**
*Risk Summary:* Fluoxymesterone is used in the treatment of various diseases, such as endometriosis, hereditary angioedema, and fibrocystic breast disease. Nevertheless, Fluoxymesterone is absolutely contraindicated during pregnancy due to the risk of developing female pseudohermaphroditism. Therefore, women planning to become pregnant should stop taking Fluoxymesterone first.

**Further Reading:**
- Dmowski, W. P., & Cohen, M. R., (1978). Antigonadotropin (danazol) in the treatment of endometriosis. Evaluation of posttreatment fertility and three-year follow-up data. *Am. J. Obstet. Gynecol., 130*, 41–48.
- *Drug Information.* Halotestin. Upjohn.
- Fayez, J. A., Collazo, L. M., & Vernon, C., (1988). Comparison of different modalities of treatment for minimal and mild endometriosis. *Am. J. Obstet. Gynecol., 159*, 927–932.

## 5.3.3   TESTOSTERONE/METHYLTESTOSTERONE

**FDA Category: X**
*Risk Summary:* Methyltestosterone is used in the treatment of various diseases, such as endometriosis, hereditary angioedema, and fibrocystic breast disease. Nevertheless, Methyltestosterone is absolutely contraindicated during pregnancy due to the risk of developing female pseudohermaphroditism. Therefore, women planning to become pregnant should stop taking Methyltestosterone first.

**Further Reading:**
- Grunwaldt, E., & Bates, T., (1957). Nonadrenal female pseudoher-maphroditism after administration of testosterone to mother during pregnancy. *Pediatrics, 20,* 503–505.
- Hayles, A. B., & Nolan, R. B., (1957). Female pseudohermaphro-ditism: Report of case in an infant born of a mother receiving methyl-testosterone during pregnancy. *Proc. Staff Meet Mayo Clin., 32,* 41–44.
- Morris, J. A., Creasy, R. K., & Hohe, P. T., (1970). Inhibition of puer-peral lactation. Double-blind comparison of chlorothianesene, testos-terone enanthate and estradiol valerate and placebo. *Obstet. Gynecol., 36,* 107–114.

## 5.4 ESTROGENIC DRUGS

### 5.4.1 CLOMIPHENE

**FDA Category: X**
***Risk Summary:*** Clomiphene is absolutely contraindicated during preg-nancy. Therefore, women planning to become pregnant should stop taking Clomiphene first.

**Further Reading:**
- Biale, Y., Leventhal, H., Altaras, M., & Ben-Aderet, N., (1978). Anen-cephaly and clomiphene-induced pregnancy. *Acta Obstet. Gynecol. Scand., 57,* 483–484.
- *Drug Information. Clomid.* Hoechst Marion Roussel.
- *Drug Information. Serophene.* Serono Laboratories.
- James, W. H., (1977). Clomiphene, anencephaly, and spina bifida. *Lancet, 1,* 603.
- Sceusa, D. K., & Klein, P. E., (1990). Ultrasound diagnosis of an acar-dius acephalic monster in a quintuplet pregnancy. *JDMS, 2,* 109–112. As cited by In: Martinez-Roman, S., Torres, P. J., & Puerto, B., Acar-dius acephalous after ovulation induction by clomiphene. *Teratology* 1995 *51,* 231–232.

## 5.4.2 DIETHYLSTILBESTROL

**FDA Category: X**
*Risk Summary:* Diethylstilbestrol is absolutely contraindicated during pregnancy. Therefore, women planning to become pregnant should stop taking Diethylstilbestrol first.

**Further Reading:**
- Robboy, S. J., Noller, K. L., Kaufman, R. H., Barnes, A. B., Townsend, D., Gundersen, J. H., & Nash, S., (1981). Information for physicians. Prenatal diethylstilbestrol (DES) exposure: Recommendations of the Diethylstilbestrol–Adenosis (DESAD) Project for the identification and management of exposed individuals. NIH Publication No. 81-2049.
- Sandberg, E. C., Riffle, N. L., Higdon, J. V., & Getman, C. E., (1981). Pregnancy outcome in women exposed to diethylstilbestrol in utero. *Am. J. Obstet. Gynecol., 140*, 194–205.
- Wilson, J. G., & Brent, R. L., (1981). Are female sex hormones teratogenic? *Am. J. Obstet. Gynecol., 141*, 567–580.

## 5.4.3 ESTRADIOL/ETHINYL ESTRADIOL

**FDA Category: X**
*Risk Summary:* Estradiol is contraindicated during pregnancy because there is usually no benefit from its use in pregnancy.

**Further Reading:**
- Luther, E. R., Roux, J., Popat, R., Gardner, A., Gray, J., Soubiran, E., & Korcaz, Y., (1980). The effect of estrogen priming on induction of labor with prostaglandins. *Am. J. Obstet. Gynecol., 137*, 351–357.
- Wiseman, R. A., & Dodds-Smith, I. C., (1984). Cardiovascular birth defects and antenatal exposure to female sex hormones: A reevaluation of some base data. *Teratology, 30*, 359–370.

## 5.4.4 COMBINED ORAL CONTRACEPTIVE (ETHINYL ESTRADIOL/ LEVONORGESTREL)

**FDA Category: X**
*Risk Summary:* Ethinyl estradiol/levonorgestrel combination is contraindicated during pregnancy because there is usually no benefit from its use in pregnancy.

**Further Reading:**
- Ambani, L. M., Joshi, N. J., Vaidya, R. A., & Devi, P. K., (1977). Are hormonal contraceptives teratogenic? *Fertil Steril., 28,* 791–797.
- Bongiovanni, A. M., & McFadden, A. J., (1960). Steroids during pregnancy and possible fetal consequences. *Fertil Steril., 11,* 181–184.
- Kasan, P. N., & Andrews, J., (1980). Oral contraceptives and congenital abnormalities. *Br. J. Obstet. Gynaecol.,* 1980 *87,* 545–551.

## 5.5 ANTI-ESTROGENIC DRUG

### *5.5.1 TAMOXIFEN*

**FDA Category: D**
*Risk Summary:* Tamoxifen is contraindicated during pregnancy, and women planning to become pregnant should stop taking Tamoxifen first. However, sometimes the necessity for Tamoxifen justifies its use during pregnancy but the mother should be notified about the potential harm on the fetus.

**Further Reading:**
- Jordan, V. C., (1992). The role of tamoxifen in the treatment and prevention of breast cancer. *Curr. Probl. Cancer, 16,* 129–176.
- Pasqualini, J. R., Gulino, A., Sumida, C., & Screpanti, I., (1984). Anti-estrogens in fetal and newborn target tissues. *J. Steroid Biochem., 20,* 121–128.
- Poulet, F. M., Roessler, M. L., & Vancutsem, P. M., (1997). Initial uterine alterations caused by developmental exposure to tamoxifen. *Reprod Toxicol., 11,* 815–822.

## 5.6 PROGESTOGENIC DRUGS

### *5.6.1 ETHYNODIOL*

**FDA Category: X**
*Risk Summary:* Ethynodiol is contraindicated during pregnancy because there is usually no benefit from its use in pregnancy.

**Further Reading:**
- Ambani, L. M., Joshi, N. J., Vaidya, R. A., & Devi, P. K., (1977). Are hormonal contraceptives teratogenic? *Fertil Steril., 28*, 791–797.
- Bongiovanni, A. M., & McFadden, A. J., (1960). Steroids during pregnancy and possible fetal consequences. *Fertil Steril., 11*, 181–184.
- Kasan, P. N., & Andrews, J., (1980). Oral contraceptives and congenital abnormalities. *Br. J. Obstet. Gynaecol., 87*, 545–551.

## 5.6.2 HYDROXYPROGESTERONE

**FDA Category: B**
*Risk Summary:* Whenever it is possible, the use of Hydroxyprogesterone should be avoided in the 1st trimester because of a small risk of hypospadias and/or ambiguous genitals in males and female masculinization.

**Further Reading:**
- Committee on Obstetric Practice, American College of Obstetricians and Gynecologists (2008). Use of progesterone to reduce preterm birth. ACOG Committee Opinion. No. 419, October 2008. *Obstet. Gynecol., 112*, 963–965.
- Katz, Z., Lancet, M., Skornik, J., Chemke, J., Mogilner, B. M., & Klinberg, M., (1985). Teratogenicity of progestogens given during the first trimester of pregnancy. *Obstet. Gynecol., 65*, 775–780.
- Kauppila, A., Hartikainen-Sorri, A. L., Janne, O., Tuimala, R., & Jarvinen, P. A., (1980). Suppression of threatened premature labor by administration of cortisol and 17α-hydroxyprogesterone caproate: A comparison with ritodrine. *Am. J. Obstet. Gynecol., 138*, 404–408.

## 5.6.3 MEDROXYPROGESTERONE

**FDA Category: X**
*Risk Summary:* Medroxyprogesterone is contraindicated during pregnancy. Therefore, women planning to become pregnant should stop taking Medroxyprogesterone first.

**Further Reading:**
- Andrew, F. D., & Staples, R. E., (1977). Prenatal toxicity of medroxyprogesterone acetate in rabbits, rats, and mice. *Teratology., 15*, 25–32.

- Prahalada, S., Carroad, E., & Hendrickx, A. G., (1985). Embryotoxicity and maternal serum concentrations of medroxyprogesterone acetate (MPA) in baboons (Papio cynocephalus). *Contraception, 32,* 497–515.

## 5.6.4 NORGESTREL

**FDA Category: X**
*Risk Summary:* Norgestrel is contraindicated during pregnancy because there is usually no benefit from its use in pregnancy.

**Further Reading:**
- Ambani, L. M., Joshi, N. J., Vaidya, R. A., & Devi, P. K., (1977). Are hormonal contraceptives teratogenic? *Fertil Steril., 28,* 791–797.
- Bongiovanni, A. M., & McFadden, A. J., (1960). Steroids during pregnancy and possible fetal consequences. *Fertil Steril., 11,* 181–184.
- Kasan, P. N., & Andrews, J., (1980). Oral contraceptives and congenital abnormalities. *Br. J. Obstet. Gynaecol., 87,* 545–551.

## 5.7 ANTI-PROGESTOGENIC DRUG

### 5.7.1 MIFEPRISTONE

**FDA Category: X**
*Risk Summary:* Mifepristone induce labor and terminate pregnancy, therefore, it is contraindicated during pregnancy.

**Further Reading:**
- Cabrol, D., Carbonne, B., Bienkiewicz, A., Dallot, E., Alj, A. E., & Cedard, L., (1991). Induction of labor and cervical maturation using mifepristone (RU 486) in the late pregnant rat. Influence of a cyclooxygenase inhibitor (diclofenac). *Prostaglandins, 42,* 71–79.
- Grimes, D. A., Mishell, D. R, Jr., Shoupe, D., & Lacarra, M., (1988). Early abortion with a single dose of the antiprogestin RU-486. *Am. J. Obstet. Gynecol., 158,* 1307–1312.
- Vervest, H. A. M., & Haspels, A. A., (1985). Preliminary results with the antiprogestational compound RU-486 (mifepristone) for interruption of early pregnancy. *Fertil Steril, 44,* 627–632.

## 5.8 THYROID DRUGS

### *5.8.1 LEVOTHYROXINE*

**FDA Category: A**
***Risk Summary:*** The reproduction studies in animals have shown no evidence of fetal harm or impaired fertility. The pregnancy experience in humans is adequate to exhibit that the embryo-fetal risk is nonexistent or very low.

**Further Reading:**
- American College of Obstetricians and Gynecologists (2002). Thyroid disease in pregnancy. ACOG Practice Bulletin. No. 37, August 2002. *Obstet. Gynecol., 100*, 387–396.
- Pekonen, F., Teramo, K., Ikonen, E., Osterlund, K., Makinen, T., & Lamberg, B. A., (1984). Women on thyroid hormone therapy: Pregnancy course, fetal outcome, and amniotic fluid thyroid hormone level. *Obstet. Gynecol., 63*, 635–638.
- Potter, J. D., (1980). Hypothyroidism and reproductive failure. *Surg. Gynecol. Obstet., 150*, 251–255.

### *5.8.2 LIOTHYRONINE*

**FDA Category: A**
***Risk Summary:*** The reproduction studies in animals have shown no evidence of fetal harm or impaired fertility. The pregnancy experience in humans is adequate to exhibit that the embryo-fetal risk is nonexistent or very low.

**Further Reading:**
- American College of Obstetricians and Gynecologists (2002). Thyroid disease in pregnancy. ACOG Practice Bulletin. No. 37, August 2002. *Obstet. Gynecol., 100*, 387–396.
- Pekonen, F., Teramo, K., Ikonen, E., Osterlund, K., Makinen, T., & Lamberg, B. A., (1984). Women on thyroid hormone therapy: Pregnancy course, fetal outcome, and amniotic fluid thyroid hormone level. *Obstet. Gynecol., 63*, 635–638.
- Potter, J. D., (1980). Hypothyroidism and reproductive failure. *Surg. Gynecol. Obstet., 150*, 251–255.

## 5.8.3 LIOTRIX

**FDA Category: A**
*Risk Summary:* Liotrix is a synthetic mixture of liothyronine and levothyroxine. The reproduction studies in animals have shown no evidence of fetal harm or impaired fertility. The pregnancy experience in humans is adequate to exhibit that the embryo-fetal risk is nonexistent or very low.

**Further Reading:**
- American College of Obstetricians and Gynecologists (2002). Thyroid disease in pregnancy. ACOG Practice Bulletin. No. 37, August 2002. *Obstet. Gynecol., 100,* 387–396.
- Pekonen, F., Teramo, K., Ikonen, E., Osterlund, K., Makinen, T., & Lamberg, B. A., (1984). Women on thyroid hormone therapy: Pregnancy course, fetal outcome, and amniotic fluid thyroid hormone level. *Obstet. Gynecol., 63,* 635–638.
- Potter, J. D., (1980). Hypothyroidism and reproductive failure. *Surg. Gynecol. Obstet., 150,* 251–255.

## 5.9  ANTI-THYROID DRUGS

### 5.9.1  CARBIMAZOLE

**FDA Category: D**
*Risk Summary:* The use of Carbimazole should be avoided in pregnant women, especially during the 1st Trimester because the pregnancy experience in humans has shown the risk of embryopathy.

**Further Reading:**
- Clementi, M., Di Gianantonio, E., Pelo, E., Mammi, I., Basile, R. T., & Tenconi, R., (1999). Methimazole embryopathy: Delineation of the phenotype. *Am. J. Med. Genet., 83,* 43–46.
- Diav-Citrin, O., & Ornoy, A., (2002). Teratogen update: Antithyroid drugs—methimazole, carbimazole, and propylthiouracil. *Teratology, 65,* 38–44.
- Milham, S. Jr., (1985). Scalp defects in infants of mothers treated for hyperthyroidism with methimazole or carbimazole during pregnancy. *Teratology, 32,* 321.

- Wilson, L. C., Kerr, B. A., Wilkinson, R., Fossard, C., & Donnai, D., (1998). Choanal atresia and hypothelia following methimazole exposure in utero: A second report. *Am. J. Med. Genet., 75*, 220–222.

## 5.9.2   METHIMAZOLE

**FDA Category: D**
*Risk Summary:* The use of Methimazole should be avoided in pregnant women, especially during the 1st Trimester because the pregnancy experience in humans has shown the risk of embryopathy.

**Further Reading:**
- Clementi, M., Di Gianantonio, E., Pelo, E., Mammi, I., Basile, R. T., & Tenconi, R., (1999). Methimazole embryopathy: Delineation of the phenotype. *Am. J. Med. Genet., 83*, 43–46.
- Diav-Citrin, O., & Ornoy, A., (2002). Teratogen update: Antithyroid drugs—methimazole, carbimazole, and propylthiouracil. *Teratology 65*, 38–44.
- Milham, S. Jr., (1985). Scalp defects in infants of mothers treated for hyperthyroidism with methimazole or carbimazole during pregnancy. *Teratology 32*, 321.
- Wilson, L. C., Kerr, B. A., Wilkinson, R., Fossard, C., & Donnai, D., (1998). Choanal atresia and hypothelia following methimazole exposure in utero: A second report. *Am. J. Med. Genet., 75*, 220–222.

## 5.9.3   SODIUM IODIDE 131I

**FDA Category: X**
*Risk Summary:* Sodium Iodide 131I has been documented to be a human teratogen. Therefore, it is absolutely contraindicated during pregnancy.

**Further Reading:**
- Berg, G. E. B., Nystrom, E. H., Jacobsson, L., Lindberg, S., Lindstedt, R. G., Mattsson, S., Niklasson, C. A., Noren, A. H., & Westphal, O, G, A., (1998). Radioiodine treatment of hyperthyroidism in a pregnant woman. *J. Nucl. Med., 39*, 357–361.
- Pauwels, E. K. J., Thomson, W. H., Blokland, J. A. K., Schmidt, M. E., Bourguignon, M., El-Maghraby, T. A. F., Broerse, J. J., & Harding, L.

K., (1999). Aspects of fetal thyroid dose following iodine-131 administration during early stages of pregnancy in patients suffering from benign thyroid disorders. *Eur. J. Nucl. Med., 26,* 1453–1457.
- Ray, E. W., Sterling, K., & Gardner, L. I., (1959). Congenital cretinism associated with [131]I therapy of the mother. *Am. J. Dis Child, 98,* 506–507.

### 5.9.4 PROPYLTHIOURACIL

**FDA Category: D**
***Risk Summary:*** Even though there is limited data from the human pregnancy experience, but the possible maternal benefit extremely outweighs the unknown or known embryo/fetal risk. Propylthiouracil is generally considered safer than the above mentioned Anti-Thyroid drugs.

**Further Reading:**
- Aaron, H. H., Schneierson, S. J., & Siegel, E., (1955). Goiter in newborn infant due to mother's ingestion of propylthiouracil. *JAMA, 159,* 848–850.
- Burrow, G. N., (1965). Neonatal goiter after maternal propylthiouracil therapy. *J. Clin. Endocrinol. Metab., 25,* 403–408.
- Diav-Citrin, O., & Ornoy, A., (2002). Teratogen update: Antithyroid drugs—methimazole, carbimazole, and propylthiouracil. *Teratology., 65,* 38–44.
- Mujtaba, Q., & Burrow, G. N., (1975). Treatment of hyperthyroidism in pregnancy with propylthiouracil and methimazole. *Obstet. Gynecol., 46,* 282–286.
- Wing, D. A., Millar, L. K., Koonings, P. P., Montoro, M. N., & Mestman, J. H., (1994). A comparison of propylthiouracil versus methimazole in the treatment of hyperthyroidism in pregnancy. *Am. J. Obstet. Gynecol., 170,* 90–95.

## 5.10 PINEAL GLAND RELATED DRUGS

### 5.10.1 MELATONIN

**FDA Category: C**
***Risk Summary:*** The pregnancy experience in humans is limited, and the reproduction studies in animals have shown moderate risk adversely

affecting the growth of the neuroendocrine-reproductive axis in female rat fetuses.

**Further Reading:**

- Colmenero, M. D., Diaz, B., Miguel, J. L., Gonzalez, M. L. I., Esqui-fino, A., & Marin, B., (1991). Melatonin administration during pregnancy retards sexual maturation of female offspring in the rat. *J. Pineal. Res., 11*, 23–27.
- Melatonin. Natural Medicines Comprehensive Database (2003). Stockton, CA: Therapeutic Research Faculty (pp. 910–915).
- Price, C. J., Marr, M. C., Myers, C. B., & Jahnke, G. D., (1998). Developmental toxicity evaluation of melatonin in rats (abstract). *Teratology, 57*, 245.


## *5.10.2   RAMELTEON*

**FDA Category: C**
***Risk Summary:*** It should be used with caution because the pregnancy experience in humans is limited and the reproduction studies in animals have shown low risk.

**Further Reading:**

- *Drug Information. Rozerem.* Takeda Pharmaceuticals North America.


## *5.10.3   TASIMELTEON*

**FDA Category: C**
***Risk Summary:*** It should be used with caution because the pregnancy experience in humans is limited and the reproduction studies in animals have shown low risk.

**Further Reading:**

- Accessdata.fda.gov. 2018. Available from: https://www.accessdata. fda.gov/drugsatfda_docs/label/2014/205677s000lbl.pdf (accessed on 31 January 2020).

## 5.11 PITUITARY DRUGS

### 5.11.1 CORTICOTROPIN (ACTH)

**FDA Category: C**
*Risk Summary:* It should be used only when the maternal benefit outweighs the fetal risk because there is very limited human pregnancy data, and animal studies are not relevant.

**Further Reading:**
- Aral, K., Kuwabara, Y., & Okinaga, S., (1972). The effect of adrenocorticotropic hormone and dexamethasone, administered to the fetus in utero, upon maternal and fetal estrogens. *Am. J. Obstet. Gynecol., 113*, 316–322.
- Johnstone, F. D., & Campbell, S., (1974). Adrenal response in pregnancy to long-acting tetracosactin. *J. Obstet. Gynaecol. Br. Commonw., 81*, 363–367.
- Potert, A. J., (1962). Pregnancy and adrenal cortical hormones. *Br. Med. J., 2*, 967–972.
- Simmer, H. H., Tulchinsky, D., Gold, E. M., Frankland, M., Greipel, M., & Gold, A. S., (1974). On the regulation of estrogen production by cortisol and ACTH in human pregnancy at term. *Am. J. Obstet. Gynecol., 119*, 283–296.

### 5.11.2 DESMOPRESSIN

**FDA Category: B**
*Risk Summary:* It should be used with caution because the pregnancy experience in humans is limited and the reproduction studies in animals have shown low risk.

**Further Reading:**
- Briet, J. W., (1998). Diabetes insipidus, Sheehan's syndrome and pregnancy. *Eur. J. Obstet. Gynecol., 77*, 201–203.
- *Drug Information. DDAVP.* Rhone-Poulenc Rorer Pharmaceuticals.
- Hamai, Y., Fujii, T., Nishina, H., Kozuma, S., Yoshikawa, H., & Taketani, Y., (1997). Differential clinical courses of pregnancies complicated by diabetes insipidus which does, or does not, pre-date the pregnancy. *Hum. Reprod., 12*, 1816–1818.

- Ray, J. G., (1998). DDAVP use during pregnancy: An analysis of its safety for mother and child. *Obstet. Gynecol. Surv., 53*, 450–455.

### 5.11.3   *VASOPRESSIN*

**FDA Category: C**
***Risk Summary:*** The reproduction studies in animals have shown no evidence of fetal harm or impaired fertility. The pregnancy experience in humans is adequate to exhibit that the embryo-fetal risk is nonexistent or very low.

**Further Reading:**
- Ford, S. M. Jr., (1986). Transient vasopressin-resistant diabetes insipidus of pregnancy. *Obstet. Gynecol., 68*, 288–289.
- Gaffney, P. R., & Jenkins, D. M., (1983). Vasopressin: Mediator of the clinical signs of fetal distress. *Br. J. Obstet. Gynaecol., 90*, 987.
- Hadi, H. A., Mashini, I. S., & Devoe, L. D., (1985). Diabetes insipidus during pregnancy complicated by preeclampsia. A case report. *J. Reprod. Med., 30*, 206–208.

### 5.11.4   *LEUPROLIDE*

**FDA Category: X**
***Risk Summary:*** Human exposures during pregnancy have been associated with an increased risk of IUGR, spontaneous abortions (SABs), or major congenital malformations.

**Further Reading:**
- *Drug Information.* Lupron. Tap Pharmaceuticals, Inc.
- Ghazi, D. M., Kemmann, E., & Hammond, J. M., (1991). Normal pregnancy outcome after early maternal exposure to gonadotropin-releasing hormone agonist. A case report. *J. Reprod. Med.,36*, 173–174.
- Wilshire, G. B., Emmi, A. M., Gagliardi, C. C., & Weiss, G., (1993). Gonadotropin-releasing hormone agonist administration in early human pregnancy is associated with normal outcomes. *Fert. Steril, 60*, 980–983.

## 5.12   VASOPRESSIN RECEPTOR ANTAGONISTS

### 5.12.1   TOLVAPTAN

**FDA Category: C**
***Risk Summary:*** It should be used with caution because the pregnancy experience in humans is limited and the reproduction studies in animals have shown low risk.

**Further Reading:**
- *Drug Information*. Samsca. Otsuka America Pharmaceutical.
- Oi, A., Morishita, K., Awogi, T., Ozaki, A., Umezato, M., Fujita, S., Hosoki, E., Morimoto, H., Ishiharada, N., Ishiyama, H., & Uesugi, T., (2011). Nonclinical safety profile of tolvaptan. *Cardiovascular Drugs and Therapy, 25*(1), 91–99.

### 5.12.2   CONIVAPTAN

**FDA Category: C**
***Risk Summary:*** The pregnancy experience in humans is limited, and the reproduction studies in animals have shown a moderate risk of developmental toxicity.

**Further Reading:**
- Ali, F., Raufi, M. A., Washington, B., & Ghali, J. K., (2007). Conivaptan: A dual receptor vasopressin v1a/v2 antagonist. *Cardiovascular Drug Reviews, 25*(3), 261–279.
- *Drug Information. Vaprisol.* Astellas Pharma US.

## 5.13   SOMATOSTATIN ANALOGS

### 5.13.1   OCTREOTIDE

**FDA Category: B**
***Risk Summary:*** It should be used with caution because the pregnancy experience in humans is limited and the reproduction studies in animals have shown low risk.

**Further Reading:**
- Caron, P., Gerbeau, C., Pradayrol, L., Cimonetta, C., & Bayard, F., (1996). Successful pregnancy in an infertile woman with a thyrotropin-secreting macroadenoma treated with somatostatin analog (octreotide). *J. Clin. Endocrinol. Metab., 81,* 1164–1168.
- *Drug Information. Sandostatin.* Novartis Pharmaceuticals.
- Mozas, J., Ocon, E., Lopez de la Torre, M., Suarez, A. M., Miranda, J. A., & Herruzo, A. J., (1999). Successful pregnancy in a woman with acromegaly treated with somatostatin analog (octreotide) prior to surgical resection. *Int. J. Gynecol. Obstet., 65,* 71–73.
- Takeuchi, K., Funakoshi, T., Oomori, S., & Maruo, T., (1999). Successful pregnancy in an acromegalic woman treated with octreotide. *Obstet. Gynecol., 93,* 848.

### 5.13.2   PASIREOTIDE

**FDA Category: C**
***Risk Summary:*** It should be used with caution because the pregnancy experience in humans is limited, and the reproduction studies in animals have shown an increased incidence of skeletal malformations associated with the use of Pasireotide during organogenesis.

**Further Reading:**
- *Drug Information. Signifor.* Novartis Pharmaceuticals.

## 5.14   DRUGS THAT AFFECT BONE MINERAL HOMEOSTASIS

### 5.14.1   METABOLITES AND ANALOGS OF VITAMIN D

#### 5.14.1.1   CHOLECALCIFEROL

**FDA Category: C**
***Risk Summary:*** The reproduction studies in animals have shown no evidence of fetal harm or impaired fertility. The pregnancy experience in humans is adequate to exhibit that the embryo-fetal risk is nonexistent or very low.

**Further Reading:**
- Brooke, O. G., Brown, I. R. F., Bone, C. D. M., Carter, N. D., Cleeve, H. J. W., Maxwell, J. D., Robinson, V. P., & Winder, S. M., (1980).

Vitamin D supplements in pregnant Asian women: Effects on calcium status and fetal growth. *Br. Med. J., 280,* 751–754.

- Cockburn, F., Belton, N. R., Purvis, R. J., Giles, M. M., Brown, J. K., Turner, T. L., Wilkinson, E. M., Forfar, J. O., Barrie, W. J. M., McKay, G. S., & Pocock, S. J., (1980). Maternal vitamin D intake and mineral metabolism in mothers and their newborn infants. *Br. Med. J., 2,* 11–14.
- Ginde, A. A., Sullivan, A. F., Mansbach, J. M., Camargo, C. A. Jr., (2010). Vitamin D insufficiency in pregnant and nonpregnant women of childbearing age in the United States. *Am. J. Obstet. Gynecol., 202,* 436, e1–8.
- Hollis, B. W., & Wagner, C. L., (2004). Assessment of dietary vitamin D requirements during pregnancy and lactation. *Am. J. Clin. Nutr., 79,* 717–726.

## 5.14.1.2 ERGOCALCIFEROL

**FDA Category: C**

***Risk Summary:*** The reproduction studies in animals have shown no evidence of fetal harm or impaired fertility. The pregnancy experience in humans is adequate to exhibit that the embryo-fetal risk is nonexistent or very low.

**Further Reading:**
- Brooke, O. G., Brown, I. R. F., Bone, C. D. M., Carter, N. D., Cleeve, H. J. W., Maxwell, J. D., Robinson, V. P., & Winder, S. M., (1980). Vitamin D supplements in pregnant Asian women: Effects on calcium status and fetal growth. *Br. Med. J., 280,* 751–754.
- Cockburn, F., Belton, N. R., Purvis, R. J., Giles, M. M., Brown, J. K., Turner, T. L., Wilkinson, E. M., Forfar, J. O., Barrie, W. J. M., McKay, G. S., & Pocock, S. J., (1980). Maternal vitamin D intake and mineral metabolism in mothers and their newborn infants. *Br. Med. J., 2,* 11–14.
- Ginde, A. A., Sullivan, A. F., Mansbach, J. M., Camargo, C. A. Jr., (2010). Vitamin D insufficiency in pregnant and nonpregnant women of childbearing age in the United States. *Am. J. Obstet. Gynecol., 202,* 436, e1–8.
- Hollis, B. W., & Wagner, C. L., (2014). Assessment of dietary vitamin D requirements during pregnancy and lactation. *Am. J. Clin. Nutr., 79,* 717–726.

## 5.14.1.3   CALCITRIOL

**FDA Category: C**
*Risk Summary:* The reproduction studies in animals have shown an indication of an increased risk of fetal damage. The pregnancy experience in humans is adequate to exhibit that the embryo-fetal risk is nonexistent or very low.

**Further Reading:**
- Brooke, O. G., Brown, I. R. F., Bone, C. D. M., Carter, N. D., Cleeve, H. J. W., Maxwell, J. D., Robinson, V. P., & Winder, S. M., (1980). Vitamin D supplements in pregnant Asian women: Effects on calcium status and fetal growth. *Br. Med. J., 280*, 751–754.
- *Drug Information. Rocaltrol.* Roche Laboratories.
- Ginde, A. A., Sullivan, A. F., Mansbach, J. M., Camargo, C. A. Jr., (2010). Vitamin D insufficiency in pregnant and nonpregnant women of childbearing age in the United States. *Am. J. Obstet. Gynecol., 202*, 436, e1–8.
- Hollis, B. W., & Wagner, C. L., (2004). Assessment of dietary vitamin D requirements during pregnancy and lactation. *Am. J. Clin. Nutr., 79*, 717–726.

## 5.14.1.4   DOXERCALCIFEROL

**FDA Category: B**
*Risk Summary:* The reproduction studies in animals have shown no evidence of fetal harm or impaired fertility. The pregnancy experience in humans is limited.

**Further Reading:**
- Brooke, O. G., Brown, I. R. F., Bone, C. D. M., Carter, N. D., Cleeve, H. J. W., Maxwell, J. D., Robinson, V. P., & Winder, S. M., (1980). Vitamin D supplements in pregnant Asian women: Effects on calcium status and fetal growth. *Br. Med. J., 280*, 751–754.
- *Drug Information. Hectorol* (doxercalciferol). Genzyme Corporation, Cambridge, MA.
- Ginde, A. A., Sullivan, A. F., Mansbach, J. M., Camargo, C. A. Jr., (2010). Vitamin D insufficiency in pregnant and nonpregnant women

of childbearing age in the United States. *Am. J. Obstet. Gynecol., 202,* 436, e1–8.

- Hollis, B. W., & Wagner, C. L., (2004). Assessment of dietary vitamin D requirements during pregnancy and lactation. *Am. J. Clin. Nutr., 79,* 717–726.

## 5.14.1.5 PARICALCITOL

**FDA Category: C**
*Risk Summary:* The reproduction studies in animals have shown no evidence of fetal harm or impaired fertility. The pregnancy experience in humans is limited.

**Further Reading:**
- Brooke, O. G., Brown, I. R. F., Bone, C. D. M., Carter, N. D., Cleeve, H. J. W., Maxwell, J. D., Robinson, V. P., & Winder, S. M., (1980). Vitamin D supplements in pregnant Asian women: Effects on calcium status and fetal growth. *Br. Med. J., 280,* 751–754.
- *Drug Information.* Zemplar. Abbott Laboratories.
- Ginde, A. A., Sullivan, A. F., Mansbach, J. M., Camargo, C. A. Jr., (2010). Vitamin D insufficiency in pregnant and nonpregnant women of childbearing age in the United States. *Am. J. Obstet. Gynecol., 202,* 436, e1–8.
- Hollis, B. W., & Wagner, C. L., (2004). Assessment of dietary vitamin D requirements during pregnancy and lactation. *Am. J. Clin. Nutr., 79,* 717–726.

## 5.14.1.6 CALCIPOTRIENE

**FDA Category: C**
*Risk Summary:* The reproduction studies in animals have shown no evidence of fetal harm or impaired fertility. The pregnancy experience in humans is limited.

**Further Reading:**
- *Drug Information. Dovonex Cream.* LEO Pharma.
- Tauscher, A. E., Fleischer, A. B. Jr., Phelps, K. C., & Feldman, S. R., (2002). Psoriasis and pregnancy. *J. Cutan. Med. Surg., 6,* 561–570.

## 5.14.2   *BISPHOSPHONATES*

### 5.14.2.1   *ALENDRONATE*

**FDA Category: C**
***Risk Summary:*** It should be used with caution because the pregnancy experience in humans is limited, and the reproduction studies in animals have shown the risk of fetal and maternal toxicity.

**Further Reading:**
- Djokanovic, N., Klieger-Grossmann, C., & Koren, G., (2008). Does treatment with bisphosphonates endanger the human pregnancy? *J. Obstet. Gynaecol. Can., 30*, 1146–1148.
- *Drug Information. Fosamax*. Merck & Co.
- Ornoy, A., Wajnberg, R., & Diav-Citrin, O., (2006). The outcome of pregnancy following pre-pregnancy or early pregnancy alendronate treatment. *Reprod. Toxicol., 22*, 578–579.

### 5.14.2.2   *ETIDRONATE*

**FDA Category: C**
***Risk Summary:*** It is better to be avoided during gestation because the pregnancy experience in humans is limited, and the reproduction studies in animals have shown a low risk.

**Further Reading:**
- Djokanovic, N., Klieger-Grossmann, C., & Koren, G., (2008). Does treatment with bisphosphonates endanger the human pregnancy? *J. Obstet. Gynaecol. Can., 30*, 1146–1148.
- *Drug Information. Didronel*. Procter & Gamble Pharmaceuticals.
- Rutgers-Verhage, A. R., deVries, T. W., & Torringa, M. J. L., (2003). No effects of bisphosphonates on the human fetus. *Birth Defects Res. A Clin. Mol. Teratol., 67*, 203–204.

### 5.14.2.3   *IBANDRONATE*

**FDA Category: C**
***Risk Summary:*** It should be used with caution because the pregnancy experience in humans is limited, and the reproduction studies in animals have shown the risk of fetal growth restriction and maternal death.

**Further Reading:**

- Djokanovic, N., Klieger-Grossmann, C., & Koren, G., (2008). Does treatment with bisphosphonates endanger the human pregnancy? *J. Obstet. Gynaecol. Can., 30*, 1146–1148.
- *Drug Information. Boniva.* Roche Pharmaceuticals.

## 5.14.2.4  PAMIDRONATE

**FDA Category: D**
***Risk Summary:*** It should be used with caution because the pregnancy experience in humans is limited, and the reproduction studies in animals have shown the risk of embryo, fetal, and maternal toxicity.

**Further Reading:**

- Cabar, E. R., Nomura, R. M. Y., & Zugaib, M., (2007). Maternal and fetal outcome of pamidronate treatment before conception: A case report. *Clin. Exp. Rheumatol., 25*, 344–345.
- Djokanovic, N., Klieger-Grossmann, C., & Koren, G., (2008). Does treatment with bisphosphonates endanger the human pregnancy? *J. Obstet. Gynaecol. Can., 30*, 1146–1148.
- *Drug Information. Aredia.* Novartis Pharmaceuticals.
- Munns, C. F. J., Rauch, F., Ward, L., & Glorieux, F. H., (2004). Maternal and fetal outcome after long-term pamidronate treatment before conception: A report of two cases. *J. Bone Miner Res., 19*, 1742–1745.

## 5.14.2.5  RISEDRONATE

**FDA Category: C**
***Risk Summary:*** It should be used with caution because the pregnancy experience in humans is limited, and the reproduction studies in animals have shown the risk of developmental toxicity.

**Further Reading:**

- Djokanovic, N., Klieger-Grossmann, C., & Koren, G., (2008). Does treatment with bisphosphonates endanger the human pregnancy? *J. Obstet. Gynaecol. Can., 30*, 1146–1148.
- *Drug Information. Actonel.* Procter & Gamble Pharmaceuticals.

## 5.14.2.6   TILUDRONATE

**FDA Category: C**
*Risk Summary:* It is better to be avoided during gestation because the pregnancy experience in humans is limited, and the reproduction studies in animals have shown the risk of maternal and developmental toxicities.

**Further Reading:**
- Djokanovic, N., Klieger-Grossmann, C., & Koren, G., (2008). Does treatment with bisphosphonates endanger the human pregnancy? *J. Obstet. Gynaecol. Can.,* 2008 *30,* 1146–1148.
- *Drug Information. Skelid.* Sanofi-Synthelabo.
- Rutgers-Verhage, A. R., deVries, T. W., & Torringa, M. J. L., (2003). No effects of bisphosphonates on the human fetus. *Birth Defects Res. A Clin. Mol. Teratol., 67,* 203–204.

## 5.14.2.7   ZOLEDRONATE (ZOLEDRONIC ACID)

**FDA Category: D**
*Risk Summary:* It should be used with caution because the pregnancy experience in humans is limited, and the reproduction studies in animals have shown the risk of fetal and maternal toxicity.

**Further Reading:**
- Andreadis, C., Charalampidou, M., Diamantopoulos, N., Chouchos, N., & Mouratidou, D., (2004). Combined chemotherapy and radiotherapy during conception and first two trimesters of gestation in a woman with metastatic breast cancer. *Gynecol. Oncol., 95,* 252–255.
- Djokanovic, N., Klieger-Grossmann, C., & Koren, G., (2008). Does treatment with bisphosphonates endanger the human pregnancy? *J. Obstet. Gynaecol. Can., 30,* 1146–1148.
- *Drug Information. Zometa.* Novartis Pharmaceuticals.

### 5.14.3   CALCIUM REGULATION HORMONES

## 5.14.3.1   TERIPARATIDE

**FDA Category: C**
*Risk Summary:* It should be used with caution because the pregnancy experience in humans is limited and the reproduction studies in animals have shown a low risk of tumorigenicity.

**Further Reading:**
- *Drug Information. Forteo.* Lilly, Eli, and Company, Indianapolis, IN.

## 5.14.3.2 CALCITONIN

**FDA Category: C**
*Risk Summary:* The reproduction studies in animals have shown no evidence of fetal harm or impaired fertility. The pregnancy experience in humans is limited.

**Further Reading:**
- *Drug Information.* Miacalcin. Novartis Pharmaceuticals.
- Kovarik, J., Woloszczuk, W., Linkesch, W., & Pavelka, R., (1980). Calcitonin in pregnancy. *Lancet, 1*, 199–200.
- Tohei, A., VandeGarde, B., Arbogast, L. A., & Voogt, J. L., (2000). Calcitonin inhibition of prolactin secretion in lactating rats: Mechanism of action. *Neuroendocrinology, 71*, 327–332.

## 5.14.4 CALCIUM RECEPTOR AGONIST

### 5.14.4.1 CINACALCET

**FDA Category: C**
*Risk Summary:* It is contraindicated in pregnancy because the pregnancy experience in humans is limited and the reproduction studies in animals have shown the significant risk of abortion.

**Further Reading:**
- *Drug Information.* Sensipar. Amgen.
- Edling, K. L., Korenman, S. G., Janzen, C., Sohsman, M. Y., Apple, S. K., Bhuta, S., & Yeh, M. W., (2013). A pregnant dilemma: Primary hyperthyroidism due to parathyromatosis in pregnancy. *Endo. Pract., 6*, 1–15.
- Horjus, C., Groot, I., Telting, D., van Setten, P., van Sorge, A., Kovacs, C. S., Hermus, A., & de Boer, H., (2009). Cincacalcet for hyperparathyroidism in pregnancy and puerperium. *J. Pediatr. Endocrinol. Metab., 22*, 741–749.

## 5.14.5   *SELECTIVE ESTROGEN RECEPTOR MODULATOR*

### 5.14.5.1   *RALOXIFENE*

**FDA Category: X**
***Risk Summary:*** It is contraindicated in pregnancy because the pregnancy experience in humans is limited and the reproduction studies in animals have shown the significant risk of abortion.

**Further Reading:**
• Buelke-Sam, J., Bryant, H. U., & Francis, P. C., (1998). The selective estrogen receptor modulator, raloxifene: An overview of nonclinical pharmacology and reproductive and developmental testing. *Reprod. Toxicol., 12,* 217–221.
• Clarke, D. O., Griffey, K. I., Buelke-Sam, J. L., & Francis, P. C., (1996). The selective estrogen receptor modulator, raloxifene: Reproductive assessments following preimplantation exposure in mated female rats. *Teratology, 53,* 103–104.
• *Drug Information. Evista.* Eli Lilly.

## 5.14.6   **RANK LIGAND (RANKL) INHIBITOR**

### 5.14.6.1   *DENOSUMAB*

**FDA Category: X**
***Risk Summary:*** It is contraindicated in pregnancy because the pregnancy experience in humans is limited and the reproduction studies in Cynomolgus monkeys have shown the significant risk of abortion, stillbirths, and postnatal mortality, along with evidence of abnormal bone growth, absent lymph nodes, and decreased neonatal growth.

**Further Reading:**
• *Drug Information.* Prolia. Amgen.

## 5.15   **PROSTAGLANDINS**

### 5.15.1   *CARBOPROST*

**FDA Category: C**
***Risk Summary:*** Carboprost is contraindicated in pregnancy unless it is intended for termination & or evacuation of pregnancy.

**Further Reading:**
- Arnon, J., & Ornoy, A., (1995). Clinical teratology counseling and consultation case report: Outcome of pregnancy after failure of early induced abortions. *Teratology, 52*, 126–1257.
- *Drug Information. Hemabate.* Pfizer.
- Pastuszak, A. L., Schuler, L., Speck-Martins, C. E., Coehlo, K. E., Cordello, S. M., Vargas, F., Brunoni, D., Schwarz, I. V., Larranda-buru, M., Safattle, H., Meloni, V. F., & Koren, G., (1998). Use of misoprostol during pregnancy and Möbius syndrome in infants. *N. Engl. J. Med., 338*, 1881–1885.

### 5.15.2  DINOPROSTONE

**FDA Category: C**
*Risk Summary:* Dinoprostone is contraindicated in pregnancy unless it is intended for termination & or evacuation of pregnancy.

**Further Reading:**
- Arnon, J., & Ornoy, A., (1995). Clinical teratology counseling and consultation case report: Outcome of pregnancy after failure of early induced abortions. *Teratology, 52*, 126,127.
- *Drug Information. Cervidil.* Forest Laboratories.

## 5.16  GROWTH HORMONE RELATED AGENTS

### 5.16.1  PEGVISOMANT

**FDA Category: C**
*Risk Summary:* It should be used with caution because the pregnancy experience in humans is limited and the reproduction studies in animals have shown low risk.

**Further Reading:**
- Brian, S. R., Bidlingmaier, M., Wajnrajch, M. P., Weinzimer, S. A., & Inzucchi, S. E., (2007). Treatment of acromegaly with pegvisomant during pregnancy: Maternal and fetal effects. *J. Clin. Endocrinol. Metab., 92*, 3374–3377.

- Cheng, S., Grasso, L., Martinez-Orozco, J. A., Al-Agha, R., Pivonello, R., Colao, A., & Ezzat, S., (2012). Pregnancy in acromegaly: Experience from two referral centers and systematic review of the literature. *Clin. Endocrinol., (Oxf)*, *76*, 264–271.
- *Drug Information. Somavert.* Pharmacia & Upjohn.

## 5.16.2   TESAMORELIN

**FDA Category: X**
***Risk Summary:*** Tesamorelin is contraindicated in pregnancy because there is no human pregnancy data, and animal reproduction studies have shown significant risks of hydrocephalus in offspring.

**Further Reading:**
- *Drug Information. Egrifta.* EMD Serono.

## 5.17   MISCELLANEOUS AGENTS

### 5.17.1   BROMOCRIPTINE

**FDA Category: B**
***Risk Summary:*** The reproduction studies in animals have shown no evidence of fetal harm or impaired fertility. The pregnancy experience in humans is adequate to exhibit that the embryo-fetal risk is nonexistent or very low.

**Further Reading:**
- *Drug Information.* Parlodel. Sandoz Pharmaceuticals.
- Konopka, P., Raymond, J. P., Merceron, R. E., & Seneze, J., (1983). Continuous administration of bromocriptine in the prevention of neurological complications in pregnant women with prolactinomas. *Am. J. Obstet. Gynecol.*, *146*, 935–938.
- Turkalj, I., Braun, P., & Krupp, P., (1982). Surveillance of bromocriptine in pregnancy. *JAMA*, *247*, 1589–1591.

## 5.17.2  CABERGOLINE

**FDA Category: B**
*Risk Summary:* It should be used with caution because the pregnancy experience in humans is limited and the reproduction studies in animals have shown low risk.

**Further Reading:**
- *Drug Information*. Dostinex. Pharmacia & Upjohn.
- Jones, T. H., & Fraser, R. B., (1994). Cabergoline treated hyperprolactinemia results in pregnancy in a bromocriptine intolerant patient after seventeen years of infertility. *Br. J. Obstet. Gynaecol., 101*, 349–350.
- Negishi, H., & Koide, S. S., (1997). Prevention and termination of pregnancy in rats by cabergoline, a dopamine agonist. *J. Reprod. Fertil., 109*, 103–107.
- Woo, I., & Ehsanipoor, R. M., (2013). Cabergoline therapy for Cushing disease throughout pregnancy. *Obstet. Gynecol., 122*, 485–487.

## 5.17.3  IVACAFTOR

**FDA Category: B**
*Risk Summary:* It should be used with caution because the pregnancy experience in humans is limited and the reproduction studies in animals have shown low risk.

**Further Reading:**
- *Drug Information. Kalydeco*. Vertex Pharmaceuticals.

## 5.17.4  CARGLUMIC ACID

**FDA Category: C**
*Risk Summary:* The pregnancy experience in humans is limited, and the reproduction studies in animals have shown a moderate risk of maternal toxicity.

**Further Reading:**
- *Drug Information. Carbaglu*. Accredo Health Group.

**KEYWORDS**

- cabergoline
- carglumic acid
- intrauterine growth restriction
- RANK Ligand
- spontaneous abortions
- tesamorelin

# CHAPTER 6

# Drugs Affecting the Respiratory System

## 6.1 ANTI-INFLAMMATORY DRUGS (INHALED)

### 6.1.1 CROMOLYN SODIUM

**FDA Category: B**

*Risk Summary:* The reproduction studies in animals have shown no evidence of fetal harm or impaired fertility. The pregnancy experience in humans is adequate to exhibit that the embryo-fetal risk is nonexistent or very low.

**Further Reading:**
- Cox, J. S. G., Beach, J. E., Blair, A. M. J. N., & Clarke, A. J., (1970). Disodium cromoglycate (Intal). *Adv. Drug. Res., 5*, 135, 136. As cited in: Shepard, T. H., Catalog of Teratogenic Agents. (6th edn., p. 174). Baltimore, MD: Johns Hopkins University Press, 1989.
- *Drug Information. Intal.* Rhone-Poulenc Rorer Pharmaceuticals.
- Dykes, M. H. M., (1974). Evaluation of an antiasthmatic agent cromolyn sodium (Aarane, Intal). *JAMA, 227*, 1061–1062.
- Wilson, J., (1982). Use of sodium cromoglycate during pregnancy: Results on 296 asthmatic women. *Acta Therap., 8*(Suppl), 45–51.

### 6.1.2 NEDOCROMIL SODIUM

**FDA Category: B**

*Risk Summary:* The reproduction studies in animals have shown no evidence of fetal harm or impaired fertility. The pregnancy experience in humans is limited.

**Further Reading:**
- Carrasco, E., & Sepulveda, R., (1988). The acceptability, safety and efficacy of nedocromil sodium in long-term clinical use in patients with perennial asthma. *J. Int. Med. Res., 16*, 394–401.
- *Drug Information*. Tilade. Rhone-Poulenc Rorer Pharmaceuticals.
- Wilton, L. V., Pearce, G. L., Martin, R. M., Mackay, F. J., & Mann, R. D. The outcomes of pregnancy in women exposed to

## 6.2   ANTITUSSIVE DRUGS

### 6.2.1   *CODEINE*

**FDA Category: C**
*Risk Summary:* It is better to be avoided during the 1st & 3rd Trimesters because the pregnancy experience in humans has shown the risk of congenital defects associated with the use of Codeine.

**Further Reading:**
- Creanga, A. A., Sabel, J. C., Ko, J. Y., Wasserman, C. R., Shapiro-Mendoza, C. K., Taylor, P., Barfield, W., Cawthon, L., & Paulozzi, L. J., (2012). Maternal drug use and its effect on neonates—a population-based study in Washington state. *Obstet. Gynecol., 119*, 924–933.
- Gill, A. C., Oei, J., Lewis, N. L., Younan, N., Kennedy, I., & Lui, K., (2003). Strabismus in infants of opiate-dependent mothers. *Acta Paediatr., 92*, 379–385.
- Nezvalova-Henriksen, K., Spigset, O., & Nordeng, H., (2011). Effects of codeine on pregnancy outcome: Results from a large population-based cohort study. *Eur. J. Clin. Pharmacol., 67*, 1253–1261.

### 6.2.2   *DEXTROMETHORPHAN*

**FDA Category: C**
*Risk Summary:* The reproduction studies in animals have shown no evidence of fetal harm or impaired fertility. The pregnancy experience in humans is adequate to exhibit that the embryo-fetal risk is nonexistent or very low.

**Further Reading:**
- Einarson, A., Lyszkiewicz, D., & Koren, G., (2001). The safety of dextromethorphan in pregnancy. Results of a controlled study. *Chest, 119*, 466–469.

- Martinez-Frias, M. L., & Rodriguez-Pinilla, E., (2001). Epidemio-logic analysis of prenatal exposure to cough medicines containing dextromethorphan: No evidence of human teratogenicity. *Teratology*, *63*, 38–41.
- Polifka, J. E., & Shepard, T. H., (1999). Studies of the fetal effects of dextromethorphan in ovo. *Teratology, 60*, 56, 57. (Originally published as an untitled letter to the editor: Pediatr Res 1998 44, 415.)

## 6.2.3  HYDROCODONE

**FDA Category: C**
*Risk Summary:* It is better to be avoided during the 1st & 3rd Trimesters because the pregnancy experience in humans has shown the risk of congenital defects associated with the use of Codeine.

**Further Reading:**
- Broussard, C. S., Rasmussen, S. A., Reefhuis, J., Friedman, J. M., Jann, M. W., Riehle-Colarusso, T., & Honein, M. A., (2011). National Birth Defects Prevention Study. Maternal treatment with opioid analgesics and risk for birth defects. *Am. J. Obstet. Gynecol., 204*, 314–317.
- Meyer, D., & Tobias, J. D., (2005). Adverse effects following the inadvertent administration of opioids to infants and children. *Clin. Pediatr., (Phil), 44*, 499–503.
- Schick, B., Hom, M., Tolosa, J., Librizzi, R., & Donnfeld, A., (1996). Preliminary Analysis of First Trimester Exposure to Oxycodone and Hydrocodone (Abstract). Presented at the Ninth International Conference of the Organization of Teratology Information Services, Salt Lake City, Utah, May 2–4, 1996. *Reprod. Toxicol., 10*, 162.

## 6.3  BRONCHODILATORS

### 6.3.1  B2-ADRENERGIC AGENTS

#### 6.3.1.1  ALBUTEROL

**FDA Category: C**
*Risk Summary:* The reproduction studies in animals have shown no evidence of fetal harm or impaired fertility. The pregnancy experience in humans is adequate to exhibit that the embryo-fetal risk is nonexistent or very low.

**Further Reading:**
- *Drug Information.* Albuterol sulfate inhalant. Actavis Mid Atlantic.
- Kuhn, R. J. P., Speirs, A. L., Pepperell, R. J., Eggers, T. R., Doyle, L. W., & Hutchison, A., (1982). Betamethasone, albuterol, and threatened premature delivery: Benefits and risks. Study of 469 pregnancies. *Obstet. Gynecol., 60,* 403–408.
- Rayburn, W. F., Atkinson, B. D., Gilbert, K. A., & Turnbull, G. L., (1994). Acute effects of inhaled albuterol (Proventil) on fetal hemodynamics (abstract). *Teratology, 49,* 370.

## 6.3.1.2  ARFORMOTEROL

**FDA Category: C**
***Risk Summary:*** The reproduction studies in animals have shown no evidence of fetal harm or impaired fertility. The pregnancy experience in humans is limited.

**Further Reading:**
- *Drug Information.* Brovana. Sepracor.
- Schaefer, C., Paul, P., & Richard, K. M., (2015). *Drugs During Pregnancy and Lactation Treatment Options and Risk Assessment.* Amsterdam: Elsevier.

## 6.3.1.3  FORMOTEROL

**FDA Category: C**
***Risk Summary:*** The reproduction studies in animals have shown no evidence of fetal harm or impaired fertility. The pregnancy experience in humans is limited.

**Further Reading:**
- *Drug Information.* Foradil Aerolizer. Schering.
- Shinkai, N., Takasuna, K., & Takayama, S., (2003). Inhibitory effects of formoterol on lipopolysaccharide-induced premature delivery through modulation of proinflammatory cytokine production in mice. *Reproduction, 125,* 199–203.

- Wilton, L. V., & Shakir, S. A., (2002). A post-marketing surveillance study of formoterol (Foradil): Its use in general practice in England. *Drug Saf., 25,* 213–223.

## 6.3.1.4 INDACATEROL

**FDA Category: C**
*Risk Summary:* The reproduction studies in animals have shown no evidence of fetal harm or impaired fertility. The pregnancy experience in humans is limited.

**Further Reading:**
- *Drug Information. Arcapta.* Novartis Pharmaceuticals.
- Schaefer, C., Paul, P., & Richard, K. M., (2015). *Drugs During Pregnancy and Lactation Treatment Options and Risk Assessment.* Amsterdam: Elsevier.

## 6.3.1.5 LEVALBUTEROL

**FDA Category: C**
*Risk Summary:* The reproduction studies in animals have shown no evidence of fetal harm or impaired fertility. The pregnancy experience in humans is limited.

**Further Reading:**
- *Drug Information.* Xopenex. Sepracor.
- Schaefer, C., Paul, P., & Richard, K. M., (2015). *Drugs During Pregnancy and Lactation Treatment Options and Risk Assessment.* Amsterdam: Elsevier.

## 6.3.1.6 METAPROTERENOL

**FDA Category: C**
*Risk Summary:* The reproduction studies in animals have shown no evidence of fetal harm or impaired fertility. The pregnancy experience in humans is adequate to exhibit that the embryo-fetal risk is nonexistent or very low.

**Further Reading:**
- *Drug Information*. Alupent. Boehringer Ingelheim.
- Freysz, H., Willard, D., Lehr, A., Messer, J., & Boog, G., (1977). A long term evaluation of infants who received a β- mimetic drug while in utero. *J. Perinat. Med., 5*, 94–99.
- Zilianti, M., & Aller, J., (1971). Action of orciprenaline on uterine contractility during labor, maternal cardiovascular system, fetal heart rate, and acid-base balance. *Am. J. Obstet. Gynecol., 109*, 1073–1079.

## 6.3.1.7   PIRBUTEROL

**FDA Category: C**
*Risk Summary:* The reproduction studies in animals have shown no evidence of fetal harm or impaired fertility. The pregnancy experience in humans is limited.

**Further Reading:**
- *Drug Information*. Maxair. Graceway Pharmaceuticals.
- Schaefer, C., Paul, P., & Richard, K. M., (2015). Drugs During Pregnancy and Lactation Treatment Options and Risk Assessment. Amsterdam: Elsevier.

## 6.3.1.8   SALMETEROL

**FDA Category: C**
*Risk Summary:* The reproduction studies in animals have shown no evidence of fetal harm or impaired fertility. The pregnancy experience in humans is limited.

**Further Reading:**
- Allergy, Asthma and Immunology (ACAAI) (2000). The use of newer asthma and allergy medications during pregnancy. Position statement. *Ann. Allergy Asthma Immunol., 84*, 475–480.
- *Drug Information. Serevent*. Glaxo Wellcome.
- Manchee, G. R., Barrow, A., Kulkarni, S., Palmer, E., Oxford, J., Colthup, P. V., Maconochie, J. G., & Tarbit, M. H., (1993). Disposition of salmeterol xinafoate in laboratory animals and humans. *Drug. Metab. Dispos., 21*, 1022–1028.

• The American College of Obstetricians and Gynecologists (ACOG) and the American College of

### 6.3.1.9    TERBUTALINE

**FDA Category: C**
*Risk Summary:* The reproduction studies in animals have shown no evidence of fetal harm or impaired fertility. The pregnancy experience in humans is limited.

**Further Reading:**
• *Drug Information.* Brethine. Novartis Pharmaceuticals.
• Haller, D. L., (1980). The use of terbutaline for premature labor. *Drug Intell. Clin. Pharm., 14,* 757–764.
• Mendez-Bauer, C., Shekarloo, A., Cook, V., & Freese, U., (1987). Treatment of acute intrapartum fetal distress by $\beta$2- sympathomimetics. *Am. J. Obstet. Gynecol.,156,* 638–642.
• Suzuki, M., Inagaki, K., Kihira, M., Matsuzawa, K., Ishikawa, K., & Ishizuka, T., 1985(). Maternal liver impairment associated with prolonged high-dose administration of terbutaline for premature labor. *Obstet. Gynecol., 66,* 14S–15S.

### 6.3.2    OTHER SYMPATHOMIMETIC AGENTS

### 6.3.2.1    EPHEDRINE

**FDA Category: C**
*Risk Summary:* The reproduction studies in animals have shown no evidence of fetal harm or impaired fertility. The pregnancy experience in humans is adequate to exhibit that the embryo-fetal risk is nonexistent or very low.

**Further Reading:**
• Datta, S., Alper, M. H., Ostheimer, G. W., & Weiss, J. B., (1982). Method of ephedrine administration and nausea and hypotension during spinal anesthesia for cesarean section. *Anesthesiology, 56,* 68–70.
• Shepard, T. H., (1980). *Catalog of Teratogenic Agents* (3rd edn., pp. 134–135). Baltimore, MD: The Johns Hopkins University Press.

- Wright, R. G., Shnider, S. M., Levinson, G., Rolbin, S. H., & Parer, J. T., (1981). The effect of maternal administration of ephedrine on fetal heart rate and variability. *Obstet. Gynecol., 57,* 734–738.

## 6.3.2.2   EPINEPHRINE

**FDA Category: C**
***Risk Summary:*** It should be used with caution because the human pregnancy experience has shown a low risk.

**Further Reading:**
- Entman, S. S., & Moise, K. J., (1984). Anaphylaxis in pregnancy. *S. Med. J., 77,* 402.
- Nishimura, H., & Tanimura, T., (1976). *Clinical Aspects of the Teratogenicity of Drugs* (p. 231). New York, NY: American Elsevier.
- Shepard, T. H., (1980). *Catalog of Teratogenic Agents* (3rd edn., pp. 134–135). Baltimore, MD: The Johns Hopkins University Press.

## 6.3.2.3   ISOPROTERENOL

**FDA Category: C**
***Risk Summary:*** The pregnancy experience in humans is limited, and the reproduction studies in animals have shown moderate risk.

**Further Reading:**
- DeSimone, C. A., Leighton, B. L., Norris, M. C., Chayen, B., & Menduke, H., (1988). The chronotropic effect of isoproterenol is reduced in term pregnant women. *Anesthesiology, 69,* 626–628.
- Entman, S. S., & Moise, K. J., (1984). Anaphylaxis in pregnancy. *S. Med. J., 77,* 402.
- Nishimura, H., & Tanimura, T., (1976). *Clinical Aspects of the Teratogenicity of Drugs* (p. 231). New York, NY: American Elsevier.
- Shepard, T. H., (1980). *Catalog of Teratogenic Agents* (3rd edn., pp. 134, 135). Baltimore, MD: The Johns Hopkins University Press.

## 6.3.3   XANTHINE DERIVATIVES

### 6.3.3.1   AMINOPHYLLINE

**FDA Category: C**
*Risk Summary:* The reproduction studies in animals have shown no evidence of fetal harm or impaired fertility. The pregnancy experience in humans is adequate to exhibit that the embryo-fetal risk is nonexistent or very low.

**Further Reading:**
- Bird, L. M., Anderson, N. C. Jr., Chandler, M. L., & Young, R. C., (1987). The effects of aminophylline and nifedipine on contractility of isolated pregnant human myometrium. *Am. J. Obstet. Gynecol., 157*, 171–177.
- Granati, B., Grella, P. V., Pettenazzo, A., Di Lenardo, L., & Rubaltelli, F. F., (1984). The prevention of respiratory distress syndrome in premature infants: Efficacy of antenatal aminophylline treatment versus prenatal glucocorticoid administration. *Pediatr Pharmacol (New York), 4*, 21–24.
- Yeh, T. F., & Pildes, R. S., (1977). Transplacental aminophylline toxicity in a neonate. *Lancet, 1*, 910.

### 6.3.3.2   DYPHYLLINE

**FDA Category: C**
*Risk Summary:* It should be used only when the maternal benefit outweighs the fetal risk because there is very limited human pregnancy data, and animal studies are not relevant.

**Further Reading:**
- *Drug Information.* Difil, G. SJ Pharmaceuticals LLC, Atlanta, GA.
- Schaefer, C., Paul, P., & Richard, K. M., (2015). *Drugs During Pregnancy and Lactation Treatment Options and Risk Assessment.* Amsterdam: Elsevier.

*6.3.3.3   THEOPHYLLINE*

**FDA Category: C**
***Risk Summary:*** The reproduction studies in animals have shown no evidence of fetal harm or impaired fertility. The pregnancy experience in humans is adequate to exhibit that the embryo-fetal risk is nonexistent or very low.

**Further Reading:**
- Dombrowski, M. P., Bottoms, S. F., Boike, G. M., & Wald, J., (1986). Incidence of preeclampsia among asthmatic patients lower with theophylline. *Am. J. Obstet. Gynecol., 155*, 265–267.
- *Drug Information. Theo-Dur.* Key Pharmaceuticals.
- Horowitz, D. A., Jablonski, W., & Mehta, K. A., (1982). Apnea associated with theophylline withdrawal in a term neonate. *Am. J. Dis. Child., 136*, 73–74.
- Lalli, C. M., & Raju, L., (1981). Pregnancy and chronic obstructive pulmonary disease. *Chest, 80*, 759–761.

## *6.3.4   ANTICHOLINERGICS*

*6.3.4.1   ACLIDINIUM BROMIDE*

**FDA Category: C**
***Risk Summary:*** The reproduction studies in animals have shown no evidence of fetal harm or impaired fertility. The pregnancy experience in humans is limited.

**Further Reading:**
- *Drug Information.* Tudorza Pressair. Forest Pharmaceuticals.
- Schaefer, C., Paul, P., & Richard, K. M., (2015). *Drugs During Pregnancy and Lactation Treatment Options and Risk Assessment.* Amsterdam: Elsevier.

*6.3.4.2   IPRATROPIUM*

**FDA Category: B**
***Risk Summary:*** The reproduction studies in animals have shown no evidence of fetal harm or impaired fertility. The pregnancy experience in humans is limited.

**Further Reading:**
- D'Alonzo, G. E., (1990). The pregnant asthmatic patient. *Semin Perinatol., 14,* 119–129.
- *Drug Information. Atrovent.* Boehringer Ingelheim Pharmaceuticals.
- Schatz, M., (1992). Asthma during pregnancy: Interrelationships and management. *Ann. Allergy, 68,* 123–133.

## 6.3.4.3 TIOTROPIUM

**FDA Category: C**
*Risk Summary:* It should be used with caution because the pregnancy experience in humans is limited and the reproduction studies in animals have shown low risk.

**Further Reading:**
- *Drug Information.* Spiriva. Boehringer Ingelheim Pharmaceuticals.
- Schaefer, C., Paul, P., & Richard, K. M., (2015). *Drugs During Pregnancy and Lactation Treatment Options and Risk Assessment.* Amsterdam: Elsevier.

## 6.4 INHALED CORTICOSTEROIDS

### 6.4.1 BECLOMETHASONE

**FDA Category: C**
*Risk Summary:* The reproduction studies in animals have shown no evidence of fetal harm or impaired fertility. The pregnancy experience in humans is adequate to exhibit that the embryo-fetal risk is nonexistent or very low.

**Further Reading:**
- *Drug Information.* Beclovent. Glaxo Wellcome.
- Namazy, J., Schatz, M., Long, L., Lipkowitz, M., Lillie, M., Voss, M., Deitz, R. J., & Petitti, D., (2004). Use of inhaled steroids by pregnant asthmatic women does not reduce intrauterine growth. *J. Allergy Clin. Immunol., 113,* 427–432.
- Rahimi, R., Nikfar, S., & Abdollahi, M., (2006). Meta-analysis finds use of inhaled corticosteroids during pregnancy safe: A systematic meta-analysis review. *Hum. Exp. Toxicol., 25,* 447–452.

## 6.4.2   BUDESONIDE

**FDA Category (Inhaled/Nasal): B**

Risk Summary (Inhaled/Nasal): The reproduction studies in animals have shown no evidence of fetal harm or impaired fertility. The pregnancy experience in humans is adequate to exhibit that the embryo-fetal risk is nonexistent or very low.

**Further Reading:**
- *Drug Information. Pulmicort* Turbuhaler. AstraZeneca.
- *Drug Information. Rhinocort.* AstraZeneca.
- Kihlstrom, I., & Lundberg, C., (1987). Teratogenicity study of the new glucocorticosteroid budesonide in rabbits. *Arzneimittelforschung, 37*, 43–46.
- Norjavaara, E., & Gerhardsson de Verdier, M., (2003). Normal pregnancy outcomes in a population-based study including 2968 pregnant women exposed to budesonide. *J. Allergy Clin. Immunol., 111*, 736–742.
- Rahimi, R., Nikfar, S., & Abdollahi, M., (2006). Meta-analysis finds use of inhaled corticosteroids during pregnancy safe: A systematic meta-analysis review. *Hum. Exp. Toxicol., 25*, 447–452.

## 6.4.3   CICLESONIDE

**FDA Category: C**
***Risk Summary:*** Although there is limited data from the human pregnancy experience, but the possible maternal benefit extremely outweighs the unknown or known embryo/fetal risk.

**Further Reading:**
- Blais, L., & Forget, A., (2008). Asthma exacerbations during the first trimester of pregnancy and the risk of congenital malformations among asthmatic women. *J. Allergy Clin. Immunol., 121*, 1379–1384.
- Derendorf, H., (2007). Pharmacokinetic and pharmacodynamic properties of inhaled ciclesonide. *J. Clin. Pharmacol., 47*, 782–789.
- *Drug Information. Alvesco.* Nycomed US.

### 6.4.4 FLUNISOLIDE

**FDA Category: C**
*Risk Summary:* It should be used with caution because the pregnancy experience in humans is limited, and the reproduction studies in animals have shown the risk of teratogenicity associated with the use of Flunisolide.

**Further Reading:**
- *Drug Information. Aerobid.* Forest Pharmaceuticals.
- Itabashi, M., Inoue, T., Yokota, M., Takehara, K., & Tajima, M., (1982). Reproductive studies on flunisolide in rats: Oral administration during the period of organogenesis. *Oyo Yakuri (Pharmacometrics), 24*, 643–659.
- Tamagawa, M., Hatori, M., Ooi, A., Nishioeda, R., & Tanaka, N., (1982). Comparative teratological study of flunisolide in mice. *Oyo Yakuri (Pharmacometrics), 24*, 741–750.

### 6.4.5 FLUTICASONE

**FDA Category: C**
*Risk Summary:* The reproduction studies in animals have shown no evidence of fetal harm or impaired fertility. The pregnancy experience in humans is adequate to exhibit that the embryo-fetal risk is nonexistent or very low.

**Further Reading:**
- Choi, J. S., Han, J. Y., Kim, M. Y., Velazquez-Armenta, E. Y., & Nava-Ocampo, A. A., (2007). Pregnancy outcomes in women using inhaled fluticasone during pregnancy: A case series. *Allergol. Immunopathol. (Madr), 35*, 239–242.
- *Drug Information. Flovent.* GlaxoSmithKline.
- Rahimi, R., Nikfar, S., & Abdollahi, M., (2006). Meta-analysis finds use of inhaled corticosteroids during pregnancy safe: A systematic meta-analysis review. *Hum. Exp. Toxicol., 25*, 447–452.

### 6.4.6 MOMETASONE

**FDA Category: C**
*Risk Summary:* The reproduction studies in animals have shown no evidence of fetal harm or impaired fertility. The pregnancy experience in humans is adequate to exhibit that the embryo-fetal risk is nonexistent or very low.

**Further Reading:**

- *Drug Information*. Nasonex. Schering Corporation.
- Lindheimer, M., Caritis, S. N., Leveno, K. J., Meis, P., Miodovnik, M., Wapner, R. J., Paul, R. H., Varner, M. W., O'Sullivan, M. J., Thurnau, G. R., & Conway, D. L., (2004). for The National Institute of Child Health and Development Maternal-Fetal Medicine Units Network and the National Heart, Lung, and Blood Institute. The relationship of asthma medication use to perinatal outcomes. *J. Allergy Clin. Immunol., 113*, 1040–1045.
- Schatz, M., Dombrowski, M. P., Wise, R., Momirova, V., Landon, M., Mabie, W., Newman, R. B., & Hauth, J. C.
- Schatz, M., Zeiger, R. S., Harden, K., Hoffman, C. C., Chilingar, L., & Petitti, D., (1997). The safety of asthma and allergy medications during pregnancy. *J. Allergy Clin. Immunol., 100*, 301–306.

### 6.4.7 TRIAMCINOLONE

**FDA Category (Local/Inhaled): B**

*Risk Summary (Local/Inhaled):* The reproduction studies in animals have shown no evidence of fetal harm or impaired fertility. The pregnancy experience in humans is adequate to exhibit that the embryo-fetal risk is nonexistent or very low.

**Further Reading:**

- *Drug Information. Azmacort*. Rhône-Poulenc Rorer Pharmaceuticals, Inc., 1994.
- Rahimi, R., Nikfar, S., & Abdollahi, M., (2006). Meta-analysis finds use of inhaled corticosteroids during pregnancy safe: A systematic meta-analysis review. *Hum. Exp. Toxicol., 25*, 447–452.
- Tarara, R. P., Cordy, D. R., & Hendrickx, A. G., (1989). Central nervous system malformations induced by triamcinolone acetonide in nonhuman primates: Pathology. *Teratology, 39*, 75–84.
- Zhou, M., & Walker, B. E., (1993). Potentiation of triamcinolone-induced cleft palate in mice by maternal high dietary fat. *Teratology, 48*, 53–57.

## 6.5 ANTIHISTAMINES

### *6.5.1 AZELASTINE*

**FDA Category: C**
*Risk Summary:* It should be used with caution because the pregnancy experience in humans is limited and the reproduction studies in animals have shown low risk.

**Further Reading:**
- American College of Allergy, Asthma and Immunology (ACAAI) (2000). The use of newer asthma and allergy medications during pregnancy. *Ann. Allergy Asthma Immunol., 84*, 475–480.
- *Drug Information. Astelin.* MedPointe Pharmaceuticals.
- Joint Committee of the American College of Obstetricians and Gynecologists (ACOG) and the

### *6.5.2 BROMPHENIRAMINE*

**FDA Category: C**
*Risk Summary:* It should be used only when the maternal benefit outweighs the fetal risk because there is very limited human pregnancy data, and animal studies are not relevant.

**Further Reading:**
- *Drug Information. Dimetane.* AH Robins Company.
- Zierler, S., & Purohit, D., (1986). Prenatal antihistamine exposure and retrolental fibroplasia. *Am. J. Epidemiol., 123*, 192–196.

### *6.5.3 CARBINOXAMINE*

**FDA Category: C**
*Risk Summary:* The reproduction studies in animals have shown no evidence of fetal harm or impaired fertility. The pregnancy experience in humans is limited.

**Further Reading:**
- *Drug Information. Arbinoxa.* Hawthorn Pharmaceuticals.

## 6.5.4   CETIRIZINE

**FDA Category: C**
*Risk Summary:* It should be used with caution because the pregnancy experience in humans is limited and the reproduction studies in animals have shown low risk.

**Further Reading:**
- *Drug Information.* Zyrtec. Pfizer.
- Weber-Schoendorfer, C., & Schaefer, C., (2008). The safety of cetirizine during pregnancy—a prospective observational cohort study. *Reprod Toxicol., 26,* 19–23.

## 6.5.5   CHLORPHENIRAMINE

**FDA Category: B**
*Risk Summary:* The reproduction studies in animals have shown no evidence of fetal harm or impaired fertility. The pregnancy experience in humans is adequate to exhibit that the embryo-fetal risk is nonexistent or very low.

**Further Reading:**
- Heinonen, O. P., Slone, D., & Shapiro, S., (1977). *Birth Defects and Drugs in Pregnancy.* Littleton, MA: Publishing Sciences Group.
- Kallen, B., (2002). Use of antihistamine drugs in early pregnancy and delivery outcome. *J. Matern Fetal Neonatal Med., 11,* 146–152.

## 6.5.6   CLEMASTINE

**FDA Category: B**
*Risk Summary:* The reproduction studies in animals have shown no evidence of fetal harm or impaired fertility. The pregnancy experience in humans is adequate to exhibit that the embryo-fetal risk is nonexistent or very low.

**Further Reading:**
- *Drug Information.* Tavist. Sandoz Pharmaceuticals.
- Kallen, B., (2002). Use of antihistamine drugs in early pregnancy and delivery outcome. *J. Matern Fetal Neonatal Med., 11,* 146–152.

## 6.5.7   CYCLIZINE

**FDA Category: B**
*Risk Summary:* The reproduction studies in animals have shown no evidence of fetal harm or impaired fertility. The pregnancy experience in humans is adequate to exhibit that the embryo-fetal risk is nonexistent or very low.

**Further Reading:**
- Heinonen, O. P., Slone, D., & Shapiro, S., (1977). *Birth Defects and Drugs in Pregnancy*. Littleton, MA: Publishing Sciences Group.
- Kallen, B., (2002). Use of antihistamine drugs in early pregnancy and delivery outcome. *J. Matern Fetal Neonatal Med., 11*, 146–152.

## 6.5.8   CYPROHEPTADINE

**FDA Category: B**
*Risk Summary:* It should be used with caution because the pregnancy experience in humans is limited and the reproduction studies in animals have shown low risk.

**Further Reading:**
- *Drug Information. Periactin*. Merck & Co.
- Kallen, B., (2002). Use of antihistamine drugs in early pregnancy and delivery outcome. *J. Matern Fetal Neonatal Med., 11*, 146–152.

## 6.5.9   DESLORATADINE

**FDA Category: C**
*Risk Summary:* It should be used with caution because the pregnancy experience in humans is limited and the reproduction studies in animals have shown low risk.

**Further Reading:**
- *Drug Information. Clarinex*. Schering Corporation.
- Gilbert, C., Mazzotta, P., Loebstein, R., & Koren, G., (2005). Fetal safety of drugs used in the treatment of allergic rhinitis: A critical review. *Drug Saf., 28*, 707–719.

### 6.5.10   DEXCHLORPHENIRAMINE

**FDA Category: B**
***Risk Summary:*** The reproduction studies in animals have shown no evidence of fetal harm or impaired fertility. The pregnancy experience in humans is adequate to exhibit that the embryo-fetal risk is nonexistent or very low.

**Further Reading:**
- *Drug Information. Polaramine.* Schering Corporation.
- Kallen, B., (2002). Use of antihistamine drugs in early pregnancy and delivery outcome. *J. Matern Fetal Neonatal Med., 11,* 146–152.

### 6.5.11   DIMENHYDRINATE

**FDA Category: B**
***Risk Summary:*** The reproduction studies in animals have shown no evidence of fetal harm or impaired fertility. The pregnancy experience in humans is adequate to exhibit that the embryo-fetal risk is nonexistent or very low.

**Further Reading:**
- Hay, T. B., & Wood, C., (1967). The effect of dimenhydrinate on uterine contractions. *Aust NZ J Obstet. Gynaecol., 1,* 81–89.
- Kallen, B., (2002). Use of antihistamine drugs in early pregnancy and delivery outcome. *J. Matern Fetal Neonatal Med., 11,* 146–152.

### 6.5.12   DIPHENHYDRAMINE

**FDA Category: B**
***Risk Summary:*** The reproduction studies in animals have shown no evidence of fetal harm or impaired fertility. The pregnancy experience in humans is adequate to exhibit that the embryo-fetal risk is nonexistent or very low.

**Further Reading:**
- Brost, B. C., Scardo, J. A., & Newman, R. B., (1996). Diphenhydramine overdose during pregnancy: Lessons from the past. *Am. J. Obstet. Gynecol., 175,* 1376–1377.
- Kallen, B., (2002). Use of antihistamine drugs in early pregnancy and delivery outcome. *J. Matern Fetal Neonatal Med.,* 2002 *11,* 146–152.

## 6.5.13   DOXYLAMINE

**FDA Category: A**
***Risk Summary:*** The reproduction studies in animals have shown no evidence of fetal harm or impaired fertility. The pregnancy experience in humans is adequate to exhibit that the embryo-fetal risk is nonexistent or very low.

**Further Reading:**
- Milkovich, L., van den Berg, B. J., (1976). An evaluation of the teratogenicity of certain antinauseant drugs. *Am. J. Obstet. Gynecol., 125,* 244–248.
- Shapiro, S., Heinonen, O. P., Siskind, V., Kaufman, D. W., Monson, R. R., & Slone, D., (1977). Antenatal exposure to doxylamine succinate and dicyclomine hydrochloride (Bendectin) in relation to congenital malformations, perinatal mortality rate, birth weight, intelligence quotient score. *Am. J. Obstet. Gynecol., 128,* 480–485.

## 6.5.14   FEXOFENADINE

**FDA Category: C**
***Risk Summary:*** There is limited pregnancy experience in humans, and the reproduction studies in animals have shown moderate risk. Therefore, it is advisable to avoid its use until the human pregnancy experience is available.

**Further Reading:**
- *Drug Information. Allegra.* Hoechst Marion Roussel.
- Joint committee of the American College of Obstetricians and Gynecologists (ACOG) and the American College of Allergy, Asthma, and Immunology (ACAAI) (2000). Position statement. The use of newer asthma and allergy medications during pregnancy. *Ann. Allergy Asthma Immunol., 84,* 475–480.
- Kallen, B., (2002). Use of antihistamine drugs in early pregnancy and delivery outcome. *J. Matern Fetal Neonatal Med.,* 2002 *11,* 146–152.

## 6.5.15  HYDROXYZINE

**FDA Category: N**
*Risk Summary:* It should be used with caution because the human pregnancy experience has shown a low risk.

**Further Reading:**
- *Drug Information. Atarax.* Pfizer.
- Prenner, B. M., (2005). Neonatal withdrawal syndrome associated with Serreau, R., Komiha, M., Blanc, F., Guillot, F., & Jacqz-Aigrain, E., (eds.). Neonatal seizures associated with maternal hydroxyzine in late pregnancy. *Reprod Toxicol., 20,* 573–574.

## 6.5.16  LEVOCETIRIZINE

**FDA Category: B**
*Risk Summary:* It should be used with caution because the pregnancy experience in humans is limited and the reproduction studies in animals have shown low risk.

**Further Reading:**
- *Drug Information.* Xyzal. Sanofi-Aventis.

## 6.5.17  LORATADINE

**FDA Category: B**
*Risk Summary:* It should be used with caution because the pregnancy experience in humans is limited and the reproduction studies in animals have shown low risk.

**Further Reading:**
- *Drug Information.* Claritin. Schering.
- McIntyre, B. S., Vancutsem, P. M., Treinen, K. A., & Morrissey, R. E., (2003). Effects of perinatal loratadine exposure on male rat reproductive organ development. *Reprod. Toxicol., 17,* 691–697.
- Moretti, M. E., Caprara, D., Coutinho, C. J., Bar-Oz, B., Berkovitch, M., Addis, A., Jovanovski, E., Schuler-Faccini, L., & Koren, G., (2003). Fetal safety of loratadine use in the first trimester of pregnancy: A multicenter study. *J. Allergy Clin. Immunol., 111,* 479–483.

### 6.5.18 MECLIZINE

**FDA Category: B**

*Risk Summary:* The reproduction studies in animals have shown no evidence of fetal harm or impaired fertility. The pregnancy experience in humans is adequate to exhibit that the embryo-fetal risk is nonexistent or very low.

**Further Reading:**
- *Drug Information.* Antivert. Pfizer.
- Pettersson, F., (1964). Meclozine and congenital malformations. *Lancet, 1,* 675.
- Shapiro, S., Kaufman, D. W., Rosenberg, L., Slone, D., Monson, R. R., Siskind, V., & Heinonen, O. P., (1978). Meclizine in pregnancy in relation to congenital malformations. *Br. Med. J., 1,* 483.

### 6.5.19 PROMETHAZINE

**FDA Category: C**

*Risk Summary:* The reproduction studies in animals have shown no evidence of fetal harm or impaired fertility. The pregnancy experience in humans is adequate to exhibit that the embryo-fetal risk is nonexistent or very low.

**Further Reading:**
- Charles, A. G., & Blumenthal, L. S., (1982). Promethazine hydrochloride therapy in severely Rh-sensitized pregnancies. *Obstet. Gynecol., 60,* 627–630.
- Vella, L., Francis, D., Houlton, P., & Reynolds, F., (1985). Comparison of the antiemetics metoclopramide and promethazine in labor. *Br. Med. J., 290,* 1173–1175.

### 6.5.20 TRIPROLIDINE

**FDA Category: C**

*Risk Summary:* The reproduction studies in animals have shown no evidence of fetal harm or impaired fertility. The pregnancy experience in humans is adequate to exhibit that the embryo-fetal risk is nonexistent or very low.

**Further Reading:**
- Findlay, J. W. A., Butz, R. F., Sailstad, J. M., Warren, J. T., & Welch, R. M., (1984). Pseudoephedrine and triprolidine in plasma and breast milk of nursing mothers. *Br. J. Clin. Pharmacol., 18*, 901–906.
- Kallen, B., (2002). Use of antihistamine drugs in early pregnancy and delivery outcome. *J. Matern. Fetal Neonatal. Med., 11*, 146–152.

## 6.6   EXPECTORANTS

### *6.6.1   AMMONIUM CHLORIDE*

**FDA Category: C**
***Risk Summary:*** The reproduction studies in animals have shown no evidence of fetal harm or impaired fertility. The pregnancy experience in humans is adequate to exhibit that the embryo-fetal risk is nonexistent or very low.

**Further Reading:**
- Goodlin, R. C., & Kaiser, I. H., (1957). The effect of ammonium chloride-induced maternal acidosis on the human fetus at term. I. pH, hemoglobin, blood gases. *Am. J. Med. Sci., 233*, 666–674.
- Heinonen, O. P., Slone, D., & Shapiro, S., (1977). *Birth Defects and Drugs in Pregnancy*. Littleton, MA: Publishing Sciences Group.
- Kaiser, I. H., & Goodlin, R. C., (1958). The effect of ammonium chloride-induced maternal acidosis on the human fetus at term. II. Electrolytes. *Am. J. Med. Sci., 235*, 549–554.

### *6.6.2   GUAIFENESIN*

**FDA Category: C**
***Risk Summary:*** The reproduction studies in animals have shown no evidence of fetal harm or impaired fertility. The pregnancy experience in humans is adequate to exhibit that the embryo-fetal risk is nonexistent or very low.

**Further Reading:**
- Aselton, P., Jick, H., Milunsky, A., Hunter, J. R., & Stergachis, A., (1985). First-trimester drug use and congenital disorders. *Obstet. Gynecol., 65*, 451–455.
- Chasnoff, I. J., Diggs, G., & Schnoll, S. H., (1981). Fetal alcohol effects and maternal cough syrup abuse. *Am. J. Dis. Child, 135*, 968.

- Heinonen, O. P., Slone, D., & Shapiro, S., (1977). *Birth Defects and Drugs in Pregnancy*. Littleton, MA: Publishing Sciences Group.

### 6.6.3 POTASSIUM IODIDE

**FDA Category: D**
*Risk Summary:* As an expectorant, it is generally contraindicated during pregnancy because of fetal toxicity, as well as the availability of much safer alternatives.

**Further Reading:**
- Ayromlooi, J., (1972). Congenital goiter due to maternal ingestion of iodides. *Obstet. Gynecol., 39*, 818–822.
- Committee on Drugs (1976). American Academy of Pediatrics. Adverse reactions to iodide therapy of asthma and other pulmonary diseases. *Pediatrics, 57,* 272–274.
- Petersen, S., & Serup, J., (1977). Case report: Neonatal thyrotoxicosis. *Acta Paediatr Scand, 66,* 639–642.
- Schaefer, C., Paul, P., & Richard, K. M., (2015). *Drugs During Pregnancy and Lactation Treatment Options and Risk Assessment*. Amsterdam: Elsevier.

### 6.6.4 SODIUM IODIDE

**FDA Category: D**
*Risk Summary:* As an expectorant, it is generally contraindicated during pregnancy because of fetal toxicity, as well as the availability of much safer alternatives.

**Further Reading:**
- Ayromlooi, J., (1972). Congenital goiter due to maternal ingestion of iodides. *Obstet. Gynecol., 39*, 818–822.
- Committee on Drugs (1976). American Academy of Pediatrics. Adverse reactions to iodide therapy of asthma and other pulmonary diseases. *Pediatrics, 57,* 272–274.
- Petersen, S., & Serup, J., (1977). Case report: Neonatal thyrotoxicosis. *Acta Paediatr. Scand., 66,* 639–642.

- Schaefer, C., Paul, P., & Richard, K. M., (2015). *Drugs During Pregnancy and Lactation Treatment Options and Risk Assessment.* Amsterdam: Elsevier.

## 6.7 LEUKOTRIENE RECEPTOR ANTAGONISTS

### 6.7.1 MONTELUKAST

**FDA Category: B**
*Risk Summary:* The reproduction studies in animals have shown no evidence of fetal harm or impaired fertility. The pregnancy experience in humans is limited.

**Further Reading:**
- Bakhireva, L. N., Jones, K. L., Schatz, M., Klonoff-Cohen, H. S., Johnson, D., Slymen, D. J., & Chambers, C. D., (2007). and the Organization of Teratology Information Specialists Collaborative Research Group. Safety of leukotriene receptor antagonists in pregnancy. *J. Allergy Clin. Immunol., 119,* 618–625.
- *Drug Information.* Singulair. Merck.
- Sarkar, M., Koren, G., Kalra, S., Ying, A., Smorlesi, C., De Santis, M., Diav-Citrin, Avgil, M., Voyer Lavigne, S., Berkovich, M., & Einarson, A., (2009). Montelukast use during pregnancy: A multicentre, prospective, comparative study of infant outcomes. *Eur. J. Clin. Pharmacol., 65,* 1259–1264.
- Schaefer, C., Paul, P., & Richard, K. M., (2015). *Drugs During Pregnancy and Lactation Treatment Options and Risk Assessment.* Amsterdam: Elsevier.

### 6.7.2 ZAFIRLUKAST

**FDA Category: B**
*Risk Summary:* It should be used with caution because the pregnancy experience in humans is limited and the reproduction studies in animals have shown low risk.

**Further Reading:**
- Bakhireva, L. N., Jones, K. L., Schatz, M., Klonoff-Cohen, H. S., Johnson, D., Slymen, D. J., & Chambers, C. D., (2007)., and the Organization of Teratology Information Specialists Collaborative Research Group. Safety of leukotriene receptor antagonists in pregnancy. *J. Allergy Clin. Immunol., 119,* 618–625.
- *Drug Information. Accolate.* AstraZeneca Pharmaceuticals.
- Joint Committee of the American College of Obstetricians and Gynecologists (ACOG) and the American College of Allergy, Asthma, and Immunology (ACAAI) (2000). The use of newer asthma and allergy medications during pregnancy. *Ann. Allergy Asthma Immunol., 84,* 475–480.

## 6.8   LEUKOTRIENE FORMATION INHIBITOR

### 6.8.1   ZILEUTON

**FDA Category: C**
*Risk Summary:* It should be used with caution because the pregnancy experience in humans is limited, and the reproduction studies in animals have shown risk.

**Further Reading:**
- Anonymous (2000). Drugs for asthma. *Med. Lett. Drugs Ther., 42,* 19–24.
- *Drug Information.* Zyflo. Abbott Laboratories.
- Schaefer, C., Paul, P., & Richard, K. M., (2015). *Drugs During Pregnancy and Lactation Treatment Options and Risk Assessment.* Amsterdam: Elsevier.

## 6.9   MONOCLONAL ANTIBODIES

### 6.9.1   OMALIZUMAB

**FDA Category: B**
*Risk Summary:* The reproduction studies in animals have shown no evidence of fetal harm or impaired fertility. The pregnancy experience in humans is limited.

**Further Reading:**
- *Drug Information*. Xolair. Genentech.
- Namazy, Jennifer, Michael, D. C., Angela, E. S., John, M. T., Hubert, C., Gillis, C., Yan, W., Joachim, V., & Elizabeth, B. A., (2015). "The Xolair Pregnancy Registry (EXPECT): The Safety of Omalizumab Use during Pregnancy." *Journal of Allergy and Clinical Immunology 135*(2), 407–412. doi: 10.1016/j.jaci.2014.08.025.

### 6.9.2  PALIVIZUMAB

**FDA Category: C**
***Risk Summary:*** It should be used only when the maternal benefit outweighs the fetal risk because there is very limited human pregnancy data, and animal studies are not relevant.

**Further Reading:**
- *Drug Information*. Synagis. MedImmune.
- Schaefer, C., Paul, P., & Richard, K. M., (2015). *Drugs During Pregnancy and Lactation Treatment Options and Risk Assessment.* Amsterdam: Elsevier.

## 6.10   MUCOLYTIC

### 6.10.1  ACETYLCYSTEINE

**FDA Category: B**
***Risk Summary:*** Although there is limited data from the human pregnancy experience regarding the use of acetylcysteine as a mucolytic, but the possible maternal benefit extremely outweighs the unknown or known embryo/fetal risk.

***FURTHER READING:***

- *Drug Information*. Acetylcysteine Solution, USP. Bedford Laboratories.

- Schaefer, C., Paul, P., & Richard, K. M., (2015). *Drugs During Pregnancy and Lactation Treatment Options and Risk Assessment.* Amsterdam: Elsevier.
- Zed, P. J., & Krenzelok, E. P., (1999). Treatment of acetaminophen overdose. *Am. J. Health-Syst. Pharm., 56,* 1081–1091.

## 6.10.2  ROMHEXINE

**FDA Category: N**
*Risk Summary:* It should be used only when the maternal benefit outweighs the fetal risk because there is very limited human pregnancy data, and animal studies are not relevant.

**Further Reading:**
- Schaefer, C., Paul, P., & Richard, K. M., (2015). *Drugs During Pregnancy and Lactation Treatment Options and Risk Assessment.* Amsterdam: Elsevier.

## 6.10.3  AMBROXOL

**FDA Category: N**
*Risk Summary:* It should be used only when the maternal benefit outweighs the fetal risk because there is very limited human pregnancy data, and animal studies are not relevant.

**Further Reading:**
- Schaefer, C., Paul, P., & Richard, K. M., (2015). *Miller. Drugs During Pregnancy and Lactation Treatment Options and Risk Assessment.* Amsterdam: Elsevier.

## 6.10.4  DORNASE ALFA

**FDA Category: B**
*Risk Summary:* The reproduction studies in animals have shown no evidence of fetal harm or impaired fertility. The pregnancy experience in humans is limited.

**Further Reading:**
- *Drug Information. Pulmozyme.* Genentech.


## 6.11    SELECTIVE PHOSPHODIESTERASE 4 INHIBITOR

- 6.11.1    Roflumilast

**FDA Category: C**
***Risk Summary:*** The pregnancy experience in humans is limited, and the reproduction studies in animals have shown moderate risk.

**Further Reading:**
- *Drug Information. Daliresp.* Forest Pharmaceuticals.
- Schaefer, C., Paul, P., & Richard, K. M., (2015*). Miller. Drugs During Pregnancy and Lactation Treatment Options and Risk Assessment.* Amsterdam: Elsevier.


## KEYWORDS

- **acetylcysteine**
- **ambroxol**
- **bromhexine**
- **dornase alfa**
- **monoclonal antibodies**
- **palivizumab**

# CHAPTER 7

# Drugs Affecting the Central Nervous System

## 7.1 ANTICONVULSANTS DRUGS

### 7.1.1 CARBAMAZEPINE

**FDA Category: D**
*Risk Summary:* Although there is a risk of congenital malformations, but the possible maternal benefit extremely outweighs the unknown or known embryo/fetal risk.

**Further Reading:**
- Diav-Citrin, O., Shechtman, S., Arnon, J., & Ornoy, A., (2001). Is carbamazepine teratogenic? A prospective controlled study of 210 pregnancies. *Neurology, 57,* 321–324.
- *Drug Information. Tegretol.* Novartis Pharmaceuticals.
- Matalon, S., Shechtman, S., Goldzweig, G., & Ornoy, A., (2002). The teratogenic effect of carbamazepine: A meta-analysis of 1255 exposures. *Reprod. Toxicol., 16,* 9–17.
- Vestermark, V., & Vestermark, S., (1991). Teratogenic effect of carbamazepine. *Arch Dis. Child, 66,* 641–642.

### 7.1.2 CLOBAZAM

**FDA Category: C**
*Risk Summary:* Because of the potential risk to the fetus, it is advisable to use it only when safer alternatives are not available or have failed.

**Further Reading:**
- *Drug Information.* Onfi. Lundbeck.
- Kulaga, S., Sheehy, O., Zargarzadeh, A. H., Moussally, K., & Bérard, A., (2011). Antiepileptic drug use during pregnancy: Perinatal outcomes. *Seizure, 20,* 667–672.
- Pundey, S. K., & Gupta, S., (2005). Neuroembryopathic effect of clobazam in rat: A histological study. *Nepal Med. Coll. J., 7,* 10–12.

### 7.1.3  CLONAZEPAM

**FDA Category: D**
*Risk Summary:* It should be used with caution because the human pregnancy experience has shown a low risk of congenital malformations.

**Further Reading:**
- *Drug Information.* Klonopin. Roche Laboratories.
- Lin, A. E., Peller, A. J., Westgate, M. N., Houde, K., Franz, A., & Holmes, L. B., (2004). Clonazepam use in pregnancy and the risk of malformations. *Birth Defects Res., (Part A), 70,* 534–536.
- Weinstock, L., Cohen, L. S., Bailey, J. W., Blatman, R., & Rosenbaum, J. F., (2001). Obstetrical and neonatal outcome following clonazepam use during pregnancy: A case series. *Psychother. Psychosom., 70,* 158–162.

### 7.1.4  CLORAZEPATE

**FDA Category: D**
*Risk Summary:* It should be used with caution because the human pregnancy experience has shown a low risk of congenital malformations.

**Further Reading:**
- *Drug Information. Clorazepate* Dipotassium. Mylan Pharmaceuticals.
- Patel, D. A., & Patel, A. R., (1980). Clorazepate and congenital malformations. *JAMA, 244,* 135, 136.

## 7.1.5   ETHOSUXIMIDE

**FDA Category: N**
***Risk Summary:*** It should be used with caution because the human pregnancy experience has shown a low risk of congenital malformations.

**Further Reading:**
- *Drug Information. Ethosuximide.* Pliva.
- Tomson, T., & Villen, T., (1994). Ethosuximide enantiomers in pregnancy and lactation. *Ther. Drug Monit., 16*, 621–623.

## 7.1.6   ETHOTOIN

**FDA Category: D**
***Risk Summary:*** Ethotoin is believed to be safer than the more potent phenytoin; also, the possible maternal benefit extremely outweighs the unknown or known embryo/fetal risk

**Further Reading:**
- Heinonen, O. P., Slone, D., & Shapiro, S., (1977). *Birth Defects and Drugs in Pregnancy* (pp. 358, 359). Littleton, MA: Publishing Sciences Group.
- Zablen, M., & Brand, N., (1978). Cleft lip and palate with the anticonvulsant ethantoin. *N. Engl. J. Med., 298*, 285.

## 7.1.7   EZOGABINE

**FDA Category: C**
***Risk Summary:*** It should be used with caution because the pregnancy experience in humans is limited and the reproduction studies in animals have shown low risk.

**Further Reading:**
- *Drug Information. Potiga.* GlaxoSmithKline.

### 7.1.8   FELBAMATE

**FDA Category: C**
*Risk Summary:* It should be used with caution because the pregnancy experience in humans is limited and the reproduction studies in animals have shown moderate risk.

**Further Reading:**
- *Drug Information*. Felbatol. Wallace Laboratories.
- Wagner, M. L., (1994). Felbamate: A new antiepileptic drug. *Am. J. Hosp. Pharm., 51*, 1657–1666.

### 7.1.9   GABAPENTIN

**FDA Category: C**
*Risk Summary:* It should be used with caution because the pregnancy experience in humans is limited and the reproduction studies in animals have shown the risk of fetotoxicity in mice.

**Further Reading:**
- *Drug Information*. Neurontin. Parke-Davis.
- Fujii, H., Goel, A., Bernard, N., Pistelli, A., Yates, L. M., Stephens, S., Han, J. Y., Matsui, D., Erwell, F., Einarson, R., Koren, G., & Einarson, A., (2013). Pregnancy outcomes following gabapentin use: Results of a prospective comparative cohort study. *Neurology, 80*, 1–6.
- Jurgens, T. P., Schaefer, C., & May, A., (2009). Treatment of cluster headache in pregnancy and lactation. *Cephalalgia, 29*, 391–400.

### 7.1.10   GABAPENTIN ENACARBIL

**FDA Category: C**
*Risk Summary:* It should be used with caution because the pregnancy experience in humans is limited and the reproduction studies in animals have shown the risk of fetotoxicity in mice.

**Further Reading:**
- *Drug Information*. Horizant. GlaxoSmithKline.

- Fujii, H., Goel, A., Bernard, N., Pistelli, A., Yates, L. M., Stephens, S., Han, J. Y., Matsui, D., Erwell, F., Einarson, R., Koren, G., & Einarson, A., (2013). Pregnancy outcomes following gabapentin use: Results of a prospective comparative cohort study. *Neurology, 80,* 1–6.
- Jurgens, T. P., Schaefer, C., & May, A., (2009). Treatment of cluster headache in pregnancy and lactation. *Cephalalgia, 29,* 391–400.

## 7.1.11  LACOSAMIDE

**FDA Category: C**
***Risk Summary:*** It should be used with caution because the pregnancy experience in humans is limited and the reproduction studies in animals have shown moderate risk.

**Further Reading:**
- *Drug Information*. Vimpat. UCB.

## 7.1.12  LAMOTRIGINE

**FDA Category: C**
***Risk Summary:*** Although there is a risk of congenital malformations, but the possible maternal benefit extremely outweighs the unknown or known embryo/fetal risk.

**Further Reading:**
- Dichter, M. A., & Brodie, M. J., (1996). New antiepileptic drugs. *N. Engl. J. Med., 334,* 1583–1590.
- *Drug Information. Lamictal.* GlaxoSmithKline.
- Holmes, L. B., & Hernandez-Diaz, S., (2012). Newer anticonvulsants: Lamotrigine, topiramate, and gabapentin. *Birth Defects Res. A Clin. Mol. Teratol., 94,* 599–606.
- Holmes, L. B., Wyszynski, D. F., Baldwin, E. J., Habecker, E., Glassman, L. H., & Smith, C. R., (2006). Increased risk for non-syndromic cleft palate among infants exposed to lamotrigine during pregnancy (abstract). *Birth Defects Res. A Clin. Mol. Teratol., 76,* 318.

### 7.1.13   LEVETIRACETAM

**FDA Category: C**
***Risk Summary:*** It should be used with caution because the pregnancy experience in humans is limited and the reproduction studies in animals have shown the risk of severe growth restriction.

**Further Reading:**
- *Drug Information. Keppra.* UCB Pharma.
- Ten Berg, K., Samren, E. B., van Oppen, A. C., Engelsman, M., & Lindhout, D., (2005). Levetiracetam use and pregnancy outcome. *Reprod. Toxicol., 20,* 175–178.

### 7.1.14   MAGNESIUM SULFATE

**FDA Category: D**
***Risk Summary:*** Magnesium sulfate is contraindicated in pregnant women with cardiovascular and renal diseases, as in these situations the absorption of magnesium ions brings on a further burden.

**Further Reading:**
- *Drug Information.* Magnesium Sulfate. Abbott Pharmaceutical, Abbott Park, IL.
- Duley, L., Henderson-Smart, D. J., & Meher, S., (2006). Drugs for treatment of very high blood pressure during pregnancy. *Cochrane Database Syst. Rev., 3,* CD001449.

### 7.1.15   METHSUXIMIDE

**FDA Category: N**
***Risk Summary:*** It should be used only when the maternal benefit outweighs the fetal risk because there is very limited human pregnancy data, and animal studies are not relevant. Nevertheless, Methsuximide is considered the treatment of choice for petit mal epilepsy during the 1st trimester.

**Further Reading:**
- Annegers, J. F., Elveback, L. R., Hauser, W. A., & Kurland, L. T., (1974). Do anticonvulsants have a teratogenic effect? *Arch Neurol., 31*, 364–373.
- Heinonen, O. P., Slone, D., & Shapiro, S., (1977). Birth Defects and Drugs in Pregnancy (pp. 358, 359). Littleton, MA: Publishing Sciences Group.
- The National Institutes of Health (1981). Anticonvulsants found to have teratogenic potential. *JAMA, 241*, 36.

### 7.1.16   OXCARBAZEPINE

**FDA Category: C**
***Risk Summary:*** It should be used with caution because the pregnancy experience in humans is limited and the reproduction studies in animals have shown the risk of fetotoxicity.

**Further Reading:**
- Andermann, E., (1994). Pregnancy and oxcarbazepine. *Epilepsia, 35* (Suppl 3), S26.
- *Drug Information. Trileptal.* Novartis Pharmaceuticals.
- Gentile, S., (2006). Prophylactic treatment of bipolar disorder in pregnancy and breastfeeding: Focus on emerging mood stabilizers. *Bipolar Disord., 8*, 207–220.

### 7.1.17   PERAMPANEL

**FDA Category: C**
***Risk Summary:*** It should be used with caution because the pregnancy experience in humans is limited and the reproduction studies in animals have shown the risk of visceral abnormalities.

**Further Reading:**
- *Drug Information.* Fycompa. Eisai.

## 7.1.18   PHENOBARBITAL

**FDA Category: D**
*Risk Summary:* The pregnancy experience in humans has shown the risk of congenital malformations, hemorrhage, and addiction in the newborn. Nevertheless, the possible maternal benefit extremely outweighs the unknown or known embryo/fetal risk.

**Further Reading:**
- Dessens, A. B., Cohen-Kettenis, P. T., Mellenbergh, G. J., Koppe, J. G., van de Poll, N. E., & Boer, K., (2000). Association of prenatal phenobarbital and phenytoin exposure with small head size at birth and with learning problems. *Acta Paediatr., 89,* 533–541.
- Gupta, C., Yaffe, S. J., & Shapiro, B. H., (1982). Prenatal exposure to phenobarbital permanently decreases testosterone and causes reproductive dysfunction. *Science, 216,* 640–642.
- Reinisch, J. M., Sanders, S. A., Mortensen, E. L., & Rubin, D. B., (1995). In utero exposure to phenobarbital and intelligence deficits in adult men. *JAMA, 274,* 1518–1525.

## 7.1.19   PHENYTOIN

**FDA Category: D**
*Risk Summary:* The pregnancy experience in humans has shown the risk of congenital malformations, and hemorrhage in the newborn. Nevertheless, the possible maternal benefit extremely outweighs the unknown or known embryo/fetal risk.

**Further Reading:**
- D'Souza, S. W., Robertson, I. G., Donnai, D., & Mawer, G., (1990). Fetal phenytoin exposure, hypoplastic nails, and jitteriness. *Arch Dis. Child, 65,* 320–324.
- Loughnan, P. M., Gold, H., & Vance, J. C., (1973). Phenytoin teratogenicity in man. *Lancet, 1,* 70–72.
- Tiboni, G. M., Iammarrone, E., Giampietro, F., Lamonaca, D., Bellati, U., & Di Ilio, C., (1999). Teratological interaction between the bistriazole antifungal agent fluconazole and the anticonvulsant drug phenytoin. *Teratology, 59,* 81–87.

## 7.1.20  PREGABALIN

**FDA Category: C**
*Risk Summary:* There is no pregnancy experience in humans, and the reproduction studies in animals have shown moderate risk. Therefore, it is advisable to avoid its use until the human pregnancy experience is available.

**Further Reading:**
- *Drug Information. Lyrica.* Parke-Davis.

## 7.1.21  PRIMIDONE

**FDA Category: D**
*Risk Summary:* The use of Primidone should be avoided in pregnant women because the pregnancy experience in humans has shown the risk of developmental toxicity associated with the use of this drug.

**Further Reading:**
- Krauss, C. M., Holmes, L. B., VanLang, Q. N., & Keith, D. A., (1984). Four siblings with similar malformations after exposure to phenytoin and primidone. *J. Pediatr., 105,* 750–755.
- Myhree, S. A., & Williams, R., (1981). Teratogenic effects associated with maternal primidone therapy. *J. Pediatr., 99,* 160–162.
- Rudd, N. L., & Freedom, R. M., (1979). A possible primidone embryopathy. *J. Pediatr., 94,* 835–837.

## 7.1.22  RUFINAMIDE

**FDA Category: C**
*Risk Summary:* It should be used with caution because the pregnancy experience in humans is limited, and the reproduction studies in animals have shown the risk of embryo-fetal toxicity.

**Further Reading:**
- *Drug Information. Banzel.* Eisai.

### 7.1.23  TIAGABINE

**FDA Category: C**
*Risk Summary:* It should be used with caution because the pregnancy experience in humans is limited, and the reproduction studies in animals have shown the risk of fetal malformations.

**Further Reading:**
- *Drug Information. Gabitril.* Cephalon.
- Leppik, I. E., Gram, L., Deaton, R., & Sommerville, K. W., (1999). Safety of tiagabine: Summary of 53 trials. *Epilepsy Res., 33,* 235–246.
- Yerby, M. S., (2003). Clinical care of pregnant women with epilepsy: Neural tube defects and folic acid supplementation. *Epilepsia, 44*(Suppl 3), 33–40.

### 7.1.24  TOPIRAMATE

**FDA Category: D**
*Risk Summary:* The use of Topiramate should be avoided in pregnant women because the pregnancy experience in humans has shown the risk of fetal malformations associated with the use of this drug.

**Further Reading:**
- Holmes, L. B., & Hernandez-Diaz, S., (2012). Newer anticonvulsants: Lamotrigine, topiramate, and gabapentin. *Birth Defects Res. A Clin. Mol. Teratol., 94,* 599–606.
- Ornoy, A., Zvi, N., Arnon, J., Wajnberg, R., Shechtman, S., & Diav-Citrin, O., (2008). The outcome of pregnancy following topiramate treatment: A study on 52 pregnancies. *Reprod. Toxicol., 25,* 388–389.
- Rihtman, T., Parush, S., & Ornoy, A., (2012). Preliminary findings of the developmental effects of in utero exposure to topiramate. *Reprod. Toxicol., 34,* 308–311.

### 7.1.25  VALPROIC ACID

**FDA Category: D (for treating convulsion)**
**FDA Category: X (for treating migraine)**
*Risk Summary:* The use of Valproic Acid should be avoided, if possible, in pregnant women because the pregnancy experience in humans has shown

the risk of congenital abnormalities, hepatotoxicity, and intrauterine growth restriction (IUGR), associated with the use of this drug.

**Further Reading:**
- Dalens, B., Raynaud, E. J, & Gaulme, J., (1980). Teratogenicity of valproic acid. *J. Pediatr., 97,* 332, 333.
- Jager-Roman, E., Deichi, A., Jakob, S., Hartmann, A. M, Koch, S., Rating, D., Steldinger, R., Nau, H., & Helge, H., (1986). Fetal growth, major malformations, and minor anomalies in infants born to women receiving Valproic acid. *J. Pediatr.,108,* 997–1004.
- Jentink, J., Loane, M. A., Dolk, H., Barisic, I., Garne, E., Morris, J. K., & de jong-van den Berg, L. T. W., (2010). for the EUROCAT Antiepileptic Study Working Group. Valproic acid monotherapy in pregnancy and major congenital malformations. *N. Engl. J. Med., 362,* 2185–2193.
- Ornoy, A., (2009). Valproic acid in pregnancy: How much are we endangering the embryo and fetus? *Reprod. Toxicol., 28,* 1–10.

### 7.1.26   ZONISAMIDE

**FDA Category: C**
*Risk Summary:* Because of the potential risk to the fetus, it is advisable to use it only when safer alternatives are not available or have failed.

**Further Reading:**
- *Drug Information.* Zonegran. Elan Biopharmaceuticals.
- Kondo, T., Kaneko, S., Amano, Y., & Egawa, I., (1996). Preliminary report on teratogenic effects of zonisamide in the offspring of treated women with epilepsy. *Epilepsia, 37,* 1242–1244.

## 7.2   ANTIDEPRESSANTS DRUGS

### 7.2.1   AMINOKETONE

#### 7.2.1.1   BUPROPION

**FDA Category: C**
*Risk Summary:* It should be used with caution because the pregnancy experience in humans is limited and the reproduction studies in animals have shown low risk.

**Further Reading:**
- *Alwan, S., Reefh*uis, J., Botto, L. D., Rasmussen, S. A., Correa, A., & Friedman, J. M., (2010). and the National Birth Defects Prevention Study. Maternal use of bupropion and risk for congenital heart defects. Am. J. Obstet. Gynecol., 203, 52, e1–6.
- Chun-Fai-Chan, B., *Koren, G., Fayez, I., Kalra*, S., Voyer-Lavigne, S., Boshier, A., Shakir, S., & Einarson, A., (2005). Pregnancy outcome of women exposed to bupropion during pregnancy: A prospective comparative study. Am. J. Obstet. Gynecol., 192, 932–936.
- Drug I*nformation. Wellbutrin. Glaxo*SmithKline.
- The Bupropion Pregnancy Registry. Final Report, 1 September 1997 through 31 March 2008. GlaxoSmithKline, August 2008.

## 7.2.2   *MONOAMINE OXIDASE INHIBITORS*

### 7.2.2.1   *ISOCARBOXAZID*

**FDA Category: C**
***Risk Summary:*** It should be used with caution because the pregnancy experience in humans is limited and the reproduction studies in animals are not relevant.

**Further Reading:**
- Heinonen, O. P., Slone, D., & Shapiro, S., (1977). *Birth Defects and Drugs in Pregnancy* (pp. 336, 337). Littleton, MA: Publishing Sciences Group.

### 7.2.2.2   *PHENELZINE*

**FDA Category: C**
***Risk Summary:*** It should be used with caution because the pregnancy experience in humans is limited, and the reproduction studies in animals have shown moderate risk.

**Further Reading:**
- *Drug Information.* Nardil. Parke-Davis.
- Frayne, J., Nguyen, T., Kohan, R., De Felice, N., & Rampono, J., (2014). The comprehensive management of pregnant women with

major mood disorders: A case study involving phenelzine, lithium, and quetiapine. *Arch Womens Ment Health, 17*, 73–75.
- Gracious, B. L., & Wisner, K. L., (1997). Phenelzine use throughout pregnancy and the puerperium: Case report, review of the literature, and management recommendations. *Depress Anxiety, 6*, 124–128.

## 7.2.2.3 *TRANYLCYPROMINE*

**FDA Category: N**
*Risk Summary:* It should be used with caution because the pregnancy experience in humans is limited, and the reproduction studies in animals have shown moderate risk.

**Further Reading:**
- *Drug Information*. Parnate. SmithKline Beecham Pharmaceuticals.
- Heinonen, O. P., Slone, D., & Shapiro, S., (1977). *Birth Defects and Drugs in Pregnancy* (pp. 336, 337). Littleton, MA: Publishing Sciences Group.
- Kennedy, D. S., Evans, N., Wang, I., & Webster, W. S., (2000). Fetal abnormalities associated with high-dose tranylcypromine in two consecutive pregnancies (abstract). *Teratology, 61*, 441.

## 7.2.3 *PHENYLPIPERAZINE*

### 7.2.3.1 *NEFAZODONE*

**FDA Category: C**
*Risk Summary:* It should be used with caution because the pregnancy experience in humans is limited and the reproduction studies in animals have shown moderate risk.

**Further Reading:**
- *Drug Information. Serzone*. Bristol-Myers Squibb.
- Einarson, A., Bonari, L., Voyer-Lavigne, S., Addis, A., Matsui, D., Johnson, Y., & Koren, G., (2003). A multicenter prospective controlled study to determine the safety of trazodone and nefazodone use during pregnancy. *Can. J. Psychiatry, 48*, 106–109.

- Einarson, A., Choi, J., Einarson, T. R., & Koren, G., (2009). Incidence of major malformations in infants following antidepressant exposure in pregnancy: Results of a large prospective cohort study. *Can. J. Psychiatry, 54*, 242–246.

## 7.2.4   SELECTIVE SEROTONIN REUPTAKE INHIBITORS

### 7.2.4.1   CITALOPRAM

**FDA Category: C**
***Risk Summary:*** It should be used with caution because the pregnancy experience in humans suggests a risk of developmental toxicities.

**Further Reading:**
- Alwan, S., Reefhuis, J., Rasmussen, S. A., Olney, R. S., Friedman, J. M., (2007). for the National Birth Defects Prevention Study. Use of selective serotonin-reuptake inhibitors in pregnancy and the risk of birth defects. *N. Engl. J. Med., 356*, 2684–2692.
- *Drug Information. Celexa.* Forest Pharmaceuticals.
- Sivojelezova, A., Shuhaiber, S., Sarkissian, L., Einarson, A., & Koren, G., (2005). Citalopram use in pregnancy: Prospective comparative evaluation of pregnancy and fetal outcome. *Am. J. Obstet. Gynecol., 193*, 2004–2009.

### 7.2.4.2   ESCITALOPRAM

**FDA Category: C**
***Risk Summary:*** It should be used with caution because the pregnancy experience in humans suggests a risk of developmental toxicities.

**Further Reading:**
- Alwan, S., Reefhuis, J., Rasmussen, S. A., Olney, R. S., Friedman, J. M., (2007). for the National Birth Defects Prevention Study. Use of selective serotonin-reuptake inhibitors in pregnancy and the risk of birth defects. *N. Engl. J. Med., 356*, 2684–2692.
- *Drug Information. Lexapro.* Forest Pharmaceuticals.
- Gentile, S., (2006). Escitalopram late in pregnancy and while breast-feeding. *Ann. Pharmacother, 40*, 1696–1697.

## 7.2.4.3  FLUOXETINE

**FDA Category: C**
*Risk Summary:* It should be used with caution because the pregnancy experience in humans suggests a risk of developmental toxicities.

**Further Reading:**
- Diav-Citrin, O., Shechtman, S., Weinbaum, D., Arnon, J., Gianantonio, E. D., Clementi, M., & Ornoy, A., (2005). Paroxetine and fluoxetine in pregnancy: A multicenter, prospective, controlled study (abstract). *Reprod. Toxicol., 20,* 459.
- *Drug Information. Prozac.* Dista Products.
- Hines, R. N., Adams, J., Buck, G. M., Faber, W., Holson, J. F., Jacobson, S. W., Keszler, M., McMartin, K., Segraves, R. T., Singer, L. T., Sipes, I. G., & Williams, P. L., (2004). NTP-CERHR expert panel report on the reproductive and developmental toxicity of fluoxetine. *Birth Defects Res. B Dev Reprod Toxicol., 71,* 193–280.

## 7.2.4.4  FLUVOXAMINE

**FDA Category: C**
*Risk Summary:* It should be used with caution because the pregnancy experience in humans suggests a risk of developmental toxicities.

**Further Reading:**
- *Drug Information. Luvox.* Solvay Pharmaceuticals.
- Gentile, S., (2006). Quetiapine-fluvoxamine combination during pregnancy and while breastfeeding. *Arch Womens Ment Health, 9,* 158, 159.

## 7.2.4.5  PAROXETINE

**FDA Category: D**
*Risk Summary:* The use of Paroxetine should be avoided in pregnant women because the pregnancy experience in humans has shown the risk of congenital malformations and cardiac defects associated with the use of this drug.

**Further Reading:**
- Berard, A., Ramos, E., Rey, E., Blais, L., St. Andre, M, & Oraichi, D., (2007). First trimester exposure to paroxetine and risk of cardiac malformations in infants: The importance of dosage. *Birth Defects Res. B Dev Reprod. Toxicol., 80*, 18–27.
- Cole, J. A., Ephross, S. A., Cosmatos, I. S., & Walker, A. M., (2007). Paroxetine in the first trimester and the prevalence of congenital malformations. *Pharmacoepidemiol Drug Saf., 16*, 1075–1085.
- *Drug Information*. Paxil. GlaxoSmithKline.
- Prescribing Information Paxil – Food and Drug Administration [Internet] (2017). Available from: https://www.accessdata.fda.gov/drugsatfda_docs/label/2017/020031s074lbl.pdf(accessed on 31 January 2020).
- Wurst, K. E., Poole, C., Ephross, S. A., & Olshan, A. F., (2010). First trimester paroxetine use and the prevalence of congenital, specifically cardiac, defects: A meta-analysis of epidemiological studies. *Birth Defects Res. A Clin. Mol. Teratol., 88*, 159–170.

## 7.2.4.6   *SERTRALINE*

**FDA Category: C**
***Risk Summary:*** It should be used with caution because the pregnancy experience in humans suggests a risk of developmental toxicities.

**Further Reading:**
- Chambers, C. D., Dick, L. M., Felix, R. J., Johnson, K. A., & Jones, K. L., (1999). Pregnancy outcome in women who use sertraline (abstract). *Teratology, 59*, 376.
- *Drug Information*. Zoloft. Pfizer.
- Kent, L. S. W., & Laidlaw, J. D. D., (1995). Suspected congenital sertraline dependence. *Br. J. Psychiatry, 167*, 412–413.

## 7.2.4.7   *VILAZODONE*

**FDA Category: C**
***Risk Summary:*** It should be used with caution because the pregnancy experience in humans suggests a risk of developmental toxicities.

**Further Reading:**
- *Drug Information.* Viibryd. Forest Pharmaceuticals.

## 7.2.5 *SEROTONIN AND NOREPINEPHRINE REUPTAKE INHIBITORS*

### 7.2.5.1 *DULOXETINE*

**FDA Category: C**
***Risk Summary:*** It should be used with caution because the pregnancy experience in humans is limited and the animal reproduction studies suggest a high risk of developmental toxicities.

**Further Reading:**
- Briggs, G. G., Ambrose, P. J., Ilett, K. F., Hackett, L. P., Nageotte, M. P., & Padilla, G., (2009). Use of duloxetine in pregnancy and lactation. *Ann. Pharmacother., 43,* 1898–1902.
- *Drug Information. Cymbalta.* Eli Lilly.
- Hoog, S. L., Cheng, Y., Elpers, J., & Dowsett, S. A., (2013). Duloxetine and pregnancy outcomes: Safety surveillance findings. *Int. J. Med. Sci., 10,* 413–419.

### 7.2.5.2 *DESVENLAFAXINE*

**FDA Category: C**
***Risk Summary:*** It should be used with caution because there is no pregnancy experience in humans and the animal reproduction studies suggest a risk of developmental toxicities.

**Further Reading:**
- *Drug Information. Pristiq.* Wyeth.
- Ilett, K. F., Watt, F., Hackett, L. P., Kohan, R., & Teoh, S., (2010). Assessment of infant dose through milk in a lactating woman taking amisulpride and desvenlafaxine for treatment-resistant depression. *Ther Drug Monit, 32,* 704–707.

### 7.2.5.3   *MILNACIPRAN*

**FDA Category: C**
*Risk Summary:* It should be used with caution because there is no pregnancy experience in humans and the animal reproduction studies suggest a risk of developmental toxicities.

**Further Reading:**
  • *Drug Information*. Savella. Forest Pharmaceuticals.


### 7.2.5.4   *VENLAFAXINE*

**FDA Category: C**
*Risk Summary:* It should be used with caution because there is no pregnancy experience in humans and the animal reproduction studies suggest a risk of developmental toxicities.

**Further Reading:**
  • *Drug Information. Effexor*. Wyeth Pharmaceuticals.
  • Ferreira, E., Carceller, A. M., Agogue, C., Martin, B. Z., St-Andre, M., Francoeur, D., & Berard, A., (2007). Effects of selective serotonin reuptake inhibitors and venlafaxine during pregnancy in term and preterm neonates. *Pediatrics, 119,* 52–59.
  • Pakalapati, R. K., Bolisetty, S., Austin, M. P., & Oei, J., (2006). Neonatal seizures from in utero venlafaxine exposure. *J. Paediatr Child Health, 42,* 737–738.


## 7.2.6   *TETRACYCLIC ANTIDEPRESSANTS*

### 7.2.6.1   *MAPROTILINE*

**FDA Category: B**
*Risk Summary:* The reproduction studies in animals have shown no evidence of fetal harm or impaired fertility. The pregnancy experience in humans is limited.

**Further Reading:**
  • *Drug Information. Ludiomil*. CIBA.

- McElhatton, P. R., Garbis, H. M., Elefant, E., Vial, T., Bellemin, B., Mastroiacovo, P., Arnon, J., Rodriguez-Pinilla, E., Schaefer, C., Pexieder, T., Merlob, P., & Dal Verme, S., (1996). The outcome of pregnancy in 689 women exposed to therapeutic doses of antidepressants. A collaborative study of the European Network of Teratology Information Services (ENTIS). *Reprod. Toxicol., 10*, 285–294.

### 7.2.6.2   MIRTAZAPINE

**FDA Category: C**
***Risk Summary:*** It should be used with caution because the pregnancy experience in humans is limited, and the reproduction studies in animals have shown moderate risk.

**Further Reading:**
- Biswas, P. N., Wilton, L. V., & Shakir, S. A. W., (2003). The pharmacovigilance of mirtazapine: Results of a prescription event monitoring study on 13,554 patients in England. *J. Psychopharmacol., 17*, 121–126.
- Djulus, J., Koren, G., Einarson, T. R., Wilton, L., Shakir, S., Diav-Citrin, O., Kennedy, D., Lavigne, S. V., De Santis, M., & Einarson, A., (2006). Exposure to mirtazapine during pregnancy: A prospective, comparative study of birth outcomes. *J. Clin. Psychiatry., 67*, 1280–1284.
- *Drug Information. Remeron.* Organon.

## 7.2.7   TRICYCLIC ANTIDEPRESSANTS

### 7.2.7.1   AMITRIPTYLINE

**FDA Category: C**
***Risk Summary:*** It should be used with caution because the human pregnancy experience has shown a low risk.

**Further Reading:**
- *Drug Information. Elavil.* AstraZeneca.

- Wertelecki, W., Purvis-Smith, S. G., & Blackburn, W. R., (1980). Amitriptyline/perphenazine maternal overdose and birth defects (abstract). *Teratology, 21,* 74A.

## 7.2.7.2   AMOXAPINE

**FDA Category: C**
*Risk Summary:* It is better to be avoided during the 1st Trimester because the pregnancy experience in humans is limited, and the reproduction studies in animals have shown the risk of stillbirths, intrauterine death, and decreased neonatal survival associated with the use of Amoxapine.

**Further Reading:**
- *Drug Information. Asendin.* Lederle Laboratories.

## 7.2.7.3   CLOMIPRAMINE

**FDA Category: C**
*Risk Summary:* It is better to be avoided during the 1st and 3rd Trimesters because the pregnancy experience in humans suggests a risk of cardiac defects linked to the use of Clomipramine.

**Further Reading:**
- Ostergaard, G. Z., & Pedersen, S. E., (1982). Neonatal effects of maternal clomipramine treatment. *Pediatrics, 69,* 233, 234.
- Schimmell, M. S., Katz, E. Z., Shaag, Y., Pastuszak, A., & Koren, G., (1991). Toxic neonatal effects following maternal clomipramine therapy. *J. Toxicol Clin. Toxicol., 29,* 479–484.
- Singh, S., Gulati, S., Narang, A., & Bhakoo, O. N., (1990). Non-narcotic withdrawal syndrome in a neonate due to maternal clomipramine therapy. *J. Pediatr. Child Health, 26,* 110.

## 7.2.7.4   DESIPRAMINE

**FDA Category: C**
*Risk Summary:* It should be used with caution because the human pregnancy experience has shown a low risk.

**Further Reading:**
- McElhatton, P. R., Garbis, H. M., Elefant, E., Vial, T., Bellemin, B., Mastroiacovo, P., Arnon, J., Rodriguez-Pinilla, E., Schaefer, C., Pexieder, T., Merlob, P., & Dal Verme, S., (1996). The outcome of pregnancy in 689 women exposed to therapeutic doses of antidepressants. A collaborative study of the European Network of Teratology Information Services (ENTIS). *Reprod. Toxicol., 10,* 285–294.
- Nulman, I., Rovet, J., Stewart, D. E., Wolpin, J., Pace-Asciak, P., Shuhaiber, S., & Koren, G., (2002). Child development following exposure to tricyclic antidepressants or fluoxetine throughout fetal life: A prospective, controlled study. *Am. J. Psychiatry., 159,* 1889–1895.

## 7.2.7.5 DOXEPIN

**FDA Category: C**
*Risk Summary:* It should be used with caution because the human pregnancy experience has shown a low risk.

**Further Reading:**
- Nulman, I., Rovet, J., Stewart, D. E., Wolpin, J., Pace-Asciak, P., Shuhaiber, S., & Koren, G., (2002). Child development following exposure to tricyclic antidepressants or fluoxetine throughout fetal life: A prospective, controlled study. *Am. J. Psychiatry 159,* 1889–1895.
- Owaki, Y., Momiyama, H., & Onodera, N., (1971). Effects of doxepin hydrochloride administered to pregnant rats upon the fetuses and their postnatal development. *Oyo Yakuri, 5,* 913–924. As cited in: Shepard, T. H., Catalog of Teratogenic Agents. (6th edn., p. 243). Baltimore, MD: Johns Hopkins University Press, 1989.

## 7.2.7.6 IMIPRAMINE

**FDA Category: N**
*Risk Summary:* It is better to be avoided during the 1st and 3rd Trimesters because the pregnancy experience in humans suggests a risk of structural anomalies linked to the use of Imipramine.

**Further Reading:**
- Eggermont, E., (1973). Withdrawal symptoms in a neonate associated with maternal imipramine therapy. *Lancet, 2,* 680.
- Kuenssberg, E. V., & Knox, J. D. E., (1972). Imipramine in pregnancy. *Br. Med. J., 2,* 29.
- Morrow, A. W., (1972). Imipramine and congenital abnormalities. *NZ. Med. J., 75,* 228–229.

## 7.2.7.7   NORTRIPTYLINE

**FDA Category: N**
*Risk Summary:* It should be used with caution because the human pregnancy experience has shown a low risk.

**Further Reading:**
- Nulman, I., Rovet, J., Stewart, D. E., Wolpin, J., Pace-Asciak, P., Shuhaiber, S., & Koren, G., (2002). Child development following exposure to tricyclic antidepressants or fluoxetine throughout fetal life: A prospective, controlled study. *Am. J. Psychiatry, 159,* 1889–1895.
- Shearer, W. T., Schreiner, R. L., & Marshall, R. E., (1972). Urinary retention in a neonate secondary to maternal ingestion of nortriptyline. *J. Pediatr., 81,* 570–572.

## 7.2.7.8   PROTRIPTYLINE

**FDA Category: N**
*Risk Summary:* The reproduction studies in animals have shown no evidence of fetal harm or impaired fertility. The pregnancy experience in humans is limited.

**Further Reading:**
- *Drug Information. Vivactil.* Merck.

## 7.2.7.9   TRIMIPRAMINE

**FDA Category: C**
*Risk Summary:* It should be used with caution because the human pregnancy experience has shown a low risk.

**Further Reading:**
- *Drug Information*. Surmontil. Odyssey Pharmaceuticals.
- McElhatton, P. R., Garbis, H. M., Elefant, E., Vial, T., Bellemin, B., Mastroiacovo, P., Arnon, J., Rodriguez-Pinilla, E., Schaefer, C., Pexieder, T., Merlob, P., & Dal Verme, S., (1996). The outcome of pregnancy in 689 women exposed to therapeutic doses of antidepressants. A collaborative study of the European Network of Teratology Information Services (ENTIS). *Reprod. Toxicol., 10*, 285–294.

## 7.2.8  TRIAZOLOPYRIDINE

### 7.2.8.1  TRAZODONE

**FDA Category: C**
*Risk Summary:* It should be used with caution because the pregnancy experience in humans is limited and the reproduction studies in animals have shown low risk.

**Further Reading:**
- Einarson, A., Bonari, L., Voyer-Lavigne, S., Addis, A., Matsui, D., Johnson, Y., & Koren, G., (2003). A multicenter prospective controlled study to determine the safety of trazodone and nefazodone use during pregnancy. *Can. J. Psychiatry, 48*, 106–109.
- Einarson, A., Choi, J., Einarson, T. R., & Koren, G., (2009). Incidence of major malformations in infants following antidepressant exposure in pregnancy: Results of a large prospective cohort study. *Can. J. Psychiatry, 54*, 242–246.

## 7.3  ANTIPSYCHOTIC DRUGS

A typical antipsychotics are listed below.

### 7.3.1  PHENYLBUTYLPIPERADINES

#### 7.3.1.1  DROPERIDOL

**FDA Category: C**
*Risk Summary:* The reproduction studies in animals have shown no evidence of fetal harm or impaired fertility. The pregnancy experience in humans is adequate to exhibit that the embryo-fetal risk is nonexistent or very low.

**Further Reading:**
*   *Drug Information. Inapsine*. Akorn.
*   Nageotte, M. P., Briggs, G. G., Towers, C. V., & Asrat, T., (1996). Droperidol and diphenhydramine in the management of hyperemesis gravidarum. *Am. J. Obstet. Gynecol., 174*, 1801–1806.

## 7.3.1.2   HALOPERIDOL

**FDA Category: C**
***Risk Summary:*** It is better to be avoided during the 1st Trimester because the pregnancy experience in humans is limited, and the reproduction studies in animals have shown the risk of increased fetal mortality associated with the use of Haloperidol.

**Further Reading:**
*   Diav-Citrin, O., Shechtman, S., Ornoy, S., Arnon, J., Schaefer, C., Garbis, H., Clementi, M., & Ornoy, A., (2005). Safety of haloperidol and penfluridol in pregnancy: A multicenter, prospective, controlled study. *J. Clin. Psychiatry, 66*, 317–322.
*   *Drug Information. Haloperidol*. Major Pharmaceuticals.
*   Kopelman, A. E., McCullar, F. W., & Heggeness, L., (1975). Limb malformations following maternal use of haloperidol. *JAMA, 231*, 62–64.

## 7.3.1.3   PIMOZIDE

**FDA Category: C**
***Risk Summary:*** It is better to be avoided during the 1st Trimester because the pregnancy experience in humans is limited and the reproduction studies in animals have shown low risk.

**Further Reading:**
*   Bjarnason, N. H., Rode, L., & Dalhoff, K., (2006). Fetal exposure to pimozide: A case report. *J. Reprod. Med., 51*, 443, 444.
*   Committee on Drugs. American Academy of Pediatrics (2000). Use of psychoactive medication during pregnancy and possible effects on the fetus and newborn. *Pediatrics, 105*, 880–887.
*   *Drug Information. Orap*. Gate Pharmaceuticals.

## 7.3.2  PHENOTHIAZINES

### 7.3.2.1  CHLORPROMAZINE

**FDA Category: N**
***Risk Summary:*** The reproduction studies in animals have shown no evidence of fetal harm or impaired fertility. The pregnancy experience in humans is adequate to exhibit that the embryo-fetal risk is nonexistent or very low. However, Chlorpromazine should be avoided near term due to the risk of maternal hypotension.

**Further Reading:**
- Ayd, F. J. Jr., (ed.) (1968). Phenothiazine therapy during pregnancy-effects on the newborn infant. *Int. Drug Ther Newslett.*, *3*, 39–40.
- Slone, D., Siskind, V., Heinonen, O. P., Monson, R. R., Kaufman, D. W., & Shapiro, S., (1977). Antenatal exposure to the phenothiazines in relation to congenital malformations, perinatal mortality rate, birth weight, and intelligence quotient score. *Am. J. Obstet. Gynecol.*, *128*, 486–488.
- Sullivan, C. L., (1957). Treatment of nausea and vomiting of pregnancy with chlorpromazine. A report of 100 cases. *Postgrad Med.*, *22*, 429–432.

### 7.3.2.2  FLUPHENAZINE

**FDA Category: N**
***Risk Summary:*** It should be used with caution during the 1st and 2nd Trimesters. However, it is better to avoid the use of Fluphenazine during the 3rd Trimester because fetal extrapyramidal and withdrawal symptoms have been associated with its use during the last Trimester of pregnancy.

**Further Reading:**
- Abdel-Hamid, H. A., Abdel-Rahman, M. S., & Abdel-Rahman, S. A., (1996). Teratogenic effect of diphenylhydantoin and/or fluphenazine in mice. *J. Appl. Toxicol.*, *16*, 221–225.
- Nath, S. P., Miller, D. A., & Muraskas, J. K., (1996). Severe rhinorrhea and respiratory distress in a neonate exposed to fluphenazine hydrochloride prenatally. *Ann. Pharmacother.*, *30*, 35–37.

- Slone, D., Siskind, V., Heinonen, O. P., Monson, R. R., Kaufman, D. W., & Shapiro, S., (1977). Antenatal exposure to the phenothiazines in relation to congenital malformations, perinatal mortality rate, birth weight, and intelligence quotient score. *Am. J. Obstet. Gynecol., 128,* 486–488.

## 7.3.2.3   PERPHENAZINE

**FDA Category: N**
*Risk Summary:* It should be used only when the maternal benefit outweighs the fetal risk because there is very limited human pregnancy data, and the animal studies are not relevant.

**Further Reading:**
- McGarry, J. M., (1971). A double-blind comparison of the anti-emetic effect during labor of metoclopramide and perphenazine. *Br. J. Anaesth., 43,* 613–615.
- Slone, D., Siskind, V., Heinonen, O. P., Monson, R. R., Kaufman, D. W., & Shapiro, S., (1977). Antenatal exposure to the phenothiazines in relation to congenital malformations, perinatal mortality rate, birth weight, and intelligence quotient score. *Am. J. Obstet. Gynecol., 128,* 486–488.

## 7.3.2.4   PROCHLORPERAZINE

**FDA Category: N**
*Risk Summary:* It should be used only when the maternal benefit outweighs the fetal risk because there is very limited human pregnancy data, and the animal studies are not relevant.

**Further Reading:**
- Rafla, N., (1987). Limb deformities associated with prochlorpera-zine. *Am. J. Obstet. Gynecol., 156,* 1557.
- Slone, D., Siskind, V., Heinonen, O. P., Monson, R. R., Kaufman, D. W., & Shapiro, S., (1977). Antenatal exposure to the phenothiazines in relation to congenital malformations, perinatal mortality rate, birth weight, and intelligence quotient score. *Am. J. Obstet. Gynecol., 128,* 486–488.

## 7.3.2.5 *THIORIDAZINE*

**FDA Category: N**
***Risk Summary:*** It should be used only when the maternal benefit outweighs the fetal risk because there is very limited human pregnancy data, and the animal studies are not relevant.

**Further Reading:**
- *Drug Information. Mellaril.* Sandoz Pharmaceutical Corporation.
- Scanlan, F. J., (1972). The use of thioridazine (Mellaril) during the first trimester. *Med. J. Aust., 1*, 1271, 1272.
- Slone, D., Siskind, V., Heinonen, O. P., Monson, R. R., Kaufman, D. W., & Shapiro, S., (1977). Antenatal exposure to the phenothiazines in relation to congenital malformations, perinatal mortality rate, birth weight, and intelligence quotient score. *Am. J. Obstet. Gynecol., 128*, 486–488.

## 7.3.2.6 *TRIFLUOPERAZINE*

**FDA Category: N**
***Risk Summary:*** It should be used with caution because the pregnancy experience in humans is limited and the reproduction studies in animals have shown low risk.

**Further Reading:**
- *Drug Information.* Stelazine. SmithKline Beecham Pharmaceuticals.
- Slone, D., Siskind, V., Heinonen, O. P., Monson, R. R., Kaufman, D. W., & Shapiro, S., (1977). Antenatal exposure to the phenothiazines in relation to congenital malformations, perinatal mortality rate, birth weight, and intelligence quotient score. *Am. J. Obstet. Gynecol., 128*, 486–488.

## 7.3.3 *PHENOTHIAZINES*

### 7.3.3.1 *THIOTHIXENE*

**FDA Category: N**
***Risk Summary:*** It should be used with caution because the pregnancy experience in humans is limited and the reproduction studies in animals have shown low risk.

**Further Reading:**
- *Drug Information*. Navane. Pfizer.
- Slone, D., Siskind, V., Heinonen, O. P., Monson, R. R., Kaufman, D. W., & Shapiro, S., (1977). Antenatal exposure to the phenothiazines in relation to congenital malformations, perinatal mortality rate, birth weight, and intelligence quotient score. *Am. J. Obstet. Gynecol., 128*, 486–488.

### 7.3.4  BENZOISOTHIAZOL

#### 7.3.4.1  LURASIDONE

**FDA Category: B**
*Risk Summary:* The reproduction studies in animals have shown no evidence of fetal harm or impaired fertility. The pregnancy experience in humans is adequate to exhibit that the embryo-fetal risk is very low.

**Further Reading:**
- *Drug Information*. Latuda. Sunovion.
- Koren, G., Cohn, T., Chitayat, D., Kapur, B., Remington, G., Myles-Reid, D., & Zipursky, R. B., (2002). Use of atypical antipsychotics during pregnancy and the risk of neural tube defects in infants. *Am. J. Psychiatry, 159*, 136, 137.

### 7.3.5  BENZISOXAZOLES

#### 7.3.5.1  ILOPERIDONE

**FDA Category: N**
*Risk Summary:* It should be used with caution because the pregnancy experience in humans is limited, and the reproduction studies in animals have shown moderate risk.

**Further Reading:**
- American College of Obstetricians and Gynecologists (2008). Use of psychiatric medications during pregnancy and lactation. ACOG Practice Bulletin. No. 92, April 2008. *Obstet. Gynecol., 111*, 1001–1019.
- *Drug Information. Fanapt*. Vanda Pharmaceuticals.

## 7.3.5.2 PALIPERIDONE

**FDA Category: C**
*Risk Summary:* It should be used with caution because the pregnancy experience in humans is limited and the reproduction studies in animals have shown low risk.

**Further Reading:**
- American College of Obstetricians and Gynecologists, (2008). Use of psychiatric medications during pregnancy and lactation. ACOG Practice Bulletin. No. 92, April 2008. *Obstet. Gynecol., 111*, 1001–1019.
- *Drug Information*. Invega. Janssen.
- Koren, G., Cohn, T., Chitayat, D., Kapur, B., Remington, G., Myles-Reid, D., & Zipursky, R. B., (2002). Use of atypical antipsychotics during pregnancy and the risk of neural tube defects in infants. *Am. J. Psychiatry, 159*, 136–137.

## 7.3.5.3 RISPERIDONE

**FDA Category: C**
*Risk Summary:* Although there is limited data from the human pregnancy experience, but the possible maternal benefit extremely outweighs the unknown or known embryo/fetal risk.

**Further Reading:**
- *Drug Information*. Risperdal. Janssen Pharmaceuticals.
- Kim, S. W., Kim, K. M., Kim, J. M., Shin, I. S., Shin, H. Y., Yang, S. J., & Yoon, J. S., (2007). Use of long-acting injectable risperidone before and throughout pregnancy in schizophrenia. *Prog. Neuropsychopharmacol Biol. Psychiatry, 31*, 543–545.
- Koren, G., Cohn, T., Chitayat, D., Kapur, B., Remington, G., Myles-Reid, D., & Zipursky, R. B., (2002). Use of atypical antipsychotics during pregnancy and the risk of neural tube defects in infants. *Am. J. Psychiatry, 159*, 136–137.

## 7.3.5.4 ZIPRASIDONE

**FDA Category: C**
*Risk Summary:* It should be used with caution because the pregnancy experience in humans is limited, and the reproduction studies in animals

have shown the risk of embryo-fetal toxicity associated with the use of Ziprasidone.

**Further Reading:**
- *Drug Information. Geodon.* Pfizer.
- Peitl, M. V., Petric, D., & Peitl, V., (2010). Ziprasidone as a possible cause of cleft palate in a newborn. *Psychiatr Danub, 22,* 117–119.

### 7.3.6   DIBENZAPINES

#### 7.3.6.1   ASENAPINE

**FDA Category: C**
*Risk Summary:* It should be used with caution because the pregnancy experience in humans is limited, and the reproduction studies in animals have shown risk associated with the use of Asenapine.

**Further Reading:**
- *Drug Information. Saphris.* Organon Pharmaceuticals USA.
- Koren, G., Cohn, T., Chitayat, D., Kapur, B., Remington, G., Myles-Reid, D., & Zipursky, R. B., (2002). Use of atypical antipsychotics during pregnancy and the risk of neural tube defects in infants. *Am. J. Psychiatry, 159,* 136–137.

#### 7.3.6.2   CLOZAPINE

**FDA Category: B**
*Risk Summary:* Although there is limited data from the human pregnancy experience, but the possible maternal benefit extremely outweighs the unknown or known embryo/fetal risk.

**Further Reading:**
- *Drug Information. Clozaril.* Novartis Pharmaceuticals.
- Mendhekar, D., (2007). Possible delayed speech acquisition with clozapine therapy during pregnancy and lactation. *J. Neuropsychiatry Clin Neurosci., 19,* 196, 197.
- Walderman, M. D., & Safferman, A. Z., (1993). Pregnancy and clozapine. *Am. J. Psychiatry, 150,* 168–169.

## 7.3.6.3   LOXAPINE

**FDA Category: C**
*Risk Summary:* It should be used with caution because the pregnancy experience in humans is limited, and the reproduction studies in animals have shown moderate risk.

**Further Reading:**
- *Drug Information. Loxitane.* Watson Laboratories.
- Koren, G., Cohn, T., Chitayat, D., Kapur, B., Remington, G., Myles-Reid, D., & Zipursky, R. B., (2002). Use of atypical antipsychotics during pregnancy and the risk of neural tube defects in infants. *Am. J. Psychiatry, 159,* 136, 137.

## 7.3.6.4   OLANZAPINE

**FDA Category: C**
*Risk Summary:* Although there is limited data from the human pregnancy experience, but the possible maternal benefit extremely outweighs the unknown or known embryo/fetal risk.

**Further Reading:**
- Biwsas, P. N., Wilton, L. V., Pearce, G. L., Freemantle, S., Shakir, S. A. W., (2001). The pharmacovigilance of olanzapine: Results of a post-marketing surveillance study on 8858 patients in England. *J. Psychopharmacol., 15,* 265–271.
- *Drug Information. Zyprexa.* Eli Lilly.
- Kirchheiner, J., Berghofer, A., & Bolk-Weischedel, D., (2000). Healthy outcome under olanzapine treatment in a pregnant woman. *Pharmacopsychiatry, 33,* 78–80.

## 7.3.6.5   QUETIAPINE

**FDA Category: C**
*Risk Summary:* Although there is limited data from the human pregnancy experience, but the possible maternal benefit extremely outweighs the unknown or known embryo/fetal risk.

**Further Reading:**
- *Drug Information. Seroquel.* AstraZeneca Pharmaceuticals.
- Taylor, T. M., O'Toole, M. S., Ohlsen, R. I., Walters, J., & Pilowsky, L. S., (2003). Safety of quetiapine during pregnancy. *Am. J. Psychiatry, 160,* 588–589.

### 7.3.7   QUINOLINONES

#### 7.3.7.1   ARIPIPRAZOLE

**FDA Category: C**
*Risk Summary:* It should be used with caution because the pregnancy experience in humans is limited, and the reproduction studies in animals have shown risk associated with the use of Aripiprazole.

**Further Reading:**
- *Drug Information. Abilify.* Bristol-Myers Squibb.
- Gentile, S., Tofani, S., & Bellantuono, C., (2011). Aripiprazole and pregnancy. A case report and literature review. *J. Clin. Psychopharmacol, 31,* 531–532.
- Mendhekar, D. N., Sharma, J. B., & Srilakshmi, P., (2006). Use of aripiprazole during late pregnancy in a woman with psychotic illness. *Ann. Pharmacother, 40,* 575.

### 7.3.8   MISCELLANEOUS PSYCHOTHERAPEUTICS

#### 7.3.8.1   LITHIUM

**FDA Category: D**
*Risk Summary:* The use of Lithium should be avoided in pregnant women because the pregnancy experience in humans has shown the risk of congenital defects associated with the use of this drug.

**Further Reading:**
- Jacobson, S. J., Jones, K., Johnson, K., Ceolin, L., Kaur, P., Sahn, D., Donnenfeld, A. E., Rieder, M., Santelli, R., Smythe, J., Pastuszak, A., Einarson, T., & Koren, G., (1992). Prospective multicentre study

of pregnancy outcome after lithium exposure during first trimester. *Lancet, 339,* 530–533.

- Pinelli, J. M., Symington, A. J., Cunningham, K. A., & Paes, B. A., (2002). Case report and review of the perinatal implications of maternal lithium use. *Am. J. Obstet. Gynecol., 187,* 245–249.

## 7.3.8.2   ATOMOXETINE

**FDA Category: D**
*Risk Summary:* It should be used with caution because the pregnancy experience in humans is limited, and the reproduction studies in animals have shown risk associated with the use of Atomoxetine.

**Further Reading:**
- *Drug Information.* Strattera. Eli Lilly.
- Heiligenstein, J., Michelson, D., Wernicke, J., Milton, D., Kratochvil, C. J., Spencer, T. J., & Newcorn, J. H., (2003). Atomoxetine and pregnancy. *J. Am. Acad Child Adolesc. Psychiatry, 42,* 884, 885.

## 7.3.8.3   SODIUM OXYBATE

**FDA Category: C**
*Risk Summary:* It should be used with caution because the pregnancy experience in humans is limited and the reproduction studies in animals have shown low risk.

**Further Reading:**
- *Drug Information. Xyrem.* Jazz Pharmaceuticals.

## 7.4   ANTIPARKINSON DRUGS

### 7.4.1   AMANTADINE

**FDA Category: C**
*Risk Summary:* It is better to be avoided during the 1st Trimester because the pregnancy experience in humans is limited, and the reproduction studies in animals have shown the risk of teratogenicity associated with the use of

Amantadine. It is believed that Rimantadine has a lower risk of harmful effects than Amantadine

**Further Reading:**
- *Drug Information. Flumadine.* Forest Pharmaceuticals.
- *Drug Information. Symmetrel.* Endo Pharmaceuticals.
- Greer, L. G., Sheffield, J. S., Rogers, V. L., Roberts, S. W., McIntire, D. D., & Wendel, G. D. Jr.,(2010). Maternal and neonatal outcomes after antepartum treatment of influenza with antiviral medications. *Obstet. Gynecol., 115*, 711–716.
- Pandit, P. B., Chitayat, D., Jefferies, A. L., Landes, A., Qamar, I. U., & Koren, G., (1994). Tibial hemimelia and tetralogy of Fallot associated with first trimester exposure to amantadine. Reprod *Toxicol, 8*, 89–92.
- Rosa, F., (1994). Amantadine pregnancy experience. *Reprod. Toxicol., 8*, 531.

### 7.4.2   CARBIDOPA/LEVODOPA

**FDA Category: C**
***Risk Summary:*** It should be used with caution because the pregnancy experience in humans is limited, and the reproduction studies in animals have shown an increased risk of fetal deaths associated with the use of Carbidopa/Levodopa.

**Further Reading:**
- Ball, M. C., & Sagar, H. J., (1995). Levodopa in pregnancy. *Mov. Disord., 10*, 115.
- *Drug Information. Sinemet.* DuPont Pharma.
- Watanabe, T., Matsubara, S., Baba, Y., Tanaka, H., Suzuki, T., & Suzuki, M., (2009). Successful management of pregnancy in a patient with Segawa disease: Case report and literature review. *J. Obstet. Gynaecol. Res., 35*, 562–564.

### 7.4.3   ENTACAPONE

**FDA Category: C**
***Risk Summary:*** It should be used with caution because the pregnancy experience in humans is limited, and the reproduction studies in animals have shown moderate risk.

**Further Reading:**
- *Drug Information.* COMTAN. Novartis Pharmaceuticals.
- Lindh, J., (2007). Short episode of seizures in a newborn of mother treated with levodopa/carbidopa/entacapone and bromocriptine. *Mod. Disord., 22,* 1515.

## 7.4.4 PRAMIPEXOLE

**FDA Category: C**
*Risk Summary:* It should be used with caution because the pregnancy experience in humans is limited, and the reproduction studies in animals have shown moderate risk.

**Further Reading:**
- *Drug Information. Mirapex.* Pharmacia & Upjohn.
- Mucchiut, M., Belgrado, E., Cutuli, D., Antonini, A., & Bergonzi, P., (2004). Pramipexole-treated Parkinson's disease during pregnancy. *Mov. Disord., 19,* 1114, 1115.

## 7.4.5 RASAGILINE

**FDA Category: C**
*Risk Summary:* It should be used with caution because the pregnancy experience in humans is limited, and the reproduction studies in animals have shown the risk of fetal toxicity associated with the use of Rasagiline.

**Further Reading:**
- *Drug Information. Azilect.* Teva Neuroscience.

## 7.4.6 ROPINIROLE

**FDA Category: C**
*Risk Summary:* It should be used with caution because the pregnancy experience in humans is limited, and the reproduction studies in animals have shown the risk of digital malformations associated with the use of Ropinirole.

**Further Reading:**
- *Drug Information. Requip.* GlaxoSmithKline.


## 7.4.7 ROTIGOTINE

**FDA Category: C**
*Risk Summary:* It should be used only when the maternal benefit outweighs the fetal risk because there is very limited human pregnancy data, and the animal studies are not relevant.

**Further Reading:**
- *Drug Information. Neupro.* Schwarz Pharma.


## 7.4.8 SELEGILINE

**FDA Category: C**
*Risk Summary:* It should be used with caution because the pregnancy experience in humans is limited and the reproduction studies in animals have shown a low risk of higher rates of stillbirths and reduced pup survival.

**Further Reading:**
- *Drug Information. Carbex.* Endo Pharmaceuticals.
- Kupsch, A., & Oertel, W. H., (1998). Selegiline, pregnancy, and Parkinson's disease. *Mov. Disord., 13*, 175–194.
- Whitaker-Azmitia, P. M., Zhang, X., & Clarke, C., (1994). Effects of gestational exposure to monoamine oxidase inhibitors in rats: Preliminary behavioral and neurochemical studies. *Neuropsychopharmacology*, 11, 125–132.


## 7.4.9 TOLCAPONE

**FDA Category: C**
*Risk Summary:* It is better to be avoided during gestation because the pregnancy experience in humans is limited, and the reproduction studies in animals have shown the risk of fetal toxicity associated with the use of Tolcapone.

**Further Reading:**
- *Drug Information. Tasmar*. Roche Pharmaceuticals.

## 7.5 ANTIMIGRAINE DRUGS

### 7.5.1 ALMOTRIPTAN

**FDA Category: C**
***Risk Summary:*** It should be used with caution because the pregnancy experience in humans is limited and the reproduction studies in animals have
shown low risk.

**Further Reading:**
- *Drug Information. Axert*. Ortho-McNeil Pharmaceutical.
- Soldin, O. P., Dahlin, J., & O'Mara, D. M., (2008). Triptans in preg-
nancy. *Ther Drug Monit., 30*, 5–9.

### 7.5.2 DIHYDROERGOTAMINE

**FDA Category: X**
***Risk Summary:*** It is contraindicated during pregnancy. Safer alternatives
are available and they should be considered for the treatment of migraines
during pregnancy.

**Further Reading:**
- *Drug Information*. Migranal. Novartis Pharmaceuticals.
- Hohmann, M., & Künzel, W., (1992). Dihydroergotamine causes fetal
growth restriction in guinea pigs. *Arch Gynecol. Obstet., 251*, 187–192.

### 7.5.3 ELETRIPTAN

**FDA Category: C**
***Risk Summary:*** It should be used with caution because the pregnancy experience in humans is limited, and the reproduction studies in animals have
shown a moderate risk of reduced fetal weights.

**Further Reading:**
- *Drug Information. Relpax.* Pfizer.
- Soldin, O. P., Dahlin, J., & O'Mara, D. M., (2008). Triptans in pregnancy. *Ther Drug Monit, 30,* 5–9.

### 7.5.4   *ERGOTAMINE*

**FDA Category: X**
*Risk Summary:* It is contraindicated during pregnancy. Safer alternatives are available and they should be considered for the treatment of migraines during pregnancy.

**Further Reading:**
- De Groot, A. N. J. A., van Dongen, P. W. J., van Roosmalen, J., Eskes, T. K. A. B., (1993). Ergotamine-induced fetal stress: Review of side effects of ergot alkaloids during pregnancy. Eur J *Obstet. Gynecol., Reprod. Biol., 51,* 73–77.
- Hughes, H. E., & Goldstein, D. A., (1988). Birth defects following maternal exposure to ergotamine, beta-blockers, and caffeine. *J. Med. Genet., 25,* 396–399.

### 7.5.5   *FROVATRIPTAN*

**FDA Category: C**
*Risk Summary:* It should be used with caution because the pregnancy experience in humans is limited and the reproduction studies in animals have shown low risk.

**Further Reading:**
- *Drug Information. Frova.* Elan Biopharmaceuticals.
- Soldin, O. P., Dahlin, J., & O'Mara, D. M., (2008). Triptans in pregnancy. *Ther Drug Monit, 30,* 5–9.

### 7.5.6   *NARATRIPTAN*

**FDA Category: C**
*Risk Summary:* It should be used with caution because the pregnancy experience in humans is limited, and the reproduction studies in animals have shown a moderate risk of developmental toxicity.

**Further Reading:**
- Nez*valova-Henriksen*, K., *Spig*set, O., & Nordeng, H., (2010). Triptan exposure during pregnancy and the risk of major congenital malformations and adverse pregnancy outcomes: Results from the Norwegian Mother and Child Cohort Study. Headache, 50, 563–575.
- Pro Drug Information. Am*erge*. *GlaxoSmithKline*.
- Soldin, O. P., Dahlin, J., & O'Mara, D. M., (2008). Triptans in pregnancy. *Ther Drug Monit*, *30*, 5–9.

### 7.5.7  RIZATRIPTAN

**FDA Category: C**
***Risk Summary:*** It should be used with caution because the pregnancy experience in humans is limited, and the reproduction studies in animals have shown a moderate risk of reduced fetal weights.

**Further Reading:**
- *Pro Drug Information*. Maxalt. Merck.
- Soldin, O. P., Dahlin, J., & O'Mara, D. M., (2008). Triptans in pregnancy. *Ther Drug Monit*, *30*, 5–9.

### 7.5.8  SUMATRIPTAN

**FDA Category: C**
***Risk Summary:*** It should be used with caution because the pregnancy experience in humans is limited, and the reproduction studies in animals have shown a moderate risk of skeletal anomalies.

**Further Reading:**
- *Drug Information. Imitrex*. GlaxoSmithKline.
- Eldridge, R. E., & Ephross, S. A., (1997). Monitoring birth outcomes in the sumatriptan pregnancy registry (abstract). *Teratology*, *55*, 48.
- Soldin, O. P., Dahlin, J., & O'Mara, D. M., (2008). Triptans in pregnancy. *Ther Drug Monit*, *30*, 5–9.

## 7.5.9   *ZOLMITRIPTAN*

**FDA Category: C**
*Risk Summary:* It should be used with caution because the pregnancy experience in humans is limited and the reproduction studies in animals have shown a low risk of increased embryo lethality.

**Further Reading:**
- *Drug Information. Zomig.* AstraZeneca.
- Soldin, O. P., Dahlin, J., & O'Mara, D. M., (20085). Triptans in pregnancy. *Ther Drug Monit, 30,* 5–9.

## 7.6   CHOLINESTERASE INHIBITORS

### 7.6.1   *DONEPEZIL*

**FDA Category: C**
*Risk Summary:* It should be used with caution because the pregnancy experience in humans is limited and the reproduction studies in animals have shown low risk.

**Further Reading:**
- *Drug Information. Aricept.* Pfizer.

### 7.6.2   *GALANTAMINE*

**FDA Category: C**
*Risk Summary:* It should be used with caution because the pregnancy experience in humans is limited and the reproduction studies in animals have shown low risk.

**Further Reading:**
- *Drug Information. Razadyne.* Janssen Pharmaceutica Products.

## 7.6.3 RIVASTIGMINE

**FDA Category: C**
*Risk Summary:* It should be used with caution because the pregnancy experience in humans is limited and the reproduction studies in animals have shown low risk.

**Further Reading:**
- *Drug Information. Exelon.* Novartis Pharmaceuticals.

## 7.7 SEDATIVES AND HYPNOTICS

### 7.7.1 ALPRAZOLAM

**FDA Category: D**
*Risk Summary:* The use of Alprazolam during the in 1st and 3rd Trimesters should be avoided because the pregnancy experience in humans, and the reproduction studies in animals have shown an increased risk of congenital abnormalities, neonatal flaccidity and withdrawal symptoms.

**Further Reading:**
- Bergman, U., Rosa, F. W., Baum, C., Wiholm, B. E., & Faich, G. A., (1992). Effects of exposure to benzodiazepine during fetal life. *Lancet, 340,* 694–696.
- Rayburn, W., Gonzalez, C., & Christensen, D., (1995). Social interactions of C57BL/6 mice offspring exposed prenatally to alprazolam (Xanax) (abstract). *Am. J. Obstet. Gynecol., 172,* 389.
- St. Clair, S. M., & Schirmer, R. G., (1992). First-trimester exposure to alprazolam. *Obstet. Gynecol., 80,* 843–846.

### 7.7.2 AMOBARBITAL

**FDA Category: N**
*Risk Summary:* It should be used only when the maternal benefit outweighs the fetal risk because there is very limited human pregnancy data, and the animal studies are not relevant.

**Further Reading:**
- Draffan, G. H., Dollery, C. T., Davies, D. S., Krauer, B., Williams, F. M., Clare, R. A., Trudinger, B. J., Darling, M., Sertel, H., & Hawkins, D. F., (1976). Maternal and neonatal elimination of amobarbital after-treatment of the mother with barbiturates during late pregnancy. *Clin. Pharmacol. Ther, 19*, 271–275.
- Heinonen, O. P., Slone, D., & Shapiro, S., (1977). *Birth Defects and Drugs in Pregnancy*. Littleton, MA: Publishing Sciences Group.

## 7.7.3  BUSPIRONE

**FDA Category: B**
*Risk Summary:* Although Buspirone has been assigned with the letter (B), according to the FDA categorization, but it should be used with caution because no human data is available and the reproduction studies in animals have shown low risk.

**Further Reading:**
- *Drug Information. Buspar*. Mead Johnson Pharmaceuticals.
- Scanlan, F. J., (1972). The use of thioridazine (Mellaril) during the first trimester. *Med. J. Aust., 1*, 1271, 1272.

## 7.7.4  CHLORAL HYDRATE

**FDA Category: C**
*Risk Summary:* It should be used only when the maternal benefit outweighs the fetal risk because there is very limited human pregnancy data, and the animal studies are not relevant.

**Further Reading:**
- Bernstine, J. B., Meyer, A. E., & Hayman, H. B., (1954). Maternal and fetal blood estimation following the administration of chloral hydrate during labor. *J. Obstet. Gynecol., Br. Emp., 61*, 683–685.
- Heinonen, O. P., Slone, D., & Shapiro, S., (1977). *Birth Defects and Drugs in Pregnancy*. Littleton, MA: Publishing Sciences Group.

## 7.7.5 CHLORDIAZEPOXIDE

**FDA Category: N**
*Risk Summary:* The use of Chlordiazepoxide during the in 1st and 3rd Trimesters should be avoided because the pregnancy experience in humans, and the reproduction studies in animals have shown an increased risk of congenital abnormalities, neonatal flaccidity and withdrawal symptoms.

**Further Reading:**
- *Drug Information. Librium.* ICN Pharmaceuticals.
- Bergman, U., Rosa, F. W., Baum, C., Wiholm, B. E., & Faich, G. A., (1992). Effects of exposure to benzodiazepine during fetal life. *Lancet, 340,* 694–696.
- Duckman, S., Spina, T., Attardi, M., & Meyer, A., (1964). Double-blind study of chlordiazepoxide in obstetrics. *Obstet. Gynecol., 24,* 601–605.

## 7.7.6 CLORAZEPATE

**FDA Category: N**
*Risk Summary:* The use of Clorazepate should be avoided during the gestational period because the pregnancy experience in humans has shown an increased risk of congenital defects.

**Further Reading:**
- *Drug Information. Clorazepate Dipotassium.* Mylan Pharmaceuticals.
- Patel, D. A., & Patel, A. R., (1980). Clorazepate and congenital malformations. *JAMA, 244,* 135–136.

## 7.7.7 DIAZEPAM

**FDA Category: D**
*Risk Summary:* The use of Diazepam during the in 1st and 3rd Trimesters should be avoided because the pregnancy experience in humans, and the reproduction studies in animals have shown an increased risk of congenital abnormalities, neonatal flaccidity and withdrawal symptoms.

**Further Reading:**
- Bergman, U., Rosa, F. W., Baum, C., Wiholm, B. E., & Faich, G. A., (1992). Effects of exposure to benzodiazepine during fetal life. *Lancet 340*, 694–696.
- Saxen, I., & Saxen, L., (1975). Association between maternal intake of diazepam and oral clefts. *Lancet, 2*, 498.
- Scher, J., Hailey, D. M., & Beard, R. W., (1972). The effects of diazepam on the fetus. *J. Obstet. Gynaecol. Br. Commonw., 79*, 635–638.

### 7.7.8   DICHLORALPHENAZONE

**FDA Category: D**
*Risk Summary:* The reproduction studies in animals have shown no evidence of fetal harm or impaired fertility. The pregnancy experience in humans is limited.

**Further Reading:**
- Heinonen, O. P., Slone, D., & Shapiro, S., (1977). *Birth Defects and Drugs in Pregnancy*. Littleton, MA: Publishing Sciences Group.
- Lewis, P. J., & Friedman, L. A., (1979). Prophylaxis of neonatal jaundice with maternal antipyrine treatment. *Lancet, 1*, 300–3002.

### 7.7.9   ESTAZOLAM

**FDA Category: X**
*Risk Summary:* The use of Estazolam during the in 1st and 3rd Trimesters should be avoided because the pregnancy experience in humans, and the reproduction studies in animals, have shown an increased risk of congenital abnormalities, neonatal flaccidity and withdrawal symptoms.

**Further Reading:**
- Bergman, U., Rosa, F. W., Baum, C., Wiholm, B. E., & Faich, G. A., (1992). Effects of exposure to benzodiazepine during fetal life. *Lancet, 340*, 694–696.
- *Drug Information. ProSom*. Abbott Laboratories.

## 7.7.10   FLURAZEPAM

**FDA Category: X**
*Risk Summary:* It is better to be avoided in pregnancy because the pregnancy experience in humans is limited and the reproduction studies in animals have shown low risk.

**Further Reading:**
- Bergman, U., Rosa, F. W., Baum, C., Wiholm, B. E, & Faich, G. A., (1992). Effects of exposure to benzodiazepine during fetal life. *Lancet, 340,* 694–696.
- *Drug Information. Dalmane.* Roche Laboratories.

## 7.7.11   FOSPROPOFOL

**FDA Category: B**
*Risk Summary:* It should be used with caution because the pregnancy experience in humans is limited and the reproduction studies in animals have shown low risk.

**Further Reading:**
- *Drug Information. Lusedra.* Eisai.

## 7.7.12   LORAZEPAM

**FDA Category: D**
*Risk Summary:* The use of Lorazepam during the in 1st and 3rd Trimesters should be avoided because the pregnancy experience in humans, and the reproduction studies in animals have shown an increased risk of congenital abnormalities, neonatal flaccidity and withdrawal symptoms.

**Further Reading:**
- Bergman, U., Rosa, F. W., Baum, C., Wiholm, B. E., & Faich, G. A., (19992). Effects of exposure to benzodiazepine during fetal life. *Lancet, 340,* 694–696.
- *Drug Information. Ativan.* Wyeth-Ayerst Pharmaceuticals.

## 7.7.13   MEPROBAMATE

**FDA Category: N**
*Risk Summary:* It should be used with caution because the human pregnancy experience has shown a low risk.

**Further Reading:**
- Belafsky, H. A., Breslow, S., Hirsch, L. M., Shangold, J. E., & Stahl, M. B., (1969). Meprobamate during pregnancy. *Obstet. Gynecol., 34,* 378–386.
- *Drug Information.* Miltown. Wallace Laboratories.

## 7.7.14   MIDAZOLAM

**FDA Category: D**
*Risk Summary:* It is better to be avoided in pregnancy because the pregnancy experience in humans is limited and the reproduction studies in animals have shown low risk.

**Further Reading:**
- Bergman, U., Rosa, F. W., Baum, C., Wiholm, B. E., & Faich, G. A., (1992). Effects of exposure to benzodiazepine during fetal life. *Lancet, 340,* 694–696.
- *Drug Information.* Versed. Roche Laboratories.
- Kelly, L. E., Poon, S., Madadi, P., & Koren, G., (2012). Neonatal benzodiazepines exposure during breastfeeding. *J. Pediatr., 161,* 448–451.

## 7.7.15   OXAZEPAM

**FDA Category: N**
*Risk Summary:* The use of Oxazepam during the in 1st and 3rd Trimesters should be avoided because the pregnancy experience in humans, and the reproduction studies in animals have shown an increased risk of congenital abnormalities, neonatal flaccidity and withdrawal symptoms.

**Further Reading:**
- Bergman, U., Rosa, F. W., Baum, C., Wiholm, B. E., & Faich, G. A., (1992). Effects of exposure to benzodiazepine during fetal life. *Lancet, 340,* 694–696.
- Drury, K. A. D., Spalding, E., Donaldson, D., & Rutherford, D., (1977). Floppy-infant syndrome: Is oxazepam the answer? *Lancet, 2,* 1126, 1127.

## *7.7.16 PHENOBARBITAL*

**FDA Category: D**
*Risk Summary:* The use of Pentobarbital should be avoided in pregnant women because the pregnancy experience in humans has shown the risk of congenital defects associated with the use of this drug.

**Further Reading:**
- Gupta, C., Yaffe, S. J., & Shapiro, B. H., (1982). Prenatal exposure to phenobarbital permanently decreases testosterone and causes reproductive dysfunction. *Science, 216,* 640–642.
- Reinisch, J. M., Sanders, S. A., Mortensen, E. L., & Rubin, D. B., (1995). In utero exposure to phenobarbital and intelligence deficits in adult men. *JAMA, 274,* 1518–1525.
- Shankaran, S., Woldt, E., Nelson, J., Bedard, M., & Delaney-Black, V., (1996). Antenatal phenobarbital therapy and neonatal outcome II: Neurodevelopmental outcome at 36 months. *Pediatrics, 97,* 649–652.

## *7.7.17 PROPOFOL*

**FDA Category: B**
*Risk Summary:* It should be used with caution because the pregnancy experience in humans is limited and the reproduction studies in animals have shown low risk.

**Further Reading:**
- Dailland, P., Jacquinot, P., Lirzin, J. D., & Jorrot, J. C., (1989). Neonatal effects of propofol administered to the mother in anesthesia in cesarean section. *Can Anesthesiol., 37,* 429–433.
- *Drug Information. Diprivan.* AstraZeneca.

## 7.7.18   QUAZEPAM

**FDA Category: X**
*Risk Summary:* The use of Oxazepam during the in 1st and 3rd Trimesters should be avoided because the pregnancy experience in humans, and the reproduction studies in animals have shown an increased risk of congenital abnormalities, neonatal flaccidity and withdrawal symptoms.

**Further Reading:**
- *Drug Information. Doral.* Wallace Laboratories.

## 7.7.19   RAMELTEON

**FDA Category: C**
*Risk Summary:* It should be used with caution because the pregnancy experience in humans is limited and the reproduction studies in animals have shown low risk.

**Further Reading:**
- *Drug Information. Rozerem.* Takeda Pharmaceuticals North America.

## 7.7.20   TEMAZEPAM

**FDA Category: X**
*Risk Summary:* It is better to be avoided in pregnancy because the pregnancy experience in humans is limited and the reproduction studies in animals have shown the risk of increased resorptions associated with the use of Temazepam.

**Further Reading:**
- *Drug Information. Restoril.* Sandoz Pharmaceuticals Corp.

## 7.7.21   TRIAZOLAM

**FDA Category: X**
*Risk Summary:* It is better to be avoided in pregnancy because the pregnancy experience in humans is limited and the reproduction studies in animals have shown low risk.

**Further Reading:**
- Bergman, U., Rosa, F. W., Baum, C., Wiholm, B. E., & Faich, G. A., (1992). Effects of exposure to benzodiazepine during fetal life. *Lancet, 340,* 694–696.
- *Drug Information. Halcion.* Pharmacia & Upjohn.


## 7.7.22 ZALEPLON

**FDA Category: C**
*Risk Summary:* It should be used with caution because the human pregnancy experience has shown a low risk.

**Further Reading:**
- *Drug Information.* Sonata. Monarch Pharmaceuticals.
- Wikner, B. N., & Kallen, B., (2011). Are hypnotic benzodiazepine receptor agonists teratogenic in humans? *J. Clin. Psychopharmacol., 31,* 356–359.


## 7.7.23 ZOLPIDEM

**FDA Category: C**
*Risk Summary:* The use of Zolpidem should be avoided in pregnant women because the pregnancy experience in humans has shown the risk of low birth weights, preterm birth, and cesarean birth associated with the use of this drug.

**Further Reading:**
- Askew, J. P., (2007). Zolpidem addiction in a pregnant woman with a history of second-trimester bleeding. *Pharmacotherapy, 27,* 306–308.
- *Drug Information. Ambien.* G.D. Searle.
- Wang, L. H., Lin, H. C., Lin, C. C., Chen, Y. H., & Lin, H. C., (2010). Increased risk of adverse pregnancy outcomes in women receiving zolpidem during pregnancy. *Clin. Pharmacol. Ther, 88,* 369–374.

## 7.8   ANESTHETICS

### 7.8.1   *LOCAL ANESTHETICS*

#### 7.8.1.1   *BENZOCAINE*

**FDA Category: C**
*Risk Summary:* The reproduction studies in animals have shown no evidence of fetal harm or impaired fertility. The pregnancy experience in humans is limited.

**Further Reading:**
- Friedman, J. M., (1988). Teratogen update: Anesthetic agents. *Teratology, 37,* 69–77.

#### 7.8.1.2   *CAMPHOR*

**FDA Category: N**
*Risk Summary:* The reproduction studies in animals have shown no evidence of fetal harm or impaired fertility. The pregnancy experience in humans is adequate to exhibit that the embryo-fetal risk is nonexistent or very low.

**Further Reading:**
- Leuschner, J., (1997). Reproductive toxicity studies of D-Camphor in rats and rabbits. *Arzneim-Forsch/Drug Res., 47,* 124–128.

#### 7.8.1.3   *LIDOCAINE*

**FDA Category: B**
*Risk Summary:* The reproduction studies in animals have shown no evidence of fetal harm or impaired fertility. The pregnancy experience in humans is adequate to exhibit that the embryo-fetal risk is nonexistent or very low.

**Further Reading:**
- Abboud, T. K., David, S., Costandi, J., Nagappala, S., Haroutunian, S., & Yeh, S. Y., (1984). Comparative maternal, fetal and neonatal effects of lidocaine versus lidocaine with epinephrine in the parturient. *Anesthesiology, 61*(Suppl), A405.

- *Drug Information. Xylocaine.* AstraZeneca.

## 7.8.1.4   PRAMOXINE

**FDA Category: N**
***Risk Summary:*** The reproduction studies in animals have shown no evidence of fetal harm or impaired fertility. The pregnancy experience in humans is adequate to exhibit that the embryo-fetal risk is nonexistent or very low.

**Further Reading:**
- Friedman, J. M., (1988). Teratogen update: Anesthetic agents. *Teratology, 37*, 69–77.

## 7.8.1.5   ROPIVACAINE

**FDA Category: B**
***Risk Summary:*** The reproduction studies in animals have shown no evidence of fetal harm or impaired fertility. The pregnancy experience in humans is adequate to exhibit that the embryo-fetal risk is nonexistent or very low.

**Further Reading:**
- *Drug Information. Naropin.* AstraZeneca.
- McCrae, A. F., Jozwiak, H., & McClure, J. H., (1995). Comparison of ropivacaine and bupivacaine in extradural analgesia for the relief of pain in labor. *Br. J. Anaesth, 74*, 261–265.

## 7.8.1.6   TETRACAINE

**FDA Category: B**
***Risk Summary:*** The reproduction studies in animals have shown no evidence of fetal harm or impaired fertility. The pregnancy experience in humans is limited.

**Further Reading:**
- *Drug Information. Synera.* Endo Pharmaceuticals.
- Sweetman, S. C., (ed.) (2005). Tetracaine. *Martindale: The Complete Drug Reference*. (34th edn., p. 1385). London: Pharmaceutical Press.

## 7.8.2   *GENERAL ANESTHETICS*

### 7.8.2.1   *DESFLURANE*

**FDA Category: B**

***Risk Summary:*** It should be used with caution because the pregnancy experience in humans is limited and the reproduction studies in animals have shown low risk.

**Further Reading:**
- *Drug Information* (2002). Suprane. Baxter Healthcare Corporation, Anesthesia & Critical Care.
- Wallace, D. H., Armstrong, A., Darras, A., Gajraj, N., Gambling, D., & White, P., (1993). The effect of desflurane or low-dose enflurane on uterine tone at cesarean delivery: Placental transfer and recovery (abstract). *Anesthesiology*, *79*, A1019.

### 7.8.2.2   *ENFLURANE*

**FDA Category: B**

***Risk Summary:*** It should be used with caution because the pregnancy experience in humans is limited and the reproduction studies in animals have shown low risk.

**Further Reading:**
- Coleman, A. J., & Downing, J. W., (1975). Enflurane anesthesia for cesarean section. *Anesthesiology*, *43*, 354–357.
- *Drug Information*. *Ethrane*. Abbott Laboratories (NZ).
- Natsume, N., Miura, S., Sugimoto, S., Nakamura, T., Horiuchi, R., Kondo, S., Furukawa, H., Inagaki, S., Kawai, T., Yamada, M., Arai, T., & Hosoda, R., (1990). Teratogenicity caused by halothane, enflurane, and sevoflurane, and changes depending on O2 concentration (abstract). *Teratology*, *42*, 30A.

### 7.8.2.3   *HALOTHANE*

**FDA Category: C**

***Risk Summary:*** It should be used with caution because the pregnancy experience in humans is limited and the reproduction studies in animals have shown low risk.

**Further Reading:**
- *Drug Information. Halothane.* Abbott Laboratories.
- Puig, N. R., Amerio, N., Piaggio, E., Barragan, J., Comba, J. O., & Elena, G. A., (1999). Effects of halothane reexposure in female mice and their offspring. *Reprod. Toxicol., 13,* 361–367.
- Quail, A. W., (1989). Modern inhalational anesthetic agents. A review of halothane, isoflurane, and enflurane. *Med. J. Aust., 150,* 95–102.

## 7.8.2.4  ISOFLURANE

**FDA Category: C**
**Risk Summary:** It should be used with caution because the pregnancy experience in humans is limited and the reproduction studies in animals have shown low risk.

**Further Reading:**
- Abboud, T. K., Zhu, J., Richardson, M., Peres Da Silva, E., & Donovan, M., (1995). Intravenous propofol vs. thiamylal-isoflurane for cesarean section, comparative maternal and neonatal effects. *Acta Anaesthesiol. Scand., 39,* 205–209.
- Quail, A. W., (1989). Modern inhalational anesthetic agents. A review of halothane, isoflurane, and enflurane. *Med. J. Aust., 150,* 95–102.

## 7.8.2.5  KETAMINE

**FDA Category: N**
**Risk Summary:** It should be used with caution because the pregnancy experience in humans is limited and the reproduction studies in animals have shown low risk.

**Further Reading:**
- Baraka, A., Louis, F., & Dalleh, R., (1990). Maternal awareness and neonatal outcome after ketamine induction of anesthesia for cesarean section. *Can. J. Anaesth., 37,* 641–644.
- *Drug Information. Ketalar.* Parke-Davis.
- Eng, M., Bonica, J. J., Akamatsu, T. J., Berges, P. U., & Ueland, K., (1975). Respiratory depression in newborn monkeys at cesarean

section following ketamine administration. *Br. J. Anaesth., 47,* 917–921.
- Maleck, W., (1995). Ketamine and thiopentone in cesarean section. *Eur. J. Anaesthesiol., 12,* 533.

## 7.8.2.6   *METHOHEXITAL SODIUM*

**FDA Category: B**
***Risk Summary:*** It should be used with caution because the pregnancy experience in humans is limited and the reproduction studies in animals have shown low risk.

**Further Reading:**
- Anderson, E. L., & Reti, I. M., (2009). ECT in pregnancy: A review of the literature from 1941 to 2007. *Psychosom. Med., 71,* 235–242.
- *Drug Information. Brevital.* JHP Pharmaceuticals.

## 7.8.2.7   *NITROUS OXIDE*

**FDA Category: N**
***Risk Summary:*** The use of Nitrous Oxide should be avoided in pregnant women because the pregnancy experience in humans has shown an increased risk of spontaneous abortions (SABs), and decreased birth weight associated with the use of this drug.

**Further Reading:**
- Ahlborg, G. Jr., Axelsson, G., & Bodin, L., (1996). Shift work, nitrous oxide exposure, and subfertility among Swedish midwives. *Int. J. Epidemiol., 25,* 783–790.
- Jevtovic-Todorovic, V., Beals, J., Benshoff, N., & Olney, J. W., (2003). Prolonged exposure to inhalational anesthetic nitrous oxide kills neurons in adult rat brain. *Neuroscience, 122,* 609–616.
- Louis-Ferdinand, R. T., (1994). Myelotoxic, neurotoxic and reproductive adverse effects of nitrous oxide. *Adverse Drug React. Toxicol. Rev., 13,* 193–206.
- Rowland, A. S., Baird, D. D., Weinberg, C. R., Shore, D. L., Shy, C. M., & Wilcox, A. J., (1992). Reduced fertility among women

employed as dental assistants exposed to high levels of nitrous oxide. *N. Engl. J. Med., 327,* 993–997.

## 7.8.2.8 SEVOFLURANE

**FDA Category: B**
*Risk Summary:* It should be used with caution because the pregnancy experience in humans is limited and the reproduction studies in animals have shown low risk.

**Further Reading:**
- Kanazawa, M., Kinefuchi, Y., Suzuki, T., Fukuyama, H., & Takiguchi, M., (1999). The use of sevoflurane anesthesia during early pregnancy. *Tokai. J. Exp. Clin. Med., 24,* 53–55.
- Natsume, N., Miura, S., Sugimoto, S., Nakamura, T., Horiuchi, R., Kondo, S., Furukawa, H., Inagaki, S., Kawai, T., Yamada, M., Arai, T., & Hosoda, R., (1990). Teratogenicity caused by halothane, enflurane, and sevoflurane, and changes depending on O2 concentration (abstract). *Teratology., 42,* 30A.

## 7.9 SKELETAL MUSCLE RELAXANTS

### 7.9.1 ATRACURIUM

**FDA Category: C**
*Risk Summary:* The reproduction studies in animals have shown no evidence of fetal harm or impaired fertility. The pregnancy experience in humans is limited.

**Further Reading:**
- *Drug Information. Tracrium.* Glaxo Wellcome.
- Mouw, R. J. C., Hermans, J., Brandenburg, H. C. R., & Kanhai, H. H. H., (1997). Effects of pancuronium or atracurium on the anemic fetus during and directly after intrauterine transfusion (IUT): A double-blind randomized study (abstract). *Am. J. Obstet. Gynecol., 176,* S18.

### 7.9.2   BACLOFEN

**FDA Category: C**
***Risk Summary:*** It should be used with caution because the pregnancy experience in humans is limited and the reproduction studies in animals have shown low risk.

**Further Reading:**
- Ali Sakr Esa, W., Toma, I., Tetzlaff, J. E., & Barsoum, S., (2009). Epidural analgesia in labor for a woman with an intrathecal baclofen pump. *Int. J. Obstet. Anesth., 18*, 64–66.
- Briner, W., (1995). Muscimol—and baclofen-induced spina bifida in the rat. *Med. Sci. Res., 24*, 639, 640.
- *Drug Information. Lioresal Intrathecal.* Medtronic.

### 7.9.3   CARISOPRODOL

**FDA Category: C**
***Risk Summary:*** It should be used only when the maternal benefit outweighs the fetal risk because there is very limited human pregnancy data, and the animal studies are not relevant.

**Further Reading:**
- Briggs, G. G., Ambrose, P. J., Nageotte, M. P., & Padilla, G., (2008). High-dose carisoprodol during pregnancy and lactation. *Ann. Pharmacother., 42*, 898–901.
- *Drug Information. Soma.* Wallace Laboratories.

### 7.9.4   CHLORZOXAZONE

**FDA Category: N**
***Risk Summary:*** It should be used only when the maternal benefit outweighs the fetal risk because there is very limited human pregnancy data, and the animal studies are not relevant.

**Further Reading:**
- Briggs, G. G., & Freeman, R. K. (2015). Drugs *in Pregnancy and Lactation: A Reference Guide to Fetal and Neonatal Risk.* Philadelphia, PA: Lippincott Williams & Wilkins.

## 7.9.5   CYCLOBENZAPRINE

**FDA Category: B**
*Risk Summary:* Although Cyclobenzaprine has been assigned with the letter (B), according to the FDA categorization, but it should be used with caution because limited human data is available and the reproduction studies in animals have shown low risk.

**Further Reading:**
- *Drug Information. Flexeril.* Merck Sharpe & Dohme.

## 7.9.6   DANTROLENE

**FDA Category: C**
*Risk Summary:* It should be used only when the maternal benefit outweighs the fetal risk because there is very limited human pregnancy data, and the animal studies are not relevant.

**Further Reading:**
- *Drug Information. Dantrium.* Norwich Eaton Pharmaceuticals.
- Shime, J., Gare, D., Andrews, J., & Britt, B., (1988). Dantrolene in pregnancy: Lack of adverse effects on the fetus and newborn infant. *Am. J. Obstet. Gynecol., 159*, 831–834.

## 7.9.7   METAXALONE

**FDA Category: B**
*Risk Summary:* Although Metaxalone has been assigned with the letter (B), according to the FDA categorization, but it should be used with caution because limited human data is available and the reproduction studies in animals have shown low risk.

**Further Reading:**
- *Drug Information. Skelaxin.* Monarch Pharmaceuticals.

### 7.9.8  METHOCARBAMOL

**FDA Category: C**
*Risk Summary:* It should be used with caution because the human pregnancy experience has shown a low risk.

**Further Reading:**
- Briggs, G. G., & Freeman, R. K. (2015). *Drugs in Pregnancy and Lactation: A Reference Guide to Fetal and Neonatal Risk.* Philadelphia, PA: Lippincott Williams & Wilkins.
- Campbell, A. D., Coles, F. K., Eubank, L. L., & Huf, E. G., (1961). Distribution and metabolism of methocarbamol. *J. Pharmacol. Exp. Ther, 131,* 18–25.

### 7.9.9  ORPHENADRINE

**FDA Category: C**
*Risk Summary:* It should be used only when the maternal benefit outweighs the fetal risk because there is very limited human pregnancy data, and the animal studies are not relevant.

**Further Reading:**
- Briggs, G. G., & Freeman, R. K. (2015). *Drugs in Pregnancy and Lactation: A Reference Guide to Fetal and Neonatal Risk.* Philadelphia, PA: Lippincott Williams & Wilkins.

### 7.9.10  PANCURONIUM

**FDA Category: C**
*Risk Summary:* It should be used with caution because the pregnancy experience in humans is limited and the reproduction studies in animals have shown low risk.

**Further Reading:**
- Horvath, L., & Seeds, J. W., (1989). Temporary arrest of fetal movement with pancuronium bromide to enable antenatal magnetic resonance imaging of holoprosencephaly. *Am. J. Perinatol., 6,* 418–420.

- Spencer, J. A. D., Ronderos-Dumit, D., & Rodeck, C. H., (1994). The effect of neuromuscular blockade on human fetal heart rate and its variation. *Br. J. Obstet. Gynaecol., 101,* 121–124.

## 7.9.11  ROCURONIUM

**FDA Category: C**
***Risk Summary:*** It should be used with caution because the pregnancy experience in humans is limited and the reproduction studies in animals have shown low risk.

**Further Reading:**
- *Drug Information. Zemuron.* Organon USA.
- Kwan, W. F., Chen, B. J., & Liao, K. T., (1995). Rocuronium for cesarean section. *Br. J. Anaesth., 74,* 347.

## 7.9.12  SUCCINYLCHOLINE

**FDA Category: C**
***Risk Summary:*** The reproduction studies in animals have shown no evidence of fetal harm or impaired fertility. The pregnancy experience in humans is adequate to exhibit that the embryo-fetal risk is nonexistent or very low.

**Further Reading:**
- Baraka, A., Haroun, S., Bassili, M., & Abu-Haider, G., (1975). Response of the newborn to succinylcholine injection in homozygotic atypical mothers. *Anesthesiology* 1975 *43,* 115,116.
- *Drug Information. Anectine.* Glaxo Wellcome.

## 7.9.13  TIZANIDINE

**FDA Category: C**
***Risk Summary:*** It should be used with caution because the pregnancy experience in humans is limited, and the reproduction studies in animals have shown a risk of increased prenatal and postnatal pup mortality associated with the use of Tizanidine.

**Further Reading:**
- *Drug Information*. Zanaflex. Elan Biopharmaceuticals.


## 7.9.14   VECURONIUM

**FDA Category: C**
*Risk Summary:* It should be used only when the maternal benefit outweighs the fetal risk because there is very limited human pregnancy data, and the animal studies are not relevant.

**Further Reading:**
- Dailey, P. A., Fisher, D. M., Shnider, S. M., Baysinger, C. L., Shinohara, Y., Miller, R. D., Abboud, T. K., & Kim, K. C., (1982). Pharmacokinetics, placental transfer, and neonatal effects of vecuronium (ORG NC45) administered prior to delivery (abstract). *Anesthesiology, 57*, A391.
- *Drug Information*. Norcuron. Organon.
- Hawkins, J. L., Johnson, T. D., Kubicek, M. A., Skjonsby, B. S., Morrow, D. H., Joyce, T. H. III., (1990). Vecuronium for rapidsequence intubation for the Cesarean section. *Anesth. Analg., 71*, 185–190.


## 7.10   ANTICHOREA

## 7.10.1   TETRABENAZINE

**FDA Category: C**
*Risk Summary:* It should be used with caution because the pregnancy experience in humans is limited, and the reproduction studies in animals have shown moderate risk.

**Further Reading:**
- *Drug Information*. Xenazine. Lundbeck.
- Lubbe, W. F., & Walker, E. B., (1983). Chorea gravidarum associated with circulating lupus anticoagulant: Successful outcome of pregnancy with prednisone and aspirin therapy. Case report. *Br. J. Obstet. Gynaecol., 90*, 487–490.

## 7.11  POTASSIUM CHANNEL BLOCKER

### 7.11.1  *DALFAMPRIDINE*

**FDA Category: C**
***Risk Summary:*** It should be used with caution because the pregnancy experience in humans is limited, and the reproduction studies in animals have shown moderate risk.

**Further Reading:**
• *Drug Information. Ampyra.* Acorda Therapeutics.

## 7.12  MISCELLANEOUS

### 7.12.1  *RILUZOLE*

**FDA Category: C**
***Risk Summary:*** Although there is limited data from the human pregnancy experience, but the possible maternal benefit extremely outweighs the unknown or known embryo/fetal risk.

**Further Reading:**
• *Drug Information.* Rilutek. Sanofi-Aventi.
• Kawamichi, Y., Makino, Y., Matsuda, Y., Miyazaki, K., Uchiyama, S., & Ohta, H., (2010). Riluzole use during pregnancy in a patient with amyotrophic lateral sclerosis: A case report. *J. Int. Med. Res., 38,* 720–726.

## KEYWORDS

- **antichorea**
- **potassium channel blocker**
- **succinylcholine**
- **tetrabenazine**
- **tizanidine**
- **vecuronium**

# CHAPTER 8

# Drugs Affecting the Autonomic Nervous System

## 8.1 CHOLINERGIC DRUGS

### 8.1.1 BETHANECHOL

**FDA Category: C**
*Risk Summary:* It should be used only when the maternal benefit outweighs the fetal risk because there is very limited human pregnancy data, and the animal studies are not relevant.

**Further Reading:**
- *Drug Information*. Urecholine. Merck.

### 8.1.2 CARBACHOL

**FDA Category: C**
*Risk Summary:* It should be used only when the maternal benefit outweighs the fetal risk because there is very limited human pregnancy data, and the animal studies are not relevant.

**Further Reading:**
- Schaefer, C., Paul, P., & Richard, K. M., (2015). *Drugs During Pregnancy and Lactation Treatment Options and Risk Assessment*. Amsterdam: Elsevier.

### 8.1.3   CEVIMELINE

**FDA Category: C**
***Risk Summary:*** It should be used only when the maternal benefit outweighs the fetal risk because there is very limited human pregnancy data, and the animal studies are not relevant.

**Further Reading:**
- *Drug Information.* Evoxaca. Daiichi Pharmaceutical.

### 8.1.4   ECHOTHIOPHATE

**FDA Category: C**
***Risk Summary:*** It should be used only when the maternal benefit outweighs the fetal risk because there is very limited human pregnancy data, and the animal studies are not relevant.

**Further Reading:**
- Birks, D. A., & Prior, V. J., (1968). Echothiophate iodide treatment of glaucoma in pregnancy. *Arch Ophthal., 79*, 283–285.

### 8.1.5   EDROPHONIUM

**FDA Category: C**
***Risk Summary:*** It should be used with caution during the 1st and 2nd Trimesters. However, it is better to avoid the use of Edrophonium during the 3rd Trimester because fetal toxicity has been associated with its use during the last Trimester.

**Further Reading:**
- McNall, P. G., & Jafarnia, M. R., (1965). Management of myasthenia gravis in the obstetrical patient. *Am. J. Obstet. Gynecol., 92*, 518–525.
- Plauche, W. C., (1979). Myasthenia gravis in pregnancy: An update. *Am. J. Obstet. Gynecol., 135*, 691–697.

## 8.1.6 NEOSTIGMINE

**FDA Category: C**
*Risk Summary:* It should be used only when the maternal benefit outweighs the fetal risk because there is very limited human pregnancy data, and the animal studies are not relevant.

**Further Reading:**
- Lefvert, A. K., & Osterman, P. O., (1983). Newborn infants to myasthenic mothers: A clinical study and an investigation of acetylcholine receptor antibodies in 17 children. *Neurology, 33*, 133–138.
- Plauche, W. C., (1979). Myasthenia gravis in pregnancy: An update. *Am. J. Obstet. Gynecol., 135*, 691–697.

## 8.1.7 PHYSOSTIGMINE

**FDA Category: C**
*Risk Summary:* It should be used only when the maternal benefit outweighs the fetal risk because there is very limited human pregnancy data, and the animal studies are not relevant.

**Further Reading:**
- Plauche, W. C., (1979). Myasthenia gravis in pregnancy: An update. *Am. J. Obstet. Gynecol., 135*, 691–697.
- Smiller, B. G., Bartholomew, E. G., Sivak, B. J., Alexander, G. D., & Brown, E. M., (1973). Physostigmine reversal of scopolamine delirium in obstetric patients. *Am. J. Obstet. Gynecol., 116*, 326–329.

## 8.1.8 PILOCARPINE

**FDA Category: C**
*Risk Summary:* The reproduction studies in animals have shown no evidence of fetal harm or impaired fertility. The pregnancy experience in humans is limited.

**Further Reading:**
- *Drug Information. Salagen.* MGI Pharma.
- Plauche, W. C., (1979). Myasthenia gravis in pregnancy: An update. *Am. J. Obstet. Gynecol., 135*, 691–697.

## *8.1.9  PYRIDOSTIGMINE*

**FDA Category: C**

*Risk Summary:* It should be used with caution because the pregnancy experience in humans is limited and the reproduction studies in animals have shown low risk.

**Further Reading:**

- Levine, B. S., & Parker, R. M., (1991). Reproductive and developmental toxicity studies of pyridostigmine bromide in rats. *Toxicology, 69*, 291–300.
- Plauche, W. C., (1979). Myasthenia gravis in pregnancy: An update. *Am. J. Obstet. Gynecol., 135*, 691–697.

## 8.2  ANTICHOLINERGIC DRUGS

### *8.2.1  ATROPINE*

**FDA Category: C**

*Risk Summary:* It should be used with caution because the human pregnancy experience has shown a low risk of a decrease in fetal breathing associated with the administration of Atropine.

**Further Reading:**

- Abboud, T., Raya, J., Sadri, S., Grobler, N., Stine, L., & Miller, F., (1983). Fetal and maternal cardiovascular effects of atropine and glycopyrrolate. *Anesth. Analg., 62*, 426–430.
- Roodenburg, P. J., Wladimiroff, J. W., & Van Weering, H. K., (1979). Effect of maternal intravenous administration of atropine (0.5 mg) on fetal breathing and heart pattern. *Contrib. Gynecol. Obstet., 6*, 92–97.

### *8.2.2  BELLADONNA*

**FDA Category: C**

*Risk Summary:* It should be used only when the maternal benefit outweighs the fetal risk because there is very limited human pregnancy data, and the animal studies are not relevant.

**Further Reading:**

- Freeman, J. J., Altieri, R. H., Baptiste, H. J., Kuo, T., Crittenden, S., Fogarty, K., Moultrie, M., Coney, E., & Kanegis, K., (1994). Evaluation and management of sialorrhea of pregnancy with concomitant hyperemesis. *J. Natl. Med. Assoc., 86*, 704–708.

### 8.2.3 BENZTROPINE

**FDA Category: N**
*Risk Summary:* It should be used only when the maternal benefit outweighs the fetal risk because there is very limited human pregnancy data, and the animal studies are not relevant.

**Further Reading:**

- Gossell-Williams, M., Fletcher, H., & Zeisel, S. H., (2008). Unexpected depletion in plasma choline and phosphatidylcholine concentrations in a pregnant woman with the bipolar affective disorder being treated with lithium, haloperidol, and benztropine: A case report. *J. Med. Case Rep., 2*, 55. doi: 10.1186/1752-1947-2-55.

### 8.2.4 CLIDINIUM

**FDA Category: N**
*Risk Summary:* It should be used only when the maternal benefit outweighs the fetal risk because there is very limited human pregnancy data, and the animal studies are not relevant.

**Further Reading:**

- Heinonen, O. P., Slone, D., & Shapiro, S., (1977). *Birth Defects and Drugs in Pregnancy* (pp. 346–353). Littleton, MA: Publishing Sciences Group.

### 8.2.5 DICYCLOMINE

**FDA Category: B**
*Risk Summary:* The reproduction studies in animals have shown no evidence of fetal harm or impaired fertility. The pregnancy experience in humans is adequate to exhibit that the embryo-fetal risk is nonexistent or very low.

**Further Reading:**
- *Drug Information. Bentyl.* Marion Merrell Dow, Inc.
- Friedman, J. M., Little, B. B., Brent, R. L., Cordero, J. F., Hanson, J. W., & Shepard, T. H., (1990). Potential human teratogenicity of frequently prescribed drugs. *Obstet. Gynecol., 75,* 594–599.

## 8.2.6   GLYCOPYRROLATE

**FDA Category: B**
*Risk Summary:* It should be used only when the maternal benefit outweighs the fetal risk because there is very limited human pregnancy data, and the animal studies are not relevant.

**Further Reading:**
- Abboud, T. K., Read, J., Miller, F., Chen, T., Valle, R., & Henriksen, E. H., (1981). Use of glycopyrrolate in the parturient: Effect on the maternal and fetal heart and uterine activity. *Obstet. Gynecol., 57,* 224–227.
- Chamchad, D., Horrow, J. C., Nakhamchik, L., Sauter, J., Roberts, N., Aronzon, B., Gerson, A., & Medved, M., (2011). Prophylactic glyco-pyrrolate prevents bradycardia after spinal anesthesia for cesarean section: A randomized, double-blind, placebo-controlled prospective trial with heart rate variability correlation. *J. Clin. Anesth., 23,* 361–366.

## 8.2.7   HOMATROPINE

**FDA Category: C**
*Risk Summary:* It should be used only when the maternal benefit outweighs the fetal risk because there is very limited human pregnancy data, and the animal studies are not relevant.

**Further Reading:**
- Heinonen, O. P., Slone, D., & Shapiro, S., (1977). *Birth Defects and Drugs in Pregnancy.* Littleton, MA: Publishing Sciences Group.

## 8.2.8   L-HYOSCYAMINE

**FDA Category: C**
*Risk Summary:* It should be used only when the maternal benefit outweighs the fetal risk because there is very limited human pregnancy data, and the animal studies are not relevant.

**Further Reading:**
- Heinonen, O. P., Slone, D., & Shapiro, S., (1977). *Birth Defects and Drugs in Pregnancy*. Littleton, MA: Publishing Sciences Group.

## 8.2.9   MEPENZOLATE

**FDA Category: B**
*Risk Summary:* It should be used only when the maternal benefit outweighs the fetal risk because there is very limited human pregnancy data, and the animal studies are not relevant.

**Further Reading:**
- Heinonen, O. P., Slone, D., & Shapiro, S., (1977). *Birth Defects and Drugs in Pregnancy*. Littleton, MA: Publishing Sciences Group.

## 8.2.10   METHSCOPOLAMINE

**FDA Category: C**
*Risk Summary:* It should be used only when the maternal benefit outweighs the fetal risk because there is very limited human pregnancy data, and the animal studies are not relevant.

**Further Reading:**
- Heinonen, O. P., Slone, D., & Shapiro, S., (1977). *Birth Defects and Drugs in Pregnancy*. Littleton, MA: Publishing Sciences Group.

## 8.2.11   *PROPANTHELINE*

**FDA Category: C**
*Risk Summary:* It should be used only when the maternal benefit outweighs the fetal risk because there is very limited human pregnancy data, and the animal studies are not relevant.

**Further Reading:**
- Heinonen, O. P., Slone, D., & Shapiro, S., (1977). *Birth Defects and Drugs in Pregnancy*. Littleton, MA: Publishing Sciences Group.

## 8.2.12   *SCOPOLAMINE*

**FDA Category: C**
*Risk Summary:* It should be used with caution because the human pregnancy experience has shown a low risk.

**Further Reading:**
- Boehm, F. H., Growdon, J. H. Jr., (1974). The effect of scopolamine on fetal heart rate baseline variability. *Am. J. Obstet. Gynecol., 120,* 1099–1104.
- *Drug Information. Transderm Scop.* Novartis Consumer Health.
- Evens, R. P., & Leopold, J. C., (1980). Scopolamine toxicity in a newborn. *Pediatrics, 66,* 329, 330.

## 8.2.13   *TRIHEXYPHENIDYL*

**FDA Category: C**
*Risk Summary:* It should be used only when the maternal benefit outweighs the fetal risk because there is very limited human pregnancy data, and the animal studies are not relevant.

**Further Reading:**
- Heinonen, O. P., Slone, D., & Shapiro, S., (1977). *Birth Defects and Drugs in Pregnancy*. Littleton, MA: Publishing Sciences Group.

## 8.3 ANTIADRENERGIC DRUGS

### *8.3.1 ACEBUTOLOL*

**FDA Category: B**

*Risk Summary:* Although Acebutolol has been assigned with the letter (B), according to the FDA categorization, but it should be used with caution because the human data is limited, and the reproduction studies in animals have shown low risk. Nevertheless, Acebutolol has Intrinsic Sympathomimetic activity, and it is expected that Acebutolol has lower fetal risks than other β-Blockers (see Atenolol and Nadolol) that lack this property.

**Further Reading:**
- *Drug Information.* Lopressor. CibaGeneva Pharmaceuticals.
- Ghanem, F. A., & Movahed, A., (2008). Use of antihypertensive drugs during pregnancy and lactation. *Cardiovascular Drug Reviews, 26*(1), 38–49.
- Kaaja, R., Hiilesmaa, V., Holma, K., & Jarvenpaa, A. L., (1992). Maternal antihypertensive therapy with beta-blockers associated with poor outcome in very low birth weight infants. *Int. J. Gynecol. Obstet., 38*, 195–199.

### *8.3.2 ATENOLOL*

**FDA Category: D**

*Risk Summary:* Atenolol is not a teratogen; however, its use during the 2nd and 3rd Trimesters is discouraged because its administration, during this period, has been linked with the incidence of reduced placental weight, and intrauterine growth restriction (IUGR).

**Further Reading:**
- *Drug Information. Tenormin.* Zeneca Pharmaceuticals.
- Lardoux, H., Gerard, J., Blazquez, G., Chouty, F., & Flouvat, B., (1983). Hypertension in pregnancy: Evaluation of two beta-blockers atenolol and labetalol. *Eur Heart J., 4*(Suppl G), 35–40.
- Woods, D. L., & Morrell, D. F., (1982). Atenolol: Side effects in a newborn infant. *Br. Med. J., 285*, 691–692.

### 8.3.3  BETAXOLOL

**FDA Category: C**
*Risk Summary:* It is not a teratogen; however, its use during the 2nd and 3rd Trimesters is discouraged because its administration, during this period, has been linked with the incidence of reduced placental weight, and IUGR.

**Further Reading:**
- Boutroy, M. J., Morselli, P. L., Bianchetti, G., Boutroy, J. L., Pepin, L., & Zipfel, A., (1990). Betaxolol: A pilot study of its pharmacological and therapeutic properties in pregnancy. Eur. *J. Clin. Pharmacol., 38*, 535–539.
- *Drug Information.* Kerlone. G.D. Searle & Co.

### 8.3.4  BISOPROLOL

**FDA Category: C**
*Risk Summary:* It is not a teratogen; however, its use during the 2nd and 3rd Trimesters is discouraged because its administration, during this period, has been linked with the incidence of reduced placental weight, and IUGR.

**Further Reading:**
- *Drug Information. Zebeta.* Lederle Laboratories.

### 8.3.5  CARTEOLOL

**FDA Category: C**
*Risk Summary:* It is not a teratogen; however, its use during the 2nd and 3rd Trimesters is discouraged because its administration, during this period, has been linked with the incidence of reduced placental weight, and IUGR.

**Further Reading:**
- *Drug Information. Cartrol.* Abbott Laboratories.
- Tamagawa, M, Namoto, T., Tanaka, N., & Hishino, H., (1979). Reproduction study of carteolol hydrochloride in mice, part 2. Perinatal and postnatal toxicity. *J. Toxicol. Sci., 4*, 59–78.

## 8.3.6   CARVEDILOL

**FDA Category: C**
*Risk Summary:* It should be used with caution because the human pregnancy experience is very limited. However, it is plausible to expect that Carvedilol has the same kind of problems associated with the use of β-Blockers during pregnancy.

**Further Reading:**
- *Drug Information. Coreg.* GlaxoSmithKline.

## 8.3.7   DIHYDROERGOTAMINE

**FDA Category: X**
*Risk Summary:* It is contraindicated during pregnancy. Safer alternatives are available and they should be considered for the treatment of migraines during pregnancy.

**Further Reading:**
- *Drug Information. Migranal.* Novartis Pharmaceuticals.
- Hohmann, M., & Künzel, W., (1992). Dihydroergotamine causes fetal growth restriction in guinea pigs. *Arch Gynecol. Obstet., 251,* 187–192.

## 8.3.8   DOXAZOSIN

**FDA Category: C**
*Risk Summary:* It is better to be avoided during the 1st Trimester because the pregnancy experience in humans is limited and the reproduction studies in animals have shown low risk.

**Further Reading:**
- Accessdata.Fda.Gov. (2015). https://www.accessdata.fda.gov/drug-satfda_docs/label/2009/019668s021lbl.pdf (accessed on 12 February 2020).
- *Drug Information.* Cardura. Pfizer.

- Pirtskhalava, N., (2012). Pheochromocytoma and pregnancy: Complications and solutions (case report). *Georgian Med News*, 208–209, 76–82.

## 8.3.9  ERGOTAMINE

**FDA Category: X**
***Risk Summary:*** It is contraindicated during pregnancy. Safer alternatives are available and they should be considered for the treatment of migraines during pregnancy.

**Further Reading:**
- De Groot, A. N. J. A., van Dongen, P. W. J., van Roosmalen, J., & Eskes, T. K. A. B., (1993). Ergotamine-induced fetal stress: Review of side effects of ergot alkaloids during pregnancy. *Eur. J. Obstet. Gynecol., Reprod Biol., 51,* 73–77.
- Hughes, H. E., & Goldstein, D. A., (1988). Birth defects following maternal exposure to ergotamine, beta-blockers, and caffeine. *J. Med. Genet., 25,* 396–399.

## 8.3.10  ESMOLOL

**FDA Category: C**
***Risk Summary:*** Although there is limited data from the human pregnancy experience, but the possible maternal benefit extremely outweighs the unknown or known embryo/fetal risk.

**Further Reading:**
- Ducey, J. P., & Knape, K. G., (1992). Maternal esmolol administration resulting in fetal distress and cesarean section in a term pregnancy. *Anesthesiology, 77,* 829–832.
- Gilson, G. J., Knieriem, K. J., Smith, J. F., Izquierdo, L., Chatterjee, M. S., & Curet, L. B., (1992). Short-acting beta-adrenergic blockade and the fetus. A case report. *J. Reprod. Med., 37,* 277–279.
- Losasso, T. J., Muzzi, D. A., & Cucchiara, R. F., (1991). Response of fetal heart rate to maternal administration of esmolol. *Anesthesiology, 74,* 782–784.

## 8.3.11 GUANETHIDINE

**FDA Category: C**
*Risk Summary:* It should be used with caution because the pregnancy experience in humans is limited and the reproduction studies in animals have shown low risk.

**Further Reading:**
- Bartolome, J., Bartolome, M., Seidler, F. J., Anderson, T. R., & Slotkin, T. A., (1976). Effects of early postnatal guanethidine administration on adrenal medulla and brain of developing rats. *Biochem. Pharmacol., 25*, 2387–2390.
- *Drug Information.* Ismelin. Ciba Pharmaceutical.
- Liuzzi, A., Foppen, F. H., & Angeletti, P. U., (1974). Adrenaline, noradrenaline and dopamine levels in brain and heart after administration of 6-hydroxydopamine and guanethidine to newborn mice. *Biochem. Pharmacol., 23*, 1041–1044.

## 8.3.12 GUANFACINE

**FDA Category: B**
*Risk Summary:* It should be used with caution because the pregnancy experience in humans is limited and the reproduction studies in animals have shown low risk.

**Further Reading:**
- *Drug Information. Tenex.* A.H. Robins Company.
- Philipp, E., (1980). Guanfacine in the treatment of hypertension due to pre-eclamptic toxemia in thirty women. *Br. J. Clin. Pharmacol., 10*(Suppl 1), 137S–140S.

## 8.3.13 LABETALOL

**FDA Category: C**
*Risk Summary:* It should be used with caution because the human pregnancy experience has shown a low risk.

**Further Reading:**
- *Drug Information. Normodyne.* Schering.
- Nylund, L., Lunell, N. O., Lewander, R., Sarby, B., & Thornstrom, S., (1984). Labetalol for the treatment of hypertension in pregnancy. *Acta Obstet. Gynecol., Scand,* 118(Suppl), 71–73.
- Plouin, P. F., Breart, G., Maillard, F., Papiernik, E., Relier, J. P., (1988). Comparison of antihypertensive efficacy and perinatal safety of labetalol and methyldopa in the treatment of hypertension in pregnancy: A randomized controlled trial. *Br. J. Obstet. Gynaecol., 95,* 868–876.

### 8.3.14   METOPROLOL

**FDA Category: C**
***Risk Summary:*** Metoprolol is not a teratogen; however, its use during the 2nd and 3rd Trimesters is discouraged because its administration, during this period, has been linked with the incidence of reduced placental weight and IUGR.

**Further Reading:**
- *Drug Information.* Lopressor. CibaGeneva Pharmaceuticals.
- Lindeberg, S., Sandstrom, B., Lundborg, P., & Regardh, C. G., (1984). Disposition of the adrenergic blocker metoprolol in the late-pregnant woman, the amniotic fluid, the cord blood, and the neonate. *Acta Obstet. Gynecol., Scand, 118*(Suppl), 61–64.
- Lundborg, P., Agren, G., Ervik, M., Lindeberg, S., & Sandstrom, B., (1981). Disposition of metoprolol in the newborn. *Br. J. Clin. Pharmacol., 12,* 598–600.
- Sandstrom, B., (1978). Antihypertensive treatment with the adrenergic beta-receptor blocker metoprolol during pregnancy. *Gynecol. Invest, 9,* 195–204.

### 8.3.15   NADOLOL

**FDA Category: C**
***Risk Summary:*** Nadolol is not a teratogen; however, its use during the 2nd and 3rd Trimesters is discouraged because its administration, during this

period, has been linked with the incidence of reduced placental weight and IUGR.

**Further Reading:**
- *Drug Information.* Corgard. Bristol Laboratories.
- Fox, R. E., Marx, C., & Stark, A. R., (1985). Neonatal effects of maternal nadolol therapy. *Am. J. Obstet. Gynecol., 152*, 1045–1046.
- Saegusa, T., Suzuki, T., & Narama, I., (1983). Reproduction studies of nadolol a new β-adrenergic blocking agent. *Yakuri to Chiryo, 11*, 5119–5138. As cited in: Shepard, T. H., & Lemire, R. J., (eds.). Catalog of Teratogenic Agents. (12th edn., p. 304). Baltimore, MD: The Johns Hopkins University Press, 2007.


## *8.3.16 NEBIVOLOL*

**FDA Category: C**
*Risk Summary:* It is not a teratogen; however, its use during the 2nd and 3rd Trimesters is discouraged because its administration, during this period, has been linked with the incidence of reduced placental weight, and IUGR.

**Further Reading:**
- *Drug Information. Bystolic.* Forest Pharmaceuticals.


## *8.3.17 PENBUTOLOL*

**FDA Category: C**
*Risk Summary:* It is not a teratogen; however, its use during the 2nd and 3rd Trimesters is discouraged because its administration, during this period, has been linked with the incidence of reduced placental weight, and IUGR.

**Further Reading:**
- *Drug Information. Levatol.* Schwarz Pharma.
- Sugisaki, T., Takagi, S., Seshimo, M., Hayashi, S., & Miyamoto, M., (1981). Reproductive studies of penbutolol sulfate given orally to mice. *Oyo Yakuri, 22*, 289–305. As cited in: Shepard, T. H., (1989). *Catalog of Teratogenic Agents* (6th edn., p. 487). Baltimore, MD: The Johns Hopkins University Press.

## 8.3.18  *PINDOLOL*

**FDA Category: C**
*Risk Summary:* Pindolol is not a teratogen; however, its use during the 2nd and 3rd Trimesters is discouraged because its administration, during this period, has been linked with the incidence of reduced placental weight and IUGR.

**Further Reading:**
- *Drug Information. Visken.* Sandoz Pharmaceuticals.
- Ghanem, F. A., & Movahed, A., (2008). Use of antihypertensive drugs during pregnancy and lactation. *Cardiovascular Drug Reviews, 26*(1), 38–49.
- Montan, S., Ingemarsson, I., Marsal, K., & Sjoberg, N. O., (1992). Randomized controlled trial of atenolol and pindolol in human pregnancy: Effects on fetal hemodynamics. *Br. Med. J., 304*, 946–949.
- Tuimala, R., & Hartikainen-Sorri, A. L., (1988). Randomized comparison of atenolol and pindolol for treatment of hypertension in pregnancy. *Curr. Ther. Res., 44*, 579–584.

## 8.3.19  *PRAZOSIN*

**FDA Category: C**
*Risk Summary:* It is better to be avoided during the 1st Trimester because the pregnancy experience in humans is limited and the reproduction studies in animals have shown low risk.

**Further Reading:**
- Bourget, P., Fernandez, H., Edouard, D., Lesne-Hulin, A., Ribou, F., Baton-Saint-Mleux, C., & Lelaidier, C., (1995). Disposition of a new rate-controlled formulation of prazosin in the treatment of hypertension during pregnancy: Transplacental passage of prazosin. *Eur. J. Drug. Metab. Pharmacokinet., 20*, 233–241.
- *Drug Information.* Minipress. Pfizer.
- Venuto, R., Burstein, P., & Schneider, R., (1984). Pheochromocytoma: Antepartum diagnosis and management with tumor resection in the puerperium. *Am. J. Obstet. Gynecol., 150*, 431, 432.

## 8.3.20   PROPRANOLOL

**FDA Category: C**
*Risk Summary:* Propranolol is not a teratogen; however, its use during the 2nd and 3rd Trimesters is discouraged because its administration, during this period, has been linked with the incidence of reduced placental weight and IUGR.

**Further Reading:**
- Barnes, A. B., (1970). Chronic propranolol administration during pregnancy: A case report. *J. Reprod. Med., 5*, 79–80.
- Fiddler, G. I., (1974). Propranolol and pregnancy. *Lancet, 2*, 722–723.
- Pruyn, S. C., Phelan, J. P., & Buchanan, G. C., (1979). Long-term propranolol therapy in pregnancy: Maternal and fetal outcome. *Am. J. Obstet. Gynecol., 135*, 485–489.

## 8.3.21   SOTALOL

**FDA Category: B**
*Risk Summary:* Although Sotalol has been assigned with the letter (B), according to the FDA categorization, but it should be used with caution because the human data is limited, and the reproduction studies in animals have shown low risk.

**Further Reading:**
- *Drug Information.* Betapace. Berlex Laboratories.
- Oudijk, M. A., Michon, M. M., Kleinman, C. S., Kapusta, L., Stoutenbeek, P., Visser, G. H. A., & Meijboom, E. J., (2000). Sotalol in the treatment of fetal dysrhythmias. *Circulation, 101*, 2721–2726.
- Wagner, X., Jouglard, J., Moulin, M., Miller, A. M., Petitjean, J., & Pisapia, A., (1990). Coadministration of flecainide acetate and sotalol during pregnancy: Lack of teratogenic effects, passage across the placenta, and excretion in human breast milk. *Am. Heart J., 119*, 700–702.

## 8.3.22   TIMOLOL

**FDA Category: C**
*Risk Summary:* Timolol is not a teratogen; however, its use during the 2nd and 3rd Trimesters is discouraged because its administration, during this

period, has been linked with the incidence of reduced placental weight and IUGR.

**Further Reading:**
- *Drug Information*. Blocadren. Merck.
- Devoe, L. D., O'Dell, B. E., Castillo, R. A., Hadi, H. A., & Searle, N., (1986). Metastatic pheochromocytoma in pregnancy and fetal biophysical assessment after maternal administration of alpha-adrenergic, beta-adrenergic, and dopamine antagonists. *Obstet. Gynecol., 68*, 15S–18S.
- Ghanem, F. A., & Movahed, A., (2008). Use of Antihypertensive Drugs during Pregnancy and Lactation. *Cardiovascular Drug Reviews, 26*(1), 38–49.
- Wagenvoort, A. M., Van Vugt, J. M. G., Sobotka, M., & Van Geijn, H. P., (1998). Topical timolol therapy in pregnancy: Is it safe for the fetus? *Teratology, 58*, 258–262.


## 8.4   ADRENERGIC DRUGS

### *8.4.1   ALBUTEROL*

**FDA Category: C**

*Risk Summary:* The reproduction studies in animals have shown no evidence of fetal harm or impaired fertility. The pregnancy experience in humans is adequate to exhibit that the embryo-fetal risk is nonexistent or very low.

**Further Reading:**
- *Drug Information. Albuterol Sulfate Inhalant*. Actavis Mid Atlantic.
- Kuhn, R. J. P., Speirs, A. L., Pepperell, R. J., Eggers, T. R., Doyle, L. W., & Hutchison, A., (1982). Betamethasone, albuterol, and threatened premature delivery: Benefits and risks. Study of 469 pregnancies. *Obstet. Gynecol., 60*, 403–408.
- Rayburn, W. F., Atkinson, B. D., Gilbert, K. A., & Turnbull, G. L., (1994). Acute effects of inhaled albuterol (Proventil) on fetal hemodynamics (abstract). *Teratology, 49*, 370.

## 8.4.2 DOBUTAMINE

**FDA Category: B**
*Risk Summary:* It should be used with caution because the pregnancy experience in humans is limited and the reproduction studies in animals have shown low risk.

**Further Reading:**
- *Drug Information.* Dobutrex. Eli Lilly and Company.
- Graves, C., Wheeler, T., & Troiano, N., (1996). The effect of dobutamine hydrochloride on ventricular function and oxygen transport in patients with severe preeclampsia (abstract). *Am. J. Obstet. Gynecol., 174,* 332.

## 8.4.3 DOPAMINE

**FDA Category: C**
*Risk Summary:* Although there is limited data from the human pregnancy experience, but the possible maternal benefit extremely outweighs the unknown or known embryo/fetal risk.

**Further Reading:**
- Fishburne, J. I. Jr., Dormer, K. J., Payne, G. G., Gill, P. S., Ashrafzadeh, A. R., & Rossavik, I. K., (1988). Effects of amrinone and dopamine on uterine blood flow and vascular responses in the gravid baboon. *Am. J. Obstet. Gynecol., 158,* 829–837.
- Nasu, K., Yoshimatsu, J., Anai, T., & Miyakawa, I., (1996). Lose-dose dopamine in treating acute renal failure caused by preeclampsia. *Gynecol. Obstet. Invest., 42,* 140,141.

## 8.4.4 EPHEDRINE

**FDA Category: C**
*Risk Summary:* The reproduction studies in animals have shown no evidence of fetal harm or impaired fertility. The pregnancy experience in humans is adequate to exhibit that the embryo-fetal risk is nonexistent or very low.

**Further Reading:**

- Datta, S., Alper, M. H., Ostheimer, G. W., & Weiss, J. B., (1982). Method of ephedrine administration and nausea and hypotension during spinal anesthesia for cesarean section. *Anesthesiology, 56,* 68–70.
- Shepard, T. H., (1980). *Catalog of Teratogenic Agents* (3rd edn., pp. 134, 135). Baltimore, MD: The Johns Hopkins University Press.
- Wright, R. G., Shnider, S. M., Levinson, G., Rolbin, S. H., & Parer, J. T., (1981). The effect of maternal administration of ephedrine on fetal heart rate and variability. *Obstet. Gynecol., 57,* 734–738.

## 8.4.5  EPINEPHRINE

**FDA Category: C**
*Risk Summary:* It should be used with caution because the human pregnancy experience has shown a low risk.

**Further Reading:**

- Entman, S. S., & Moise, K. J., (1984). Anaphylaxis in pregnancy. *S. Med. J., 77,* 402.
- Nishimura, H., & Tanimura, T., (1976). *Clinical Aspects of the Teratogenicity of Drugs* (p. 231). New York, NY: American Elsevier.
- Shepard, T. H., (1980). *Catalog of Teratogenic Agents* (3rd edn., pp. 134, 135). Baltimore, MD: The Johns Hopkins University Press.

## 8.4.6  ISOPROTERENOL

**FDA Category: C**
*Risk Summary:* The pregnancy experience in humans is limited, and the reproduction studies in animals have shown moderate risk.

**Further Reading:**

- DeSimone, C. A., Leighton, B. L., Norris, M. C., Chayen, B., & Menduke, H., (1988). The chronotropic effect of isoproterenol is reduced in term pregnant women. *Anesthesiology, 69,* 626–8.
- Entman, S. S., & Moise, K. J., (1984). Anaphylaxis in pregnancy. *S. Med. J., 77,* 402.

- Nishimura, H., & Tanimura, T., (1976). *Clinical Aspects of the Teratogenicity of Drugs* (p. 231). New York, NY: American Elsevier.
- Shepard, T. H., (1980). *Catalog of Teratogenic Agents* (3rd edn., pp. 134, 135). Baltimore, MD: The Johns Hopkins University Press.

## *8.4.7 ISOXSUPRINE*

**FDA Category: C**
*Risk Summary:* It should be used only when the maternal benefit outweighs the fetal risk because there is very limited human pregnancy data, and the animal studies are not relevant.

**Further Reading:**
- Allen, H. H., Short, H., & Fraleigh, D. M., (1965). The use of isoxsuprine in the management of premature labor. *Appl. Ther., 7*, 544–547.
- Brazy, J. E., Little, V., Grimm, J., & Pupkin, M., (1981). Risk: benefit considerations for the use of isoxsuprine in the treatment of premature labor. *Obstet. Gynecol., 58*, 297–303.

## *8.4.8 NOREPINEPHRINE*

**FDA Category: C**
*Risk Summary:* The use of Norepinephrine should be avoided in pregnant women because the pregnancy experience in humans has shown the risk of fetal hypoxia associated with the use of this drug.

**Further Reading:**
- Pitel, M., & Lerman, S., (1962). Studies on the fetal rat lens. Effects of intrauterine adrenalin and noradrenalin. *Invest. Ophthalmol., 1*, 406–412. As cited in: Shepard, T. H., (ed). Catalog of Teratogenic Agents (9th edn., p. 340). Baltimore, MD: The Johns Hopkins University Press, 1998.
- Smith, N. T., & Corbascio, A. N., (1970). The use and misuse of pressor agents. *Anesthesiology, 33*, 58–101.
- Stevens, A. D., & Lumbers, E. R., (1995). Effects of intravenous infusions of noradrenaline into the pregnant ewe on uterine blood flow, fetal renal function, and lung liquid flow. *Can. J. Physiol. Pharmacol., 73*, 202–208.

## 8.4.9   OXYMETAZOLINE

**FDA Category: N**
*Risk Summary:* It should be used only when the maternal benefit outweighs the fetal risk because there is limited human pregnancy data, and the animal studies are not relevant.

**Further Reading:**
- Rayburn, W. F., Anderson, J. C., Smith, C. V., Appel, L. L., & Davis, S. A., (1990). Uterine and fetal Doppler flow changes from a single dose of a long-acting intranasal decongestant. *Obstet. Gynecol., 76,* 180–182.
- Baxi, L. V., Gindoff, P. R., Pregenzer, G. J., & Parras, M. K., (1985). Fetal heart rate changes following maternal administration of a nasal decongestant. *Am. J. Obstet. Gynecol., 153,* 799–800.

## 8.4.10   PHENYLEPHRINE

**FDA Category: C**
*Risk Summary:* The use of Phenylephrine should be avoided in pregnant women because the pregnancy experience in humans has shown the risk of fetal hypoxia associated with the use of this drug.

**Further Reading:**
- Kallen, B. A. J., & Olausson, P. O., (2006). Use of oral decongestants during pregnancy and delivery outcome. *Am. J. Obstet. Gynecol., 194,* 480–485.
- Shepard, T. H., (1980). *Catalog of Teratogenic Agents* (3rd edn., p. 134, 135). Baltimore, MD: The Johns Hopkins University Press.
- Smith, N. T., & Corbascio, A. N., (1970). The use and misuse of pressor agents. *Anesthesiology, 33,* 58–101.

## 8.4.11   PSEUDOEPHEDRINE

**FDA Category: C**
*Risk Summary:* The use of Pseudoephedrine should be avoided in pregnant women because the pregnancy experience in humans has shown a low risk of fetal gastroschisis and small intestinal atresia after exposure to Pseudo-ephedrine during the 1st trimester.

**Further Reading:**

- Kallen, B. A. J., & Olausson, P. O., (2006). Use of oral decongestants during pregnancy and delivery outcome. *Am. J. Obstet. Gynecol., 194*, 480–485.
- Werler, M. M., Mitchell, A. A., & Shapiro, S., (1992). First-trimester maternal medication use in relation to gastroschisis. *Teratology, 45*, 361–367.

## 8.4.12  TERBUTALINE

**FDA Category: C**
***Risk Summary:*** The reproduction studies in animals have shown no evidence of fetal harm or impaired fertility. The pregnancy experience in humans is limited.

**Further Reading:**

- *Drug Information. Brethine.* Novartis Pharmaceuticals.
- Haller, D. L., (1980). The use of terbutaline for premature labor. *Drug Intell. Clin. Pharm., 14*, 757–764.
- Mendez-Bauer, C., Shekarloo, A., Cook, V., & Freese, U., (1987). Treatment of acute intrapartum fetal distress by β2-sympathomimetics. *Am. J. Obstet. Gynecol., 156*, 638–642.
- Suzuki, M., Inagaki, K., Kihira, M., Matsuzawa, K., Ishikawa, K., & Ishizuka, T., (1985). Maternal liver impairment associated with prolonged high-dose administration of terbutaline for premature labor. *Obstet. Gynecol., 66*, 14S–15S.

## KEYWORDS

- **intrauterine growth restriction**
- **isoproterenol**
- **norepinephrine**
- **oxymetazoline**
- **phenylephrine**
- **pseudoephedrine**

# CHAPTER 9

# Drugs Affecting the Gastrointestinal System

## 9.1 ANTACIDS

### 9.1.1 CALCIUM CARBONATE

**FDA Category: N**

*Risk Summary:* The reproduction studies in animals have shown no evidence of fetal harm or impaired fertility. The pregnancy experience in humans is adequate to exhibit that the embryo-fetal risk is nonexistent or very low.

**Further Reading:**
- Kleinman, G. E., Rodriquez, H., Good, M. C., & Caudle, M. R., (1991). Hypercalcemic crisis in pregnancy associated with excessive ingestion of calcium carbonate antacid (milk-alkali syndrome): Successful treatment with hemodialysis. *Obstet. Gynecol., 78,* 496–499.
- Thomas, M., & Weisman, S. M., (2006). Calcium supplementation during pregnancy and lactation: Effects on the mother and fetus. *Am. J. Obstet. Gynecol., 194,* 937–945.

### 9.1.2 SODIUM BICARBONATE

**FDA Category: C**

*Risk Summary:* It should be used with caution because the pregnancy experience in humans is limited and the reproduction studies in animals have shown a low risk of increased structural anomalies.

**Further Reading:**
- Khera, K. S., (1991). Chemically induced alterations in maternal homeostasis and histology of conceptus: Their etiologic significance in rat fetal anomalies. *Teratology, 44*, 259–297.
- Nakatsuka, T., Fujikake, N., Hasebe, M., & Ikeda, H., (1993). Effects of sodium bicarbonate and ammonium chloride on the incidence of a furosemide-induced fetal skeletal anomaly, wavy rib, in rats. *Teratology, 48*, 139–147.


## 9.2 ANTIDIARRHEAL DRUGS

### 9.2.1 ALOSETRON

**FDA Category: B**
*Risk Summary:* Although Alosetron has been assigned with the letter (B), according to the FDA categorization, but it should be used with caution because limited human data is available and the reproduction studies in animals have shown low risk.

**Further Reading:**
- *Drug Information*. Lotronex. GlaxoSmithKline.


### 9.2.2 BISMUTH SUBSALICYLATE

**FDA Category: N**
*Risk Summary:* It is better to be avoided after the second half of the gestation because the human pregnancy experience has shown a low risk.

**Further Reading:**
- Friedman, J. M., Little, B. B., Brent, R. L., Cordero, J. F., Hanson, J. W., & Shepard, T. H., (1990). Potential human teratogenicity of frequently prescribed drugs. *Obstet. Gynecol., 75*, 594–599.
- Hasking, G. J., & Duggan, J. M., (1982). Encephalopathy from bismuth subsalicylate. *Med. J. Aust., 2*, 167.

### 9.2.3 CROFELEMER

**FDA Category: C**
*Risk Summary:* The reproduction studies in animals have shown no evidence of fetal harm or impaired fertility. The pregnancy experience in humans is limited.

**Further Reading:**
- *Drug Information. Fulyzaq.* Salix Pharmaceuticals.


### 9.2.4 DIPHENOXYLATE

**FDA Category: C**
*Risk Summary:* It should be used with caution because the pregnancy experience in humans is limited and the reproduction studies in animals have shown low risk.

**Further Reading:**
- *Drug Information. Lomotil.* G.D. Searle and Company.
- Stewart, J. J., (1981). Gastrointestinal drugs. In: Wilson, J. T., (ed.) *Drugs in Breast Milk* (p. 71). Balgowlah, Australia: ADIS Press.


### 9.2.5 KAOLIN/PECTIN

**FDA Category: C**
*Risk Summary:* The reproduction studies in animals have shown no evidence of fetal harm or impaired fertility. The pregnancy experience in humans is limited.

**Further Reading:**
- Patterson, E. C., & Staszak, D. J., (1977). Effects of geophagia (kaolin ingestion) on the maternal blood and embryonic development in the pregnant rat. *J Nutr., 107*, 2020–2025.
- Mengel, C. E., Carter, W. A., & Horton, E. S., (1964). Geophagia with iron deficiency and hypokalemia: Cachexia africana. *Arch Intern. Med., 114*, 470–474.

### 9.2.6  LOPERAMIDE

**FDA Category: C**

*Risk Summary:* It should be used with caution because the pregnancy experience in humans is limited and the reproduction studies in animals have shown low risk.

**Further Reading:**
- *Drug Information. Imodium.* McNeil Consumer.


## 9.3  ANTIEMETIC DRUGS

### 9.3.1  ALOSETRON

**FDA Category: B**

*Risk Summary:* Although Alosetron has been assigned with the letter (B), according to the FDA categorization, but it should be used with caution because limited human data is available and the reproduction studies in animals have shown low risk.

**Further Reading:**
- *Drug Information. Lotronex.* GlaxoSmithKline.

### 9.3.2  APREPITANT

**FDA Category: B**

*Risk Summary:* It should be used with caution because the pregnancy experience in humans is limited and the reproduction studies in animals have shown low risk.

**Further Reading:**
- *Drug Information. Emend.* Merck.

### 9.3.3  CYCLIZINE

**FDA Category: B**

*Risk Summary:* The reproduction studies in animals have shown no evidence of fetal harm or impaired fertility. The pregnancy experience in humans is adequate to exhibit that the embryo-fetal risk is nonexistent or very low.

## Further Reading:
- Milkovich, L., & Van den Berg, B. J., (1976). An evaluation of the teratogenicity of certain antinauseant drugs. *Am. J. Obstet. Gynecol., 125*, 244–248.
- Nelson, M. M., & Forfar, J. O., (1971). Associations between drugs administered during pregnancy and congenital abnormalities of the fetus. *Br. Med. J., 1*, 523–527.

### 9.3.4   DIMENHYDRINATE

**FDA Category: B**
*Risk Summary:* The reproduction studies in animals have shown no evidence of fetal harm or impaired fertility. The pregnancy experience in humans is adequate to exhibit that the embryo-fetal risk is nonexistent or very low.

## Further Reading:
- Scott, R. S., Wallace, K. H., Badley, D. N., & Watson, B. H., (1962). Use of dimenhydrinate in labor. *Am. J. Obstet. Gynecol., 83*, 25–28.
- Watt, L. O., (1961). Oxytocic effects of dimenhydrinate in obstetrics. *Can. Med. Assoc. J., 84*, 533, 534.

### 9.3.5   DOLASETRON

**FDA Category: B**
*Risk Summary:* It should be used with caution because the pregnancy experience in humans is limited and the reproduction studies in animals have shown low risk.

## Further Reading:
- *Drug Information. Anzemet.* Aventis Pharmaceuticals.

### 9.3.6   DOXYLAMINE

**FDA Category: A**
*Risk Summary:* The reproduction studies in animals have shown no evidence of fetal harm or impaired fertility. The pregnancy experience in

humans is adequate to exhibit that the embryo-fetal risk is nonexistent or very low.

**Further Reading:**
- Milkovich, L., & van den Berg, B. J., (1976). An evaluation of the teratogenicity of certain antinauseant drugs. *Am. J. Obstet. Gynecol., 125*, 244–248.
- Shapiro, S., Heinonen, O. P., Siskind, V., Kaufman, D. W., Monson, R. R., & Slone, D., (1977). Antenatal exposure to doxylamine succinate and dicyclomine hydrochloride (Bendectin) in relation to congenital malformations, perinatal mortality rate, birth weight, intelligence quotient score. *Am. J. Obstet. Gynecol., 128*, 480–485.

## 9.3.7 DRONABINOL

**FDA Category: C**
*Risk Summary:* It should be used with caution because the pregnancy experience in humans is limited and the reproduction studies in animals have shown low risk.

**Further Reading:**
- *Drug Information*. Marinol. Abbott Laboratories.
- Farooq, M. U., Ducommun, E., & Goudreau, J., (2009). Treatment of a hyperkinetic movement disorder during pregnancy with dronabinol. *Parkinsonism. Relat. Disord., 15*, 249–251.

## 9.3.8 DROPERIDOL

**FDA Category: C**
*Risk Summary:* The reproduction studies in animals have shown no evidence of fetal harm or impaired fertility. The pregnancy experience in humans is adequate to exhibit that the embryo-fetal risk is nonexistent or very low.

**Further Reading:**
- *Drug Information*. Inapsine. Akorn.
- Nageotte, M. P., Briggs, G. G., Towers, C. V., & Asrat, T., (1996). Droperidol and diphenhydramine in the management of hyperemesis gravidarum. *Am. J. Obstet. Gynecol., 174*, 1801–1806.

## 9.3.9 GRANISETRON

**FDA Category: B**
*Risk Summary:* It should be used with caution because the pregnancy experience in humans is limited and the reproduction studies in animals have shown low risk.

**Further Reading:**
- *Drug Information.* Kytril. SmithKline Beecham Pharmaceuticals.
- Merimsky, O., Le Chevalier, T., Missenard, G., Lepechoux, C., Cojean-Zelek, I., Mesurolle, B., Le & Cesne, A., (1999). Management of cancer in pregnancy: A case of Ewing's sarcoma of the pelvis in the third trimester. *Ann. Oncol., 10,* 345–350.

## 9.3.10 MECLIZINE

**FDA Category: B**
*Risk Summary:* The reproduction studies in animals have shown no evidence of fetal harm or impaired fertility. The pregnancy experience in humans is adequate to exhibit that the embryo-fetal risk is nonexistent or very low.

**Further Reading:**
- *Drug Information.* Antivert. Pfizer.
- Shapiro, S., Kaufman, D. W., Rosenberg, L., Slone, D., Monson, R. R., Siskind, V., & Heinonen, O. P., (1978). Meclizine in pregnancy in relation to congenital malformations. *Br. Med. J., 1,* 483.
- Yerushalmy, J., & Milkovich, L., (1965). Evaluation of the teratogenic effect of meclizine in man. *Am. J. Obstet. Gynecol., 93,* 553–562.

## 9.3.11 METOCLOPRAMIDE

**FDA Category: B**
*Risk Summary:* The reproduction studies in animals have shown no evidence of fetal harm or impaired fertility. The pregnancy experience in humans is adequate to exhibit that the embryo-fetal risk is nonexistent or very low.

**Further Reading:**
- Guikontes, E., Spantideas, A., & Diakakis, J., (1992). Ondansetron and hyperemesis gravidarum. *Lancet, 340,* 1223.
- Messinis, I. E., Lolis, D. E., Dalkalitsis, N., Kanaris, C., & Souvat-zoglou, A., (1982). Effect of metoclopramide on maternal and fetal prolactin secretion during labor. *Obstet. Gynecol., 60,* 686–688.
- Sorensen, H. T., Nielsen, G. L., Christensen, K., Tage-Jensen, U., Ekborn, A., & Baron, J., (2000). and the Euromap study group. Birth outcome following maternal use of metoclopramide. *Br. J. Clin. Pharmacol., 49,* 264–268.

### 9.3.12   ONDANSETRON

**FDA Category: B**
*Risk Summary:* It is better to be avoided during the 1st Trimester because the pregnancy experience in humans has shown a low risk of birth defects associated with the use of Ondansetron.

**Further Reading:**
- Andersen, J. T., Jimenez-Solem, E., Andersen, N. L., et al., (2014). Ondansetron use in early pregnancy and the risk of congenital malformations—a registry-based nationwide control study. International Society of Pharmaco-epidemiology. Montreal, Canada; 2013. Abstract 25, Pregnancy Session 1. As cited in: Koren, G., (ed.). Scary science: Ondansetron safety in pregnancy—two opposing results from the same Danish registry. *Ther. Drug Monit., 36,* 1–2.
- *Drug Information. Zofran.* GlaxoSmithKline.
- Pasternak, B., Svanstrom, H., & Hviid, A., (2013). Ondansetron in pregnancy and risk of adverse fetal outcomes. *NEJM, 368,* 814–823.

### 9.3.13   PALONOSETRON

**FDA Category: B**
*Risk Summary:* It should be used with caution because the pregnancy expe-rience in humans is limited and the reproduction studies in animals have shown low risk.

**Further Reading:**
- *Drug Information. Aloxi.* MGI Pharma.

### 9.3.14 PROCHLORPERAZINE

**FDA Category: N**
*Risk Summary:* The reproduction studies in animals have shown no evidence of fetal harm or impaired fertility. The pregnancy experience in humans is adequate to exhibit that the embryo-fetal risk is nonexistent or very low.

**Further Reading:**
- Farag, R. A., & Ananth, J., (1978). Thanatophoric dwarfism associated with prochlorperazine administration. *N Y State J. Med., 78,* 279–282.
- Rafla, N., (1987). Limb deformities associated with prochlorperazine. *Am. J. Obstet. Gynecol., 156,* 1557.

### 9.3.15 PROMETHAZINE

**FDA Category: C**
*Risk Summary:* The reproduction studies in animals have shown no evidence of fetal harm or impaired fertility. The pregnancy experience in humans is adequate to exhibit that the embryo-fetal risk is nonexistent or very low.

**Further Reading:**
- Charles, A. G., & Blumenthal, L. S., (1982). Promethazine hydrochloride therapy in severely Rh-sensitized pregnancies. *Obstet. Gynecol., 60,* 627–630.
- Vella, L., Francis, D., Houlton, P., & Reynolds, F., (1985). Comparison of the antiemetics metoclopramide and promethazine in labor. *Br. Med. J., 290,* 1173–1175.

### 9.3.16 TRIMETHOBENZAMIDE

**FDA Category: N**
*Risk Summary:* It should be used with caution because the human pregnancy experience has shown low embryo-fetal risk.

**Further Reading:**
- *Drug Information. Tigan.* Roberts Pharmaceutical.
- Milkovich, L., & van den Berg, B. J., (1976). An evaluation of the teratogenicity of certain antinauseant drugs. *Am. J. Obstet. Gynecol., 125,* 244–248.

## 9.4   ANTIFLATULENTS

### 9.4.1   SIMETHICONE

**FDA Category: N**
***Risk Summary:*** The reproduction studies in animals have shown no evidence of fetal harm or impaired fertility. The pregnancy experience in humans is adequate to exhibit that the embryo-fetal risk is nonexistent or very low.

**Further Reading:**
- Briggs, G., Freeman, R., Towers, C., & Forninash, A., (2017). Drugs in pregnancy and lactation: A reference guide to fetal and neonatal risk. Philadelphia, Pa: Wolters Kluwer Health.

## 9.5   ANTI-INFLAMMATORY BOWEL DISEASE DRUGS

### 9.5.1   BALSALAZIDE

**FDA Category: B**
***Risk Summary:*** Although there is limited data from the human pregnancy experience, but the possible maternal benefit extremely outweighs the unknown or known embryo/fetal risk.

**Further Reading:**
- *Drug Information. Colazal.* Salix Pharmaceuticals.
- Schroeder, K. W., (2002). Role of mesalazine in the acute and long-term treatment of ulcerative colitis and its complications. *Scand. J. Gastroentrol. Suppl., 236,* 42–47.

## 9.5.2 INFLIXIMAB

**FDA Category: B**
*Risk Summary:* Although there is limited data from the human pregnancy experience, but the possible maternal benefit extremely outweighs the unknown or known embryo/fetal risk.

**Further Reading:**
- El Mourabet, M., El-Hachem, S., Harrison, J. R., & Binion, D. G., (2010). Anti-TNF antibody therapy for inflammatory bowel disease during pregnancy: A clinical review. *Curr Drug Targets,* 234–241.
- Gisbert, J. P., (2010). Safety of immunomodulators and biologics for the treatment of inflammatory bowel disease during pregnancy and breast-feeding. *Inflamm. Bowel Dis., 16,* 881–895.

## 9.5.3 MESALAMINE

**FDA Category: B**

**\* FDA Category: C (For the Delayed-Release Dosage form—Asacol®)**
*Risk Summary:* The reproduction studies in animals have shown no evidence of fetal harm or impaired fertility. The pregnancy experience in humans is adequate to exhibit that the embryo-fetal risk is nonexistent or very low.

*\*Dibutyl phthalate is an inactive excipient in Asacol's enteric coating. High doses of Dibutyl phthalate, given to pregnant rats was associated with increased incidences of developmental abnormalities in the offspring.

**Further Reading:**
- Diav-Citrin, O., Park, Y. H, Veerasuntharam, G., Polachek, H., Bologa, M., Pastuszak, A., & Koren, G., (1998). The safety of mesa-lamine in human pregnancy: A prospective controlled cohort study. *Gastroenterology., 114,* 23–28.
- *Drug Information. Asacol.* Procter & Gamble Pharmaceuticals.
- *Drug Information. Pentasa.* Hoechst Marion-Roussel Inc.

### 9.5.4  OLSALAZINE

**FDA Category: C**
**Risk Summary:** It should be used with caution because the pregnancy experience in humans is limited and the reproduction studies in animals have shown low risk.

**Further Reading:**
- *Drug Information. Dipentum.* Pharmacia & Upjohn.
- Segars, L. W., & Gales, B. J., (1992). Mesalamine and olsalazine: 5-aminosalicylic acid agents for the treatment of inflammatory bowel disease. *Clin. Pharm., 11,* 514–528.

### 9.5.5  SULFASALAZINE

**FDA Category: B**
**Risk Summary:** Although Sulfasalazine has been assigned with the letter (B) by the FDA categorization, however, it should be used with caution because the available human data have shown a low risk of congenital malformations.

**Further Reading:**
- Craxi, A., & Pagliarello, F., (1980). Possible embryotoxicity of sulfasalazine. *Arch Intern. Med., 140,* 1674.
- Hoo, J. J., Hadro, T. A., & Von Behren, P., (1988). Possible teratogenicity of sulfasalazine. *N. Engl. J. Med., 318,* 1128.
- Mogadam, M., Dobbins, W. O. III., Korelitz, B. I., & Ahmed, S. W., (1981). Pregnancy in inflammatory bowel disease: Effect of sulfasalazine and corticosteroids on fetal outcome. *Gastroenterology, 80,* 72–76.

## 9.6  ANTI-SECRETORY DRUGS

### 9.6.1  H2-RECEPTOR ANTAGONISTS

#### 9.6.1.1  CIMETIDINE

**FDA Category: B**
**Risk Summary:** The reproduction studies in animals have shown no evidence of fetal harm or impaired fertility. The pregnancy experience in humans is adequate to exhibit that the embryo-fetal risk is nonexistent or very low.

**Further Reading:**
- *Drug Information. Tagamet.* SmithKline Beecham Pharmaceuticals.
- Ruigomez, A., Rodriguez, L. A. G., Cattaruzzi, C., Troncon, M. G., Agostinis, L., Wallander, M. A., & Johansson, S., (1999). Use of cimetidine, omeprazole, and ranitidine in pregnant women and pregnancy outcomes. *Am. J. Epidemiol, 150,* 476–481.
- Shapiro, B. H., Hirst, S. A., Babalola, G. O., & Bitar, M. S., (1988). Prospective study on the sexual development of male and female rats perinatally exposed to maternally administered cimetidine. *Toxicol. Lett., 44,* 315–329.

## 9.6.1.2  FAMOTIDINE

**FDA Category: B**
***Risk Summary:*** The reproduction studies in animals have shown no evidence of fetal harm or impaired fertility. The pregnancy experience in humans is adequate to exhibit that the embryo-fetal risk is nonexistent or very low.

**Further Reading:**
- Dehlink, E., Yen, E., Leichtner, A. M., Hait, E. J., & Fiebiger, E., (2009). First evidence of a possible association between gastric acid suppression during pregnancy and childhood asthma: A population-based register study. *Clin. Exp. Allergy, 39,* 246–253.
- *Drug Information. Pepcid.* Merck Sharp & Dohme.
- Magee, L. A., Inocencion, G., Kamboj, L., Rosetti, F., & Koren, G., (1996). Safety of first-trimester exposure to histamine H2 blockers. A prospective cohort study. *Dig. Dis. Sci., 41,* 1145–1149.

## 9.6.1.3  NIZATIDINE

**FDA Category: B**
***Risk Summary:*** It should be used with caution because the pregnancy experience in humans is limited and the reproduction studies in animals have shown low risk.

**Further Reading:**
- *Drug Information.* Nizatidine. Genpharm.

- Neubauer, B. L., Goode, R. L., Best, K. L., Hirsch, K. S., Lin, T. M., Pioch, R. P., Probst, K. S., Tinsley, F. C., & Shaar, C. J., (1990). Endocrine effects of new histamine H2-receptor antagonist, nizatidine (LY139037), in the male rat. *Toxicol. Appl. Pharmacol., 102,* 219–232.
- Gill, S. K., O'Brien, L., & Koren, G., (2009). The safety of histamine 2 (H2) blockers in pregnancy: A meta-analysis. *Dig. Dis. Sci., 54,* 1835–1838.

## 9.6.1.4   RANITIDINE

**FDA Category: B**
***Risk Summary:*** The reproduction studies in animals have shown no evidence of fetal harm or impaired fertility. The pregnancy experience in humans is adequate to exhibit that the embryo-fetal risk is nonexistent or very low.

**Further Reading:**
- *Drug Information. Zantac.* Glaxo Wellcome.
- Gill, S. K., O'Brien, L., & Koren, G., (2009). The safety of histamine 2 (H2) blockers in pregnancy: A meta-analysis. *Dig. Dis. Sci., 54,* 1835–1838.

## 9.6.2   PROTON PUMP INHIBITORS

### 9.6.2.1   DEXLANSOPRAZOLE

**FDA Category: B**
***Risk Summary:*** It should be used with caution because the pregnancy experience in humans is limited and the reproduction studies in animals have shown low risk.

**Further Reading:**
- Dehlink, E., Yen, E., Leichtner, A. M., Hait, E. J., & Fiebiger, E., (2009). First evidence of a possible association between gastric acid suppression during pregnancy and childhood asthma: A population-based register study. *Clin. Exp. Allergy, 39,* 246–253.
- *Drug Information.* Kapidex. Takeda Pharmaceuticals America.

- Gill, S. K., O'Brien, L., Einarson, T. R., & Koren, G., (2009). The safety of proton pump inhibitors (PPIs) in pregnancy: A meta-analysis. *Am. J. Gastroenterol., 104*, 1541–1545.

### 9.6.2.2 *ESOMEPRAZOLE*

**FDA Category: C**
***Risk Summary:*** It should be used with caution because the pregnancy experience in humans, and animals, have shown low risk.

**Further Reading:**
- Dehlink, E., Yen, E., Leichtner, A. M., Hait, E. J., & Fiebiger, E., (2009). First evidence of a possible association between gastric acid suppression during pregnancy and childhood asthma: A population-based register study. *Clin. Exp. Allergy, 39*, 246–253.
- *Drug Information. Nexium.* AstraZeneca.
- Gill, S. K., O'Brien, L., Einarson, T. R., & Koren, G., (2009). The safety of proton pump inhibitors (PPIs) in pregnancy: A meta-analysis. *Am. J. Gastroenterol., 104*, 1541–1545.

### 9.6.2.3 *LANSOPRAZOLE*

**FDA Category: B**
***Risk Summary:*** It should be used with caution because the pregnancy experience in humans, and animals, have shown low risk.

**Further Reading:**
- Dehlink, E., Yen, E., Leichtner, A. M., Hait, E. J., & Fiebiger, E., (2009). First evidence of a possible association between gastric acid suppression during pregnancy and childhood asthma: A population-based register study. *Clin. Exp. Allergy, 39*, 246–253.
- *Drug Information. Prevacid.* Tap Pharmaceuticals.
- Gill, S. K., O'Brien, L., Einarson, T. R., & Koren, G., (2009). The safety of proton pump inhibitors (PPIs) in pregnancy: A meta-analysis. *Am. J. Gastroenterol., 104*, 1541–1545.
- Mayer, A., Sheiner, E., & Holcherg, G., (2007). Zollinger Ellison syndrome, treated with lansoprazole, during pregnancy. *Arch Gynecol. Obstet., 276*, 171–173.

## 9.6.2.4   OMEPRAZOLE

**FDA Category: C**
***Risk Summary:*** It should be used with caution because the pregnancy experience in humans, and animals, have shown low risk.

**Further Reading:**
- Dehlink, E., Yen, E., Leichtner, A. M., Hait, E. J., & Fiebiger, E., (2009). First evidence of a possible association between gastric acid suppression during pregnancy and childhood asthma: A population-based register study. *Clin. Exp. Allergy, 39*, 246–53.
- *Drug Information*. Prilosec. AstraZeneca.
- Matok, I., Levy, A., Wiznitzer, A., Uziel, E., Koren, G., & Gorodischer, R., (2012). The safety of fetal exposure to proton-pump inhibitors during pregnancy. *Dig. Dis. Sci., 57*, 699–705.

## 9.6.2.5   PANTOPRAZOLE

**FDA Category: C**
***Risk Summary:*** It should be used with caution because the pregnancy experiences in humans and animals have shown low risk.

**Further Reading:**
- Dehlink, E., Yen, E., Leichtner, A. M., Hait, E. J., & Fiebiger, E., (2009). First evidence of a possible association between gastric acid suppression during pregnancy and childhood asthma: A population-based register study. *Clin. Exp. Allergy, 39*, 246–253.
- *Drug Information*. Protonix. Wyeth-Ayerst Pharmaceuticals.
- Matok, I., Levy, A., Wiznitzer, A., Uziel, E., Koren, G., & Gorodischer, R., (2012). The safety of fetal exposure to proton-pump inhibitors during pregnancy. *Dig. Dis. Sci., 57*, 699–705.

## 9.6.2.6   RABEPRAZOLE

**FDA Category: C**
***Risk Summary:*** It should be used with caution because the pregnancy experiences in humans and animals have shown low risk.

**Further Reading:**
- Dehlink, E., Yen, E., Leichtner, A. M., Hait, E. J., & Fiebiger, E., (2009). First evidence of a possible association between gastric acid suppression during pregnancy and childhood asthma: A population-based register study. *Clin. Exp. Allergy, 39,* 246–253.
- *Drug Information. Rabeprazole.* Eisai.
- Pasternak, B., & Hviid, A., (2010). Use of proton-pump inhibitors in early pregnancy and the risk of birth defects. *N. Engl. J. Med., 363,* 2114–2123.

### 9.6.3 MISCELLANEOUS

#### 9.6.3.1 MISOPROSTOL

**FDA Category: X**
*Risk Summary:* It is contraindicated in early pregnancy because it is considered as a potent abortifacient drug.

**Further Reading:**
- Baird, D. T., Norman, J. E., Thong, K. J., & Glasier, A. F., (1992). Misoprostol, mifepristone, and abortion. *Lancet, 339,* 313.
- De Silva Dal Pizzol, T., Knop, F. P., & Mengu, S. S., (2006). Prenatal exposure to misoprostol and congenital anomalies: Systematic review and meta-analysis. *Reprod. Toxicol., 22,* 666–671.
- *Drug Information. Cytotec.* G.D. Searle.
- Shepard, T. H., (1995). Möbius syndrome after misoprostol: A possible teratogenic mechanism. *Lancet, 346,* 780.

#### 9.6.3.2 SUCRALFATE

**FDA Category: B**
*Risk Summary:* It should be used with caution because the pregnancy experience in humans is limited and the reproduction studies in animals have shown low risk.

**Further Reading:**
- Dehlink, E., Yen, E., Leichtner, A. M., Hait, E. J., & Fiebiger, E., (2009). First evidence of a possible association between gastric acid

suppression during pregnancy and childhood asthma: A population-based register study. *Clin. Exp. Allergy, 39,* 246–253.
- *Drug Information. Carafate.* Hoechst Marion Roussel.

## 9.7  GALLSTONE SOLUBILIZING DRUGS

### 9.7.1  CHENODIOL

**FDA Category: X**
*Risk Summary:* It is contraindicated in early pregnancy because of its observed dose-related hepatotoxicity.

**Further Reading:**
- Heywood, R., Palmer, A. K., Foll, C. V., & Lee, M. R., (1973). Pathological changes in fetal rhesus monkey induced by oral chenodeoxycholic acid. *Lancet, 2,*1021.
- McSherry, C. K., Morrissey, K. P., Swarm, R. L., May, P. S., Niemann, W. H., & Glenn, F., (1976). Chenodeoxycholic acid-induced liver injury in pregnant and neonatal baboons. Ann. Surg., *184,* 490–499.

### 9.7.2  URSODIOL

**FDA Category: B**
*Risk Summary:* The reproduction studies in animals have shown no evidence of fetal harm or impaired fertility. The pregnancy experience in humans is adequate to exhibit that the embryo-fetal risk is nonexistent or very low.

**Further Reading:**
- *Drug Information. Urso.* Axcan Pharma, US.
- Nicastri, P. L., Diaferia, A., Taartagni, M., Loizzi, P., & Fanelli, M., (1998). A randomized placebo-controlled trial of ursodeoxycholic acid and S-adenosylmethionine in the treatment of intrahepatic cholestasis of pregnancy. *Br. J. Obstet. Gynaecol., 105,* 1205–1207.
- Palma, J., Reyes, H., Ribalta, J., Hernandez, I., Sandoval, L., Almuna, R., Liepins, J., Lira, F., Sedano, M., Silva, O., Toha, D., & Silva, J. J., (1997). Ursodeoxycholic acid in the treatment of cholestasis of pregnancy: A randomized, double-blind study controlled with placebo. *J. Hepatol., 27,* 1022–1028.

## 9.8 GLUCAGON-LIKE PEPTIDE-2 ANALOG

### 9.8.1 *TEDUGLUTIDE*

**FDA Category: B**
*Risk Summary:* The reproduction studies in animals have shown no evidence of fetal harm or impaired fertility. The pregnancy experience in humans is limited.

**Further Reading:**
- *Drug Information. Gattex.* NPS Pharmaceuticals.


## 9.9 LAXATIVES/PURGATIVES

### 9.9.1 *BISACODYL*

**FDA Category: C**
*Risk Summary:* The reproduction studies in animals have shown no evidence of fetal harm or impaired fertility. The pregnancy experience in humans is limited.

**Further Reading:**
- Lewis, J. H., & Weingold, A. B., (1985). and The Committee on FDA-Related Matters, American College of Gastroenterology. The use of gastrointestinal drugs during pregnancy and lactation. *Am. J. Gastroenterol., 80,* 912–923.
- Onnis, A., & Grella, P., (1984). *The Biochemical Effects of Drugs in Pregnancy* (Vol. 2, p. 48–49). Chichester, UK: Ellis Horwood Limited.


### 9.9.2 *CASANTHRANOL*

**FDA Category: C**
*Risk Summary:* The reproduction studies in animals have shown no evidence of fetal harm or impaired fertility. The pregnancy experience in humans is adequate to exhibit that the embryo-fetal risk is nonexistent or very low.

**Further Reading:**
- Heinonen, O. P., Slone, D., & Shapiro, S., (1977). *Birth Defects and Drugs in Pregnancy* (pp. 384–387, 442). Littleton, MA: Publishing Sciences Group.

## 9.9.3   CASCARA SAGRADA

**FDA Category: N**
*Risk Summary:* It is better to be avoided during gestation because the pregnancy experience in humans is very limited.

**Further Reading:**
- Heinonen, O. P., Slone, D., & Shapiro, S., (1977). *Birth Defects and Drugs in Pregnancy* (pp. 384–377, 442). Littleton, MA: Publishing Sciences Group.
- Ernst, E., (2002). Herbal medicinal products during pregnancy: Are they safe? *Br. J. Obstet. Gynaecol., 109*, 227–235.

## 9.9.4   CASTOR OIL

**FDA Category: X**
*Risk Summary:* It is contraindicated in pregnancy because of its abortifacient effect. Nowadays, the use of Castor Oil as an oxytocic agent has been greatly decreased due to the emergence of safer alternatives like Misoprostol.

**Further Reading:**
- Ernst, E., (2002). Herbal medicinal products during pregnancy: Are they safe? *Br. J. Obstet. Gynaecol., 109*, 227–235.
- Mauhoub, M. E., Khalifa, M. M., Jaswal, O. B., & Garrah, M. S., (1983). "Ricin syndrome." A possible new teratogenic syndrome associated with ingestion of castor oil seed in early pregnancy: A case report. *Ann. Trop. Paediatr., 3*, 57–61.
- Sicuranza, G. B., & Figueroa, R., (2003). Uterine rupture associated with castor oil ingestion. *J. Matern Fetal Neonatal Med., 13*, 133–134.

## 9.9.5 DOCUSATE SODIUM

**FDA Category: N**
*Risk Summary:* The reproduction studies in animals have shown no evidence of fetal harm or impaired fertility. The pregnancy experience in humans is adequate to exhibit that the embryo-fetal risk is nonexistent or very low.

**Further Reading:**
- Heinonen, O. P., Slone, D., & Shapiro, S., (1977). *Birth Defects and Drugs in Pregnancy* (pp. 384–7, 442). Littleton, MA: Publishing Sciences Group.
- Schindler, A. M., (1984). Isolated neonatal hypomagnesemia associated with maternal overuse of stool softener. *Lancet, 2*, 822.

## 9.9.6 GLYCERIN

**FDA Category: C**
*Risk Summary:* The reproduction studies in animals have shown no evidence of fetal harm or impaired fertility. The pregnancy experience in humans is limited.

**Further Reading:**
- Yoshida, M., Matsuda, H., & Furuya, K., (2013). Successful prognosis of brain abscess during pregnancy. *J. Reprod. Infertil., 14*, 152–155.

## 9.9.7 LACTULOSE

**FDA Category: B**
*Risk Summary:* The reproduction studies in animals have shown no evidence of fetal harm or impaired fertility. The pregnancy experience in humans is limited.

**Further Reading:**
- *Drug Information. Duphalac.* Solvay Pharmaceuticals.

### 9.9.8   LINACLOTIDE

**FDA Category: C**
*Risk Summary:* The reproduction studies in animals have shown no evidence of fetal harm or impaired fertility. The pregnancy experience in humans is limited.

**Further Reading:**
- *Drug Information*. Linzess. Forest Pharmaceuticals.

### 9.9.9   LUBIPROSTONE

**FDA Category: C**
*Risk Summary:* The reproduction studies in animals have shown no evidence of fetal harm or impaired fertility. The pregnancy experience in humans is limited.

**Further Reading:**
- Anonymous (2006). Lubiprostone (Amitiza) for chronic constipation. *Med. Lett. Drugs Ther., 48*, 428. As cited in *Obstet. Gynecol., 108*, 1026–10267.
- *Drug Information. Amitiza.* Takeda Pharmaceuticals America.
- Ginzburg, R., & Ambizas, E. M., (2008). Clinical pharmacology of lubiprostone, a chloride channel activator in defecation disorders. *Expert Opin. Drug Metab. Toxicol., 4*, 1091–1097.

### 9.9.10   MAGNESIUM SULFATE

**FDA Category: D**
*Risk Summary:* Magnesium sulfate is contraindicated in pregnant women with cardiovascular and renal diseases, as in these situations the absorption of magnesium ions brings on a further burden.

**Further Reading:**
- *Drug Information. Magnesium Sulfate.* Abbott Pharmaceutical, Abbott Park, IL.
- Duley, L., Henderson-Smart, D. J., & Meher, S., (2006). Drugs for treatment of very high blood pressure during pregnancy. *Cochrane Database Syst. Rev., 3*, CD001449.

## 9.9.11 MINERAL OIL

**FDA Category: N**
*Risk Summary:* The reproduction studies in animals have shown no evidence of fetal harm or impaired fertility. The pregnancy experience in humans is adequate to exhibit that the embryo-fetal risk is nonexistent or very low.

**Further Reading:**
- Briggs, G., Freeman, R., Towers, C., & Forninash, A., (2017). *Drugs in Pregnancy and Lactation: A Reference Guide to Fetal and Neonatal Risk*. Philadelphia, Pa: Wolters Kluwer Health.

## 9.9.12 POLYETHYLENE GLYCOL

**FDA Category: C**
*Risk Summary:* The reproduction studies in animals have shown no evidence of fetal harm or impaired fertility. The pregnancy experience in humans is adequate to exhibit that the embryo-fetal risk is nonexistent or very low.

**Further Reading:**
- *Drug Information. Trilyte.* Alaven Pharmaceutical.
- Neri, I., Blasi, I., Castro, P., Grandinetti, G., Ricchi, A., & Facchinetti, F., (2004). Polyethylene glycol electrolyte solution (Isocolan) for constipation during pregnancy: An observational open-label study. *J. Midwifery Women's Health, 49*, 355–358.

## 9.9.13 SENNA

**FDA Category: C**
*Risk Summary:* The reproduction studies in animals have shown no evidence of fetal harm or impaired fertility. The pregnancy experience in humans is adequate to exhibit that the embryo-fetal risk is nonexistent or very low.

**Further Reading:**
- Acs, N., Banhidy, F., Puho, E. H., & Czeizel, A. E., ()2009. Senna treatment in pregnant women and congenital abnormalities in their offspring—a population-based case-control study. *Reprod. Toxicol., 28*, 100–104.

## 9.10   LIPASE INHIBITOR

### *9.1.1   ORLISTAT*

**FDA Category: X**
***Risk Summary:*** Orlistat appears to present a very low risk, if any, to the embryo or fetus because the systemic bioavailability of orlistat is negligible. However, it may lead to the maternal deficiency of fat-soluble vitamins (vitamins A, D, and E) if a daily vitamin supplement is not taken. This could lead to a direct harmful effect on the embryo or fetus.

**Further Reading:**
- *Drug Information*. Xenical. Roche Laboratories.
- Kalyoncu, N. I., Yaris, F., Kadioglu, M., Kesim, M., Ulku, C., Yaris, E., Unsal, M., & Dikici, M., (2005). Pregnancy outcome following exposure to orlistat, ramipril, glimepiride in a woman with metabolic syndrome. *Saudi. Med. J., 26*, 497–499.

## 9.11   PERIPHERAL OPIOID ANTAGONIST

### *9.11.1   ALVIMOPAN*

**FDA Category: B**
***Risk Summary:*** It should be used with caution because the pregnancy experience in humans is limited and the reproduction studies in animals have shown low risk.

**Further Reading:**
- *Drug Information. Entereg.* GlaxoSmithKline.

## 9.12   STIMULANTS

### *9.12.1   DEXPANTHENOL*

**FDA Category: C**
***Risk Summary:*** It should be used with caution because the pregnancy experience in humans is limited and the reproduction studies in animals have shown low risk.

**Further Reading:**
- *Drug Information. Ilopan.* Adria Laboratories.
- Nolan, T. E., & Schilder, J. M., (2006). Lower gastrointestinal tract disorders. Clinical Updates in Women's Health Care. *Am. Coll. Obstetricians Gynecologists, 5*(1), 5.

### 9.12.2  METOCLOPRAMIDE

**FDA Category: B**
***Risk Summary:*** The reproduction studies in animals have shown no evidence of fetal harm or impaired fertility. The pregnancy experience in humans is adequate to exhibit that the embryo-fetal risk is nonexistent or very low.

**Further Reading:**
- Guikontes, E., Spantideas, A., & Diakakis, J., (1992). Ondansetron and hyperemesis gravidarum. *Lancet, 340,* 1223.
- Messinis, I. E., Lolis, D. E., Dalkalitsis, N., Kanaris, C., & Souvat-zoglou, A., (1982). Effect of metoclopramide on maternal and fetal prolactin secretion during labor. *Obstet. Gynecol., 60,* 686–688.
- Sorensen, H. T., Nielsen, G. L., Christensen, K., Tage-Jensen, U., Ekborn, A., & Baron, J., (2000). and the Euromap study group. Birth outcome following maternal use of metoclopramide. *Br. J. Clin. Pharmacol., 49,* 264–268.

### KEYWORDS

- **dexpanthenol**
- **lipase inhibitor**
- **metoclopramide**
- **peripheral opioid antagonist**
- **polyethylene glycol**
- **senna**

# CHAPTER 10

# Drugs Affecting the Musculoskeletal System

## 10.1 NARCOTIC AGONIST ANALGESICS

### 10.1.1 ALFENTANIL

**FDA Category: C**
*Risk Summary:* It should be used with caution during the 1st and 2nd Trimesters. However, it is better to avoid the use of Alfentanil near term because of the risk of neonatal respiratory depression if used close to delivery.

**Further Reading:**
- *Drug Information. Alfenta.* Janssen Pharmaceutica, Inc.
- Giesecke, A. H. Jr., Rice, L. J., & Lipton, J. M., (1985). Alfentanil in colostrum. *Anesthesiology, 63*, A284.
- Rout, C. C., & Rocke, D. A., (1990). Effects of alfentanil and fentanyl on induction of anesthesia in patients with severe pregnancy-induced hypertension. *Br. J. Anaesth., 65*, 468–474.

### 10.1.2 CODEINE

**FDA Category: C**
*Risk Summary:* The use of Codeine should be avoided, if possible, in pregnant women because the pregnancy experience in humans has shown a low risk of congenital birth defects associated with the use of this drug. Furthermore, its use near delivery is associated with a risk of neonatal respiratory depression.

**Further Reading:**
- Bracken, M. B., & Holford, T. R., (1981). Exposure to prescribed drugs in pregnancy and association with congenital malformations. *Obstet. Gynecol., 58*, 336–44.
- Creanga, A. A., Sabel, J. C., Ko, J. Y., Wasserman, C. R., Shapiro-Mendoza, C. K., Taylor, P., Barfield, W., Cawthon, L., & Paulozzi, L. J., (2012). Maternal drug use and its effect on neonates—a population-based study in Washington state. *Obstet. Gynecol., 119*, 924–933.
- Khan, K., & Chang, J., (1997). Neonatal abstinence syndrome due to codeine. *Arch. Dis. Child, 76*, F59–60.
- Nezvalova-Henriksen, K., Spigset, O., & Nordeng, H., (2011). Effects of codeine on pregnancy outcome: Results from a large population-based cohort study. *Eur. J. Clin. Pharmacol., 67*, 1253–1261.

### 10.1.3   DIHYDROCODEINE

**FDA Category: C**
***Risk Summary:*** It should be used with caution during the 1st and 2nd Trimesters. However, it is better to avoid the use of Dihydrocodeine near term because of the risk of neonatal respiratory depression if used close to delivery.

**Further Reading:**
- Myers, J. D., (1958). A preliminary clinical evaluation of dihydro-codeine bitartrate in normal parturition. *Am. J. Obstet. Gynecol., 75*, 1096–1100.
- Sliom, C. M., (1970). Analgesia during labor: A comparison between dihydrocodeine and pethidine. *S. Afr. Med. J., 44*, 317–319.

### 10.1.4   FENTANYL

**FDA Category: C**
***Risk Summary:*** The use of Fentanyl should be avoided, if possible, in pregnant women because the pregnancy experience in humans has shown a low risk of congenital birth defects associated with the use of this drug. Furthermore, its use near delivery is associated with a risk of neonatal respiratory depression.

**Further Reading:**

- Benlabed, M., Dreizzen, E., Ecoffey, C., Escourrou, P., Migdal, M., & Gaultier, C., (1990). Neonatal patterns of breathing after cesarean section with or without epidural fentanyl. *Anesthesiology, 73,* 1110–1113.
- Broussard, C. S., Rasmussen, S. A., Reefhuis, J., Friedman, J. M., Jann, M. W., Riehle-Colarusso, T., & Honein, M. A., (2011). National Birth Defects Prevention Study. Maternal treatment with opioid analgesics and risk for birth defects. *Am. J. Obstet. Gynecol., 204,* 314–317.
- *Drug Information. Duragesic.* Janssen Pharmaceutica.

### 10.1.5  HYDROCODONE

**FDA Category: C**
***Risk Summary:*** The use of Hydrocodone should be avoided, if possible, in pregnant women because the pregnancy experience in humans has shown a low risk of congenital birth defects associated with the use of this drug. Furthermore, its use near delivery is associated with a risk of neonatal respiratory depression.

**Further Reading:**

- Broussard, C. S., Rasmussen, S. A., Reefhuis, J., Friedman, J. M., Jann, M. W., Riehle-Colarusso, T., & Honein, M. A., (2011). National Birth Defects Prevention Study. Maternal treatment with opioid analgesics and risk for birth defects. *Am. J. Obstet. Gynecol., 204,* 314–317.
- Schick, B., Hom, M., Tolosa, J., Librizzi, R., & Donnfeld, A., (1996). Preliminary analysis of first-trimester exposure to oxycodone and hydrocodone (Abstract). Presented at the Ninth International Conference of the Organization of Teratology Information Services, Salt Lake City, Utah, May 2–4, 1996. *Reprod. Toxicol., 10,* 162.

### 10.1.6  HYDROMORPHONE

**FDA Category: C**
***Risk Summary:*** The use of Hydromorphone should be avoided, if possible, in pregnant women because the pregnancy experience in humans has shown

a low risk of congenital birth defects associated with the use of this drug. Furthermore, its use near delivery is associated with a risk of neonatal respiratory depression.

**Further Reading:**
- Broussard, C. S., Rasmussen, S. A., Reefhuis, J., Friedman, J. M., Jann, M. W., Riehle-Colarusso, T., & Honein, M. A., (2011). National Birth Defects Prevention Study. Maternal treatment with opioid analgesics and risk for birth defects. *Am. J. Obstet. Gynecol., 204,* 314–317.
- *Drug Information. Dilaudid.* Purdue Pharma.

### *10.1.7 LEVORPHANOL*

**FDA Category: C**
*Risk Summary:* It should be used with caution during the 1st and 2nd Trimesters. However, it is better to avoid the use of Levorphanol near term because of the risk of neonatal respiratory depression if used close to delivery.

**Further Reading:**
- Broussard, C. S., Rasmussen, S. A., Reefhuis, J., Friedman, J. M., Jann, M. W., Riehle-Colarusso, T., & Honein, M. A., (2011). National Birth Defects Prevention Study. Maternal treatment with opioid analgesics and risk for birth defects. *Am. J. Obstet. Gynecol., 204,* 314–317.
- *Drug Information. Levo-Dromoran.* ICN Pharmaceuticals.

### *10.1.8 MEPERIDINE*

**FDA Category: C**
*Risk Summary:* The use of Meperidine should be avoided, if possible, in pregnant women because the pregnancy experience in humans has shown a low risk of congenital birth defects associated with the use of this drug. Furthermore, its use near delivery is associated with a risk of neonatal respiratory depression.

**Further Reading:**
- Broussard, C. S., Rasmussen, S. A., Reefhuis, J., Friedman, J. M., Jann, M. W., Riehle-Colarusso, T., & Honein, M. A., (2011). National Birth Defects Prevention Study. Maternal treatment with opioid analgesics and risk for birth defects. *Am. J. Obstet. Gynecol., 204*, 314–317.
- Hodgkinson, R., Bhatt, M., & Wang, C. N., (1978). Double-blind comparison of the neurobehaviour of neonates following the administration of different doses of meperidine to the mother. *Can. Anaesth. Soc. J., 25*, 405–411.

### 10.1.9 METHADONE

**FDA Category: C**
*Risk Summary:* The use of Methadone should be avoided, if possible, in pregnant women because the pregnancy experience in humans has shown a low risk of congenital birth defects associated with the use of this drug. Furthermore, its use near delivery is associated with a risk of neonatal respiratory depression.

**Further Reading:**
- Cleary, B. J., Donnelly, J. M., Strawbridge, J. D., Gallagher, P. J., Fahey, T., White, M. J., & Murphy, D. J., (2011). Methadone and perinatal outcomes: A retrospective cohort study. *Am. J. Obstet. Gynecol., 204*, 139–141.
- Kandall, S. R., & Gartner, L. M., (1973). Delayed presentation of neonatal methadone withdrawal. *Pediatr. Res., 7*, 320.
- Smialek, J. E., Monforte, J. R., Aronow, R., & Spitz, W. U., (1977). Methadone deaths in children—a continuing problem. *JAMA, 238*, 2516, 2517.

### 10.1.10 MORPHINE

**FDA Category: C**
*Risk Summary:* The use of Morphine should be avoided, if possible, in pregnant women because the pregnancy experience in humans has shown a low risk of congenital birth defects associated with the use of this drug.

Furthermore, its use near delivery is associated with a risk of neonatal respiratory depression.

**Further Reading:**
- Brizgys, R. V., & Shnider, S. M., (1984). Hyperbaric intrathecal morphine analgesia during labor in a patient with Wolff-Parkinson-White syndrome. *Obstet. Gynecol., 64,* 44S–46S.
- Broussard, C. S., Rasmussen, S. A., Reefhuis, J., Friedman, J. M., Jann, M. W., Riehle-Colarusso, T., & Honein, M. A., (2011). National Birth Defects Prevention Study. Maternal treatment with opioid analgesics and risk for birth defects. *Am. J. Obstet. Gynecol., 204,* 314–317.
- *Drug Information. Duramorph.* Elkins-Sinn, 2000.

### 10.1.11   OXYCODONE

**FDA Category: C**
***Risk Summary:*** The use of Oxycodone should be avoided, if possible, in pregnant women because the pregnancy experience in humans has shown a low risk of congenital birth defects associated with the use of this drug. Furthermore, its use near delivery is associated with a risk of neonatal respiratory depression.

**Further Reading:**
- *Drug Information.* Oxycontin. Endo Pharmaceuticals.
- Broussard, C. S., Rasmussen, S. A., Reefhuis, J., Friedman, J. M., Jann, M. W., Riehle-Colarusso, T., & Honein, M. A., (2011). National Birth Defects Prevention Study. Maternal treatment with opioid analgesics and risk for birth defects. *Am. J. Obstet. Gynecol., 204,* 314–317.

### 10.1.12   OXYMORPHONE

**FDA Category: C**
***Risk Summary:*** The use of Oxymorphone should be avoided, if possible, in pregnant women because the pregnancy experience in humans has shown a low risk of congenital birth defects associated with the use of this drug.

Furthermore, its use near delivery is associated with a risk of neonatal respiratory depression.

**Further Reading:**
- *Drug Information. Opana.* Endo Pharmaceuticals.
- Ransom, S., (1966). Oxymorphone as an obstetric analgesia. A clinical trial. *Anesthesia., 21,* 464–471.


## 10.1.13 REMIFENTANIL

**FDA Category: C**
*Risk Summary:* It should be used with caution during the 1st and 2nd Trimesters. However, it is better to avoid the use of Remifentanil near term because of the risk of neonatal respiratory depression if used close to delivery.

**Further Reading:**
- Broussard, C. S., Rasmussen, S. A., Reefhuis, J., Friedman, J. M., Jann, M. W., Riehle-Colarusso, T., & Honein, M. A., (2011). National Birth Defects Prevention Study. Maternal treatment with opioid analgesics and risk for birth defects. *Am. J. Obstet. Gynecol., 204,* 314–317.
- *Drug Information. Ultiva.* Abbott Laboratories.


## 10.1.14 SUFENTANIL

**FDA Category: C**
*Risk Summary:* It should be used with caution during the 1st and 2nd Trimesters. However, it is better to avoid the use of Sufentanil near term because of the risk of neonatal respiratory depression if used close to delivery.

**Further Reading:**
- Broussard, C. S., Rasmussen, S. A., Reefhuis, J., Friedman, J. M., Jann, M. W., Riehle-Colarusso, T., & Honein, M. A., (2011). National Birth Defects Prevention Study. Maternal treatment with opioid analgesics and risk for birth defects. *Am. J. Obstet. Gynecol., 204,* 314–317.
- *Drug Information. Sufenta.* Janssen Pharmaceutica.

342

## 10.1.15  TAPENTADOL

**FDA Category: C**
*Risk Summary:* The reproduction studies in animals have shown no evidence of fetal harm or impaired fertility. The pregnancy experience in humans is limited.

**Further Reading:**
- *Drug Information. Nucynta.* PriCara (Division of Ortho-McNeil-Janssen Pharmaceuticals), 2009.

## 10.1.16  TRAMADOL

**FDA Category: C**
*Risk Summary:* The use of Tramadol should be avoided, if possible, in pregnant women because the pregnancy experience in humans has shown a low risk of congenital birth defects associated with the use of this drug. Furthermore, its use near delivery is associated with a risk of neonatal respiratory depression.

**Further Reading:**
- Bloor, M., Paech, M. J., & Kaye, R., (2012). Tramadol in pregnancy and lactation. *Int. J. Obstet. Anesth., 21*, 163–167.
- *Drug Information. Ultram.* Janssen Pharmaceuticals.
- Khooshideh, M., & Shahriari, A., (2009). A comparison of tramadol and pethidine analgesia on the duration of labor: A randomized clinical trial. *Aust. N. Z. J. Obstet. Gynaecol., 49*, 59–63.

## 10.2  NARCOTIC AGONIST-ANTAGONIST ANALGESICS

### 10.2.1  BUPRENORPHINE

**FDA Category: C**
*Risk Summary:* It should be used with caution because the pregnancy experience in humans is limited and the reproduction studies in animals have shown a low risk of fetal toxicity.

**Further Reading:**
- Barron, S., & Chung, V. M., (1997). Prenatal buprenorphine exposure and sexually dimorphic nonreproductive behaviors in rats. *Pharmacol. Biochem. Behav., 58*, 337–343.
- *Drug Information. Buprenex.* Reckitt & Colman Pharmaceuticals.
- Marquet, P., Chevrel, J., Lavignasse, P., Merle, L., & Lachatre, G., (1997). Buprenorphine withdrawal syndrome in a newborn. *Clin. Pharmacol. Ther., 62*, 569–571.

## 10.2.2  BUTORPHANOL

**FDA Category: C**
*Risk Summary:* It should be used with caution during the 1st and 2nd Trimesters. However, it is better to avoid the use of Butorphanol during labor because there is a risk of transient neonatal depression and a sinusoidal fetal heart rate pattern.

**Further Reading:**
- *Drug Information.* Stadol NS. Bristol-Myers Squibb.
- Weintraub, S. J., & Naulty, J. S., (1985). Acute abstinence syndrome after epidural injection of butorphanol. *Anesth. Analg., 64*, 452–453.

## 10.2.3  NALBUPHINE

**FDA Category: C**
*Risk Summary:* It should be used with caution during the 1st and 2nd Trimesters. However, it is better to avoid the use of Nalbuphine during labor because there is a risk of transient neonatal depression and a sinusoidal fetal heart rate pattern.

**Further Reading:**
- *Drug Information.* Nalbuphine hydrochloride. Hospira.
- Feinstein, S. J., Lodeiro, J. G., Vintzileos, A. M., Campbell, W. A., Montgomery, J. T., & Nochimson, D. J., (1986). Sinusoidal fetal heart rate pattern after administration of nalbuphine hydrochloride: A case report. *Am. J. Obstet. Gynecol., 154*, 159, 160.

- Sgro, C., Escousse, A., Tennenbaum, D., & Gouyon, J. B., (1990). Perinatal adverse effects of nalbuphine given during labor. *Lancet, 336,* 1070.

## 10.2.4   PENTAZOCINE

**FDA Category: C**
*Risk Summary:* The use of Pentazocine should be avoided, if possible, in pregnant women because the pregnancy experience in humans has shown a low risk of congenital birth defects associated with the use of this drug. Furthermore, its use near delivery is associated with a risk of neonatal respiratory depression.

**Further Reading:**
- Broussard, C. S., Rasmussen, S. A., Reefhuis, J., Friedman, J. M., Jann, M. W., Riehle-Colarusso, T., & Honein, M. A., (2011). National Birth Defects Prevention Study. Maternal treatment with opioid analgesics and risk for birth defects. *Am. J. Obstet. Gynecol., 204,* 314–317.
- Debooy, V. D., Seshia, M. M. K., Tenenbein, M., & Casiiro, O. G., (1993). Intravenous pentazocine and methylphenidate abuse during pregnancy. Maternal lifestyle and infant outcome. *Am. J. Dis. Child, 147,* 1062–1065.
- *Drug Information.* Talwin. Hospira.
- Refstad, S. O., & Lindbaek, E., (1980). Ventilatory depression of the newborn of women receiving pethidine or pentazocine. *Br. J. Anaesth., 52,* 265–270.

## 10.3   NARCOTIC ANTAGONISTS

### 10.3.1   METHYLNALTREXONE

**FDA Category: C**
*Risk Summary:* It should be used with caution because the pregnancy experience in humans is limited and the reproduction studies in animals have shown low risk.

**Further Reading:**
- *Drug Information.* Relistor. Progenics Pharmaceuticals.

## 10.3.2 NALOXONE

**FDA Category: C**
***Risk Summary:*** The reproduction studies in animals have shown no evidence of fetal harm or impaired fertility. The pregnancy experience in humans is adequate to exhibit that the embryo-fetal risk is nonexistent or very low.

**Further Reading:**
- Bonta, B. W., Gagliardi, J. V., Williams, V., & Warshaw, J. B., (1979). Naloxone reversal of mild neurobehavioral depression in normal newborn infants after routine obstetric analgesia. *J. Pediatr., 94,* 102–105.
- *Drug Information. Narcan.* Endo Pharmaceuticals.
- Wiener, P. C., Hogg, M. I. J., & Rosen, M., (1977). Effects of naloxone on pethidine-induced neonatal depression. II. Intramuscular naloxone. *Br. Med. J., 2,* 229–231.

## 10.3.3 NALTREXONE

**FDA Category: C**
***Risk Summary:*** The pregnancy experience in humans is limited, and the reproduction studies in animals have shown moderate risk. Therefore, it is advisable to use naltrexone only if naloxone is not available.

**Further Reading:**
- Caba, M., Poindron, P., Krehbiel, D., Levy, F., Romeyer, A., & Venier, G., (1995). Naltrexone delays the onset of maternal behavior in primiparous parturient ewes. *Pharmacol. Biochem. Behav., 52,* 743–748.
- *Drug Information. Revia.* Duramed Pharmaceuticals.
- McLaughlin, P. J., Tobias, S. W., Lang, C. M., & Zagon, I. S., (1997). Chronic exposure to the opioid antagonist naltrexone during pregnancy: Maternal and offspring effects. *Physiol. Behav., 62,* 501–508.

## 10.4   NONSTEROIDAL ANTI-INFLAMMATORY DRUGS

### 10.4.1   ASPIRIN

**FDA Category: N**

*Risk Summary:* At doses for antiplatelet activity: The reproduction studies in animals have shown no evidence of fetal harm or impaired fertility. The pregnancy experience in humans is adequate to exhibit that the embryo-fetal risk is nonexistent or very low.

At doses used for analgesic and/or anti-inflammatory action: It is better to be avoided during the 1$^{st}$ and 3$^{rd}$ trimesters because the pregnancy experience in humans suggests a risk of intrauterine growth restriction (IUGR), increased perinatal mortality, and teratogenic effects linked to the use of Aspirin.

**Further Reading:**
- Elder, M. G., DeSwiet, M., Robertson, A., Elder, M. A., Flloyd, E., & Hawkins, D. F., (1988). Low-dose aspirin in pregnancy. *Lancet, 1,* 410.
- Rumack, C. M., Guggenheim, M. A., Rumack, B. H., Peterson, R. G., Johnson, M. L., & Braithwaite, W. R., (1981). Neonatal intracranial hemorrhage and maternal use of aspirin. *Obstet. Gynecol., 58*(Suppl), 52S–56S.
- Slone, D., Heinonen, O. P., Kaufman, D. W., Siskind, V., Monson, R. R., & Shapiro, S., (1976). Aspirin and congenital malformations. *Lancet, 1,* 1373–1375.
- Uzan, S., Beaufils, M., Bazin, B., & Danays, T., (1989). Idiopathic recurrent fetal growth retardation and aspirin dipyridamole therapy. *Am. J. Obstet. Gynecol., 160,* 763.
- Werler, M. M., Mitchell, A. A., & Shapiro, S., (1989). The relation of aspirin use during the first trimester of pregnancy to congenital cardiac defects. *N. Engl. J. Med., 321,* 1639–1642.

### 10.4.2   CELECOXIB

**FDA Category: C**

*Risk Summary:* It is better to be avoided during the 1st and 3rd Trimesters because the pregnancy experience in humans suggests a risk of pulmonary hypertension of the newborn, spontaneous abortions (SABs), and congenital malformations linked to the use of Celecoxib.

**Further Reading:**
- Borna, S., & Saeidi, F. M., (2007). Celecoxib versus magnesium sulfate to arrest preterm labor: Randomized trial. *J. Obstet. Gynaecol. Res., 33*, 631–634.
- Dawood, M. Y., (1993). Nonsteroidal anti-inflammatory drugs and reproduction. *Am. J. Obstet. Gynecol., 169*, 1255–1265.
- *Drug Information. Celebrex.* G.D. Searle.
- Nielsen, G. L., Sorensen, H. T., Larsen, H., & Pedersen, L., (2001). Risk of adverse birth outcome and miscarriage in pregnant users of non-steroidal anti-inflammatory drugs: Population-based observational study and case-control study. *Br. Med. J., 322*, 266–270.

### 10.4.3   DICLOFENAC

**FDA Category: C**
***Risk Summary:*** It is better to be avoided during the 1st and 3rd Trimesters because the pregnancy experience in humans suggests a risk of pulmonary hypertension of the newborn, SABs, and congenital malformations linked to the use of Diclofenac.

**Further Reading:**
- *Drug Information. Voltaren.* Geigy Pharmaceuticals.
- Levin, D. L., (1980). Effects of inhibition of prostaglandin synthesis on fetal development, oxygenation, and fetal circulation. *Semin. Perinatol., 4*, 35–44.
- Mas, C., & Menahem, S., (1999). Premature in utero closure of the ductus arteriosus following maternal ingestion of sodium diclofenac. *Aust NZ J Obstet. Gynaecol., 39*, 106–107.
- Siu, K. L., & Lee, W. H., (2004). Maternal diclofenac sodium ingestion and severe neonatal pulmonary hypertension. *J. Paediatr Child Health, 40*, 152–153.

## 10.4.4   DIFLUNISAL

**FDA Category: C**
*Risk Summary:* It is better to be avoided during the 1st and 3rd Trimesters because the pregnancy experience in humans suggests a risk of pulmonary hypertension of the newborn, SABs, and congenital malformations linked to the use of Diflunisal.

**Further Reading:**
- *Drug Information. Dolobid.* Merck Sharpe & Dohme.
- Levin, D. L., (1980). Effects of inhibition of prostaglandin synthesis on fetal development, oxygenation, and fetal circulation. *Semin. Perinatol., 4*, 35–44.

## 10.4.5   ETODOLAC

**FDA Category: C**
*Risk Summary:* It is better to be avoided during the 1st and 3rd Trimesters because the pregnancy experience in humans suggests a risk of pulmonary hypertension of the newborn, SABs, and congenital malformations linked to the use of Etodolac.

**Further Reading:**
- Dawood, M. Y., (1993). Nonsteroidal anti-inflammatory drugs and reproduction. *Am. J. Obstet. Gynecol., 169*, 1255–1265.
- *Drug Information. Lodine.* Wyeth-Ayerst Laboratories.
- Levin, D. L., (1980). Effects of inhibition of prostaglandin synthesis on fetal development, oxygenation, and the fetal circulation. *Semin Perinatol., 4*, 35–44.
- Matt, D. W., & Borzelleca, J. F., (1995). Toxic effects on the female reproductive system during pregnancy, parturition, and lactation. In: Witorsch, R. J., (ed.) *Reproductive Toxicology.* (2nd edn., pp. 175–193). New York, NY: Raven Press.
- Van Marter, L. J., Leviton, A., Allred, E. N., Pagano, M., Sullivan, K. F., Cohen, A., & Epstein, M. F., (1996). Persistent pulmonary hypertension of the newborn and smoking and aspirin and nonsteroidal anti-inflammatory drug consumption during pregnancy. *Pediatrics, 97*, 658–663.

## 10.4.6 FENOPROFEN

**FDA Category: C (Prior to 30 Weeks of Gestation)**

**FDA Category: D (After 30 Weeks of Gestation)**

*Risk Summary:* It is better to be avoided during the 1st and 3rd Trimesters because the pregnancy experience in humans suggests a risk of pulmonary hypertension of the newborn, SABs, and congenital malformations linked to the use of Fenoprofen. Furthermore, Fenoprofen has been found to inhibit labor and to prolong the length of pregnancy.

**Further Reading:**
- Dawood, M. Y., (1993). Nonsteroidal anti-inflammatory drugs and reproduction. *Am. J. Obstet. Gynecol., 169*, 1255–1265.
- *Drug Information. Nalfon.* Dista Products.
- Levin, D. L., (1980). Effects of inhibition of prostaglandin synthesis on fetal development, oxygenation, and the fetal circulation. *Semin. Perinatol., 4*, 35–44.
- Matt, D. W., & Borzelleca, J. F., (1995). Toxic effects on the female reproductive system during pregnancy, parturition, and lactation. In: Witorsch, R. J., (ed.) *Reproductive Toxicology* (2nd ed., p. 175–193). New York, NY: Raven Press.
- Van Marter, L. J., Leviton, A., Allred, E. N., Pagano, M., Sullivan, K. F., Cohen, A., & Epstein, M. F., (1996). Persistent pulmonary hypertension of the newborn and smoking and aspirin and nonsteroidal anti-inflammatory drug consumption during pregnancy. *Pediatrics, 97*, 658–663.

## 10.4.7 FLURBIPROFEN

**FDA Category: C**

*Risk Summary:* It is better to be avoided during the 1st and 3rd Trimesters because the pregnancy experience in humans suggests a risk of pulmonary hypertension of the newborn, SABs, and congenital malformations linked to the use of Flurbiprofen. Furthermore, Flurbiprofen has been found to inhibit labor and to prolong the length of pregnancy.

**Further Reading:**
- Dawood, M. Y., (1993). Nonsteroidal anti-inflammatory drugs and reproduction. *Am. J. Obstet. Gynecol., 169*, 1255–1265.

- *Drug Information*. Ansaid. The Upjohn Company.
- Levin, D. L., (1980). Effects of inhibition of prostaglandin synthesis on fetal development, oxygenation, and the fetal circulation. *Semin. Perinatol., 4*, 35–44.
- Matt, D. W., & Borzelleca, J. F., (1995). Toxic effects on the female reproductive system during pregnancy, parturition, and lactation. In: Witorsch, R. J., (ed.) *Reproductive Toxicology* (2nd ed., p. 175–193). New York, NY: Raven Press.
- Van Marter, L. J., Leviton, A., Allred, E. N., Pagano, M., Sullivan, K. F., Cohen, A., & Epstein, M. F., (1996). Persistent pulmonary hypertension of the newborn and smoking and aspirin and nonsteroidal anti-inflammatory drug consumption during pregnancy. *Pediatrics, 97*, 658–663.

### 10.4.8   IBUPROFEN

**FDA Category: C**

***Risk Summary:*** It is better to be avoided during the 1st and 3rd Trimesters because the pregnancy experience in humans suggests a risk of pulmonary hypertension of the newborn, SABs, and congenital malformations linked to the use of Ibuprofen. Furthermore, Ibuprofen has been found to inhibit labor and to prolong the length of pregnancy.

**Further Reading:**

- Dawood, M. Y., (1993). Nonsteroidal anti-inflammatory drugs and reproduction. *Am. J. Obstet. Gynecol., 169*, 1255–1265.
- *Drug Information*. Motrin. McNeil Consumer.
- Levin, D. L., (1980). Effects of inhibition of prostaglandin synthesis on fetal development, oxygenation, and the fetal circulation. *Semin. Perinatol., 4*, 35–44.
- Matt, D. W., & Borzelleca, J. F., (1995). Toxic effects on the female reproductive system during pregnancy, parturition, and lactation. In: Witorsch, R. J., (ed.) *Reproductive Toxicology* (2nd ed., p. 175–193). New York, NY: Raven Press.
- Van Marter, L. J., Leviton, A., Allred, E. N., Pagano, M., Sullivan, K. F., Cohen, A., & Epstein, M. F., (1996). Persistent pulmonary hypertension of the newborn and smoking and aspirin and nonsteroidal anti-inflammatory drug consumption during pregnancy. *Pediatrics, 97*, 658–663.

## 10.4.9 INDOMETHACIN

**FDA Category: C**
*Risk Summary:* It is better to be avoided during the 1st and 3rd Trimesters because the pregnancy experience in humans suggests a risk of pulmonary hypertension of the newborn, SABs, and congenital malformations linked to the use of Indomethacin. Its use has been associated with Necrotizing Enterocolitis in the newborn.

**Further Reading:**
- Atad, J., David, A., Moise, J., & Abramovici, H., (1980). Classification of threatened premature labor related to treatment with a prostaglandin inhibitor: Indomethacin. *Biol. Neonate, 37,* 291–296.
- Dawood, M. Y., (1993). Nonsteroidal anti-inflammatory drugs and reproduction. *Am. J. Obstet. Gynecol., 169,* 1255–1265.
- Levin, D. L., (1980). Effects of inhibition of prostaglandin synthesis on fetal development, oxygenation, and the fetal circulation. *Semin. Perinatol., 4,* 35–44.
- Matt, D. W., & Borzelleca, J. F., (1995). Toxic effects on the female reproductive system during pregnancy, parturition, and lactation. In: Witorsch, R. J., (ed.) *Reproductive Toxicology* (2nd ed., p. 175–193). New York, NY: Raven Press.
- Norton, M. E., Merrill, J., Cooper, B. A. B., Kuller, J. A., & Clyman, R. I., (1993). Neonatal complications after the administration of indomethacin for preterm labor. *N. Engl. J. Med., 329,* 1602–1607.
- Van Marter, L. J., Leviton, A., Allred, E. N., Pagano, M., Sullivan, K. F., Cohen, A., & Epstein, M. F., (1996). Persistent pulmonary hypertension of the newborn and smoking and aspirin and nonsteroidal anti-inflammatory drug consumption during pregnancy. *Pediatrics, 97,* 658–663.

## 10.4.10 KETOPROFEN

**FDA Category: C**
*Risk Summary:* It is better to be avoided during the 1st and 3rd Trimesters because the pregnancy experience in humans suggests a risk of pulmonary hypertension of the newborn, SABs, and congenital malformations linked to

the use of Ketoprofen. Furthermore, Ketoprofen has been found to inhibit labor and to prolong the length of pregnancy.

**Further Reading:**
- Dawood, M. Y., (1993). Nonsteroidal anti-inflammatory drugs and reproduction. *Am. J. Obstet. Gynecol., 169*, 1255–1265.
- *Drug Information. Ketoprofen.* Mylan Pharmaceuticals.
- Levin, D. L., (1980). Effects of inhibition of prostaglandin synthesis on fetal development, oxygenation, and the fetal circulation. *Semin. Perinatol., 4*, 35–44.
- Matt, D. W., & Borzelleca, J. F., (1995). Toxic effects on the female reproductive system during pregnancy, parturition, and lactation. In: Witorsch, R. J., (ed.) *Reproductive Toxicology* (2nd ed., p. 175–193). New York, NY: Raven Press.
- Van Marter, L. J., Leviton, A., Allred, E. N., Pagano, M., Sullivan, K. F., Cohen, A., & Epstein, M. F., (1996). Persistent pulmonary hypertension of the newborn and smoking and aspirin and nonsteroidal anti-inflammatory drug consumption during pregnancy. *Pediatrics, 97*, 658–663.

### *10.4.11   KETOROLAC*

**FDA Category: C**
***Risk Summary:*** It is better to be avoided during the 1st and 3rd Trimesters because the pregnancy experience in humans suggests a risk of pulmonary hypertension of the newborn, SABs, and congenital malformations linked to the use of Ketorolac.

**Further Reading:**
- Dawood, M. Y., (1993). Nonsteroidal anti-inflammatory drugs and reproduction. *Am. J. Obstet. Gynecol., 169*, 1255–1265.
- *Drug Information. Toradol.* Roche Laboratories.
- Levin, D. L., (1980). Effects of inhibition of prostaglandin synthesis on fetal development, oxygenation, and the fetal circulation. *Semin. Perinatol., 4*, 35–44.
- Matt, D. W., & Borzelleca, J. F., (1995). Toxic effects on the female reproductive system during pregnancy, parturition, and lactation. In: Witorsch, R. J., (ed.) *Reproductive Toxicology* (2nd ed., p. 175–193). New York, NY: Raven Press.

- Van Marter, L. J., Leviton, A., Allred, E. N., Pagano, M., Sullivan, K. F., Cohen, A., & Epstein, M. F., (1996). Persistent pulmonary hypertension of the newborn and smoking and aspirin and nonsteroidal anti-inflammatory drug consumption during pregnancy. *Pediatrics, 97,* 658–663.

## 10.4.12   *MECLOFENAMATE*

**FDA Category: C**
*Risk Summary:* It is better to be avoided during the 1st and 3rd Trimesters because the pregnancy experience in humans suggests a risk of pulmonary hypertension of the newborn, SABs, and congenital malformations linked to the use of Meclofenamate.

**Further Reading:**
- Dawood, M. Y., (1993). Nonsteroidal anti-inflammatory drugs and reproduction. *Am. J. Obstet. Gynecol., 169,* 1255–1265.
- *Drug Information. Meclomen.* Parke-Davis.
- Levin, D. L., (1980). Effects of inhibition of prostaglandin synthesis on fetal development, oxygenation, and the fetal circulation. *Semin. Perinatol., 4,* 35–44.
- Matt, D. W., & Borzelleca, J. F., (1995). Toxic effects on the female reproductive system during pregnancy, parturition, and lactation. In: Witorsch, R. J., (ed.) *Reproductive Toxicology* (2nd ed., p. 175–193). New York, NY: Raven Press.
- Van Marter, L. J., Leviton, A., Allred, E. N., Pagano, M., Sullivan, K. F., Cohen, A., & Epstein, M. F., (1996). Persistent pulmonary hypertension of the newborn and smoking and aspirin and nonsteroidal anti-inflammatory drug consumption during pregnancy. *Pediatrics, 97,* 658–663.

## 10.4.13   *MEFENAMIC ACID*

**FDA Category: N**
*Risk Summary:* It is better to be avoided during the 1st and 3rd Trimesters because the pregnancy experience in humans suggests a risk of pulmonary hypertension of the newborn, SABs, and congenital malformations linked to the use of Mefenamic Acid.

**Further Reading:**
- Dawood, M. Y., (1993). Nonsteroidal anti-inflammatory drugs and reproduction. *Am. J. Obstet. Gynecol., 169*, 1255–1265.
- *Drug Information.* Ponstel. Parke-Davis.
- Levin, D. L., (1980). Effects of inhibition of prostaglandin synthesis on fetal development, oxygenation, and the fetal circulation. *Semin. Perinatol., 4*, 35–44.
- Matt, D. W., & Borzelleca, J. F., (1995). Toxic effects on the female reproductive system during pregnancy, parturition, and lactation. In: Witorsch, R. J., (ed.) *Reproductive Toxicology* (2nd ed., p. 175–193). New York, NY: Raven Press.
- Van Marter, L. J., Leviton, A., Allred, E. N., Pagano, M., Sullivan, K. F., Cohen, A., & Epstein, M. F., (1996). Persistent pulmonary hypertension of the newborn and smoking and aspirin and nonsteroidal anti-inflammatory drug consumption during pregnancy. *Pediatrics, 97*, 658–663.

## 10.4.14   MELOXICAM

**FDA Category: C**
***Risk Summary:*** It is better to be avoided during the 1st and 3rd Trimesters because the pregnancy experience in humans suggests a risk of pulmonary hypertension of the newborn, SABs, and congenital malformations linked to the use of Meloxicam.

**Further Reading:**
- Dawood, M. Y., (1993). Nonsteroidal anti-inflammatory drugs and reproduction. *Am. J. Obstet. Gynecol., 169*, 1255–1265.
- *Drug Information.* Mobic. Boehringer Ingelheim Pharmaceuticals.
- Levin, D. L., (1980). Effects of inhibition of prostaglandin synthesis on fetal development, oxygenation, and the fetal circulation. *Semin. Perinatol., 4*, 35–44.
- Matt, D. W., & Borzelleca, J. F., (1995). Toxic effects on the female reproductive system during pregnancy, parturition, and lactation. In: Witorsch, R. J., (ed.) *Reproductive Toxicology* (2nd ed., p. 175–193). New York, NY: Raven Press.
- Van Marter, L. J., Leviton, A., Allred, E. N., Pagano, M., Sullivan, K. F., Cohen, A., & Epstein, M. F., (1996). Persistent pulmonary hypertension of the newborn and smoking and aspirin and nonsteroidal

anti-inflammatory drug consumption during pregnancy. *Pediatrics*, *97*, 658–663.

## 10.4.15 NABUMETONE

**FDA Category: C**
*Risk Summary:* It is better to be avoided during the 1st and 3rd Trimesters because the pregnancy experience in humans suggests a risk of pulmonary hypertension of the newborn, SABs, and congenital malformations linked to the use of Nabumetone.

**Further Reading:**
- Dawood, M. Y., (1993). Nonsteroidal anti-inflammatory drugs and reproduction. *Am. J. Obstet. Gynecol., 169*, 1255–1265.
- *Drug Information. Relafen.* SmithKline Beecham Pharmaceuticals.
- Levin, D. L., (1980). Effects of inhibition of prostaglandin synthesis on fetal development, oxygenation, and the fetal circulation. *Semin. Perinatol., 4*, 35–44.
- Matt, D. W., & Borzelleca, J. F., (1995). Toxic effects on the female reproductive system during pregnancy, parturition, and lactation. In: Witorsch, R. J., (ed.) *Reproductive Toxicology* (2nd ed., p. 175–193). New York, NY: Raven Press.
- Van Marter, L. J., Leviton, A., Allred, E. N., Pagano, M., Sullivan, K. F., Cohen, A., & Epstein, M. F., (1996). Persistent pulmonary hypertension of the newborn and smoking and aspirin and nonsteroidal anti-inflammatory drug consumption during pregnancy. *Pediatrics*, *97*, 658–663.

## 10.4.16 NAPROXEN

**FDA Category: C**
*Risk Summary:* It is better to be avoided during the 1st and 3rd Trimesters because the pregnancy experience in humans suggests a risk of pulmonary hypertension of the newborn, SABs, and congenital malformations linked to the use of Naproxen. Furthermore, Naproxen has been found to inhibit labor and to prolong the length of pregnancy.

**Further Reading:**

- Dawood, M. Y., (1993). Nonsteroidal anti-inflammatory drugs and reproduction. *Am. J. Obstet. Gynecol., 169*, 1255–1265.
- *Drug Information. Naprosyn*. Roche Laboratories.
- Levin, D. L., (1980). Effects of inhibition of prostaglandin synthesis on fetal development, oxygenation, and the fetal circulation. *Semin. Perinatol., 4*, 35–44.
- Matt, D. W., & Borzelleca, J. F., (1995). Toxic effects on the female reproductive system during pregnancy, parturition, and lactation. In: Witorsch, R. J., (ed.) *Reproductive Toxicology* (2nd ed., p. 175–193). New York, NY: Raven Press.
- Van Marter, L. J., Leviton, A., Allred, E. N., Pagano, M., Sullivan, K. F., Cohen, A., & Epstein, M. F., (1996). Persistent pulmonary hypertension of the newborn and smoking and aspirin and nonsteroidal anti-inflammatory drug consumption during pregnancy. *Pediatrics, 97*, 658–663.

### 10.4.17   OXAPROZIN

**FDA Category: C**

*Risk Summary:* It is better to be avoided during the 1st and 3rd Trimesters because the pregnancy experience in humans suggests a risk of pulmonary hypertension of the newborn, SABs, and congenital malformations linked to the use of Oxaprozin. Furthermore, Oxaprozin has been found to inhibit labor and to prolong the length of pregnancy.

**Further Reading:**

- Dawood, M. Y., (1993). Nonsteroidal anti-inflammatory drugs and reproduction. *Am. J. Obstet. Gynecol., 169*, 1255–1265.
- *Drug Information*. Daypro. G.D. Searle.
- Levin, D. L., (1980). Effects of inhibition of prostaglandin synthesis on fetal development, oxygenation, and the fetal circulation. *Semin. Perinatol., 4*, 35–44.
- Matt, D. W., & Borzelleca, J. F., (1995). Toxic effects on the female reproductive system during pregnancy, parturition, and lactation. In: Witorsch, R. J., (ed.) *Reproductive Toxicology* (2nd ed., p. 175–193). New York, NY: Raven Press.
- Van Marter, L. J., Leviton, A., Allred, E. N., Pagano, M., Sullivan, K. F., Cohen, A., & Epstein, M. F., (1996). Persistent pulmonary

hypertension of the newborn and smoking and aspirin and nonsteroidal anti-inflammatory drug consumption during pregnancy. *Pediatrics, 97,* 658–663.

### 10.4.18 *PIROXICAM*

**FDA Category: C**
***Risk Summary:*** It is better to be avoided during the 1st and 3rd Trimesters because the pregnancy experience in humans suggests a risk of pulmonary hypertension of the newborn, SABs, and congenital malformations linked to the use of Piroxicam.

**Further Reading:**
- Dawood, M. Y., (1993). Nonsteroidal anti-inflammatory drugs and reproduction. *Am. J. Obstet. Gynecol., 169,* 1255–1265.
- *Drug Information. Feldene.* Pfizer.
- Levin, D. L., (1980). Effects of inhibition of prostaglandin synthesis on fetal development, oxygenation, and the fetal circulation. *Semin. Perinatol., 4,* 35–44.
- Matt, D. W., & Borzelleca, J. F., (1995). Toxic effects on the female reproductive system during pregnancy, parturition, and lactation. In: Witorsch, R. J., (ed.) *Reproductive Toxicology* (2nd ed., p. 175–193). New York, NY: Raven Press.
- Van Marter, L. J., Leviton, A., Allred, E. N., Pagano, M., Sullivan, K. F., Cohen, A., & Epstein, M. F., (1996). Persistent pulmonary hypertension of the newborn and smoking and aspirin and nonsteroidal anti-inflammatory drug consumption during pregnancy. *Pediatrics, 97,* 658–663.

### 10.4.19 *SULINDAC*

**FDA Category: C**
***Risk Summary:*** It is better to be avoided during the 1st and 3rd Trimesters because the pregnancy experience in humans suggests a risk of pulmonary hypertension of the newborn, SABs, and congenital malformations linked to the use of Sulindac.

**Further Reading:**
- Dawood, M. Y., (1993). Nonsteroidal anti-inflammatory drugs and reproduction. *Am. J. Obstet. Gynecol., 169,* 1255–1265.
- Levin, D. L., (1980). Effects of inhibition of prostaglandin synthesis on fetal development, oxygenation, and the fetal circulation. *Semin. Perinatol., 4,* 35–44.
- Matt, D. W., & Borzelleca, J. F., (1995). Toxic effects on the female reproductive system during pregnancy, parturition, and lactation. In: Witorsch, R. J., (ed.) *Reproductive Toxicology* (2nd ed., p. 175–193). New York, NY: Raven Press.
- Van Marter, L. J., Leviton, A., Allred, E. N., Pagano, M., Sullivan, K. F., Cohen, A., & Epstein, M. F., (1996). Persistent pulmonary hypertension of the newborn and smoking and aspirin and nonsteroidal anti-inflammatory drug consumption during pregnancy. *Pediatrics, 97,* 658–663.

### *10.4.20   TOLMETIN*

**FDA Category: C**
***Risk Summary:*** It is better to be avoided during the 1st and 3rd Trimesters because the pregnancy experience in humans suggests a risk of pulmonary hypertension of the newborn, SABs, and congenital malformations linked to the use of Tolmetin.

**Further Reading:**
- Dawood, M. Y., (1993). Nonsteroidal anti-inflammatory drugs and reproduction. *Am. J. Obstet. Gynecol., 169,* 1255–1265.
- *Drug Information. Tolectin.* Ortho-McNeil Pharmaceutical.
- Levin, D. L., (1980). Effects of inhibition of prostaglandin synthesis on fetal development, oxygenation, and the fetal circulation. *Semin. Perinatol., 4,* 35–44.
- Matt, D. W., & Borzelleca, J. F., (1995). Toxic effects on the female reproductive system during pregnancy, parturition, and lactation. In: Witorsch, R. J., (ed.) *Reproductive Toxicology* (2nd ed., p. 175–193). New York, NY: Raven Press.
- Van Marter, L. J., Leviton, A., Allred, E. N., Pagano, M., Sullivan, K. F., Cohen, A., & Epstein, M. F., (1996). Persistent pulmonary hypertension of the newborn and smoking and aspirin and nonsteroidal

anti-inflammatory drug consumption during pregnancy. *Pediatrics*, *97*, 658–663.

## 10.5 DISEASE-MODIFYING ANTI-RHEUMATIC DRUGS (DMARDS)

### 10.5.1 *CONVENTIONAL DMARDS*

#### 10.5.1.1 *AURANOFIN*

**FDA Category: C**
***Risk Summary:*** It should be used with caution because the pregnancy experience in humans is limited and the reproduction studies in animals have shown low risk.

**Further Reading:**
- *Drug Information*. Ridaura. Prometheus Laboratories.

#### 10.5.1.2 *AZATHIOPRINE*

**FDA Category: D**
***Risk Summary:*** It should be used with caution during the 1st and 2nd Trimesters. However, it is better to avoid the use of Azathioprine during the 3rd Trimester because it has been associated with immunosuppression and bone marrow suppression of the newborn. However, sometimes the maternal benefit from using Azathioprine outweighs the fetal risk.

**Further Reading:**
- Alstead, E. M., Ritchie, J. K., Lennard-Jones, J. E., Farthing, M. J. G., & Clark, M. L., (1990). Safety of azathioprine in pregnancy in inflammatory bowel disease. *Gastroenterology*, *99*, 443–446.
- Cararach, V., Carmona, F., Monleón, F. J., & Andreu, J., (1993). Pregnancy after renal transplantation: 25 years of experience in Spain. *Br. J. Obstet. Gynaecol.*, *100*, 122–125.
- Davison, J. M., Dellagrammatikas, H., & Parkin, J. M., (1985). Maternal azathioprine therapy and depressed hemopoiesis in the babies of renal allograft patients. *Br. J. Obstet. Gynaecol.*, *92*, 233–239.

- DeWitte, D. B., Buick, M. K., Cyran, S. E., & Maisels, M. J., (1984). Neonatal pancytopenia and severe combined immunodeficiency associated with antenatal administration of azathioprine and prednisone. *J. Pediatr., 105*, 625–628.
- *Drug Information. Imuran.* FARO Pharmaceuticals.

## 10.5.1.3   CHLOROQUINE

**FDA Category: N**
***Risk Summary:*** Although there is limited data from the human pregnancy experience, but the possible maternal benefit from Chloroquine, as an antimalarial drug, extremely outweighs the unknown or known embryo/fetal risk. However, it is better to avoid its use in pregnant women with rheumatic diseases, and to look for safer alternative(s).

**Further Reading:**
- *Drug Information. Aralen.* Sanofi Pharmaceuticals.
- Ross, J. B., & Garatsos, S., (1974). Absence of chloroquine induced ototoxicity in a fetus. *Arch Dermatol., 109*, 573.
- Wolfe, M. S., & Cordero, J. F., (1985). Safety of chloroquine in chemosuppression of malaria during pregnancy. *Br. Med. J., 290*, 1466–1467.

## 10.5.1.4   HYDROXYCHLOROQUINE

**FDA Category: N**
***Risk Summary:*** Although there is limited data from the human pregnancy experience, but the possible maternal benefit from Hydroxychloroquine, as an antimalarial drug, extremely outweighs the unknown or known embryo/fetal risk. However, it is better to avoid its use in pregnant women with rheumatic diseases, and to look for safer alternative(s).

**Further Reading:**
- Buchanan, N. M. M., Toubi, E., Khamashta, M. A., Lima, F., Kerslake, S., & Hughes, G. R. V., (1995). The safety of hydroxychloroquine in lupus pregnancy: Experience in 27 pregnancies (abstract). *Br. J. Rheumatol., 34*(Suppl 1),14.
- *Drug Information. Plaquenil.* Sanofi Winthrop Pharmaceuticals.

- Suhonen, R., (1983). Hydroxychloroquine administration in pregnancy. *Arch Dermatol., 119*, 185–186.

## 10.5.1.5   CYCLOPHOSPHAMIDE

**FDA Category: D**
***Risk Summary:*** It is contraindicated during the 1st Trimester. Furthermore, its use later in pregnancy has been associated with fetal bone marrow suppression.

**Further Reading:**
- Coates, A., (1970). Cyclophosphamide in pregnancy. *Aust N-Z J. Obstet. Gynaecol., 10*, 33, 34.
- Hardin, J. A., (1972). Cyclophosphamide treatment of lymphoma during third trimester of pregnancy. *Obstet. Gynecol., 39*, 850–851.
- Kirshon, B., Wasserstrum, N., Willis, R., Herman, G. E., McCabe, E. R. B., (1988). Teratogenic effects of first-trimester cyclophosphamide therapy. *Obstet. Gynecol., 72*, 462–464.
- Tolchin, S. F., Winkelstein, A., Rodnan, G. P., Pan, S. F., & Nankin, H. R., (1974). Chromosome abnormalities from cyclophosphamide therapy in rheumatoid arthritis and progressive systemic sclerosis (scleroderma) *Arthritis. Rheum., 17*, 375–382.

## 10.5.1.6   CYCLOSPORINE

**FDA Category: C**
***Risk Summary:*** It should be used with caution because the pregnancy experience in humans is limited and the reproduction studies in animals have shown low risk.

**Further Reading:**
- *Drug Information. Neoral, Sandimmune.* Novartis Pharmaceuticals.
- Ziegenhagen, D. J., Grombach, G., Dieckmann, M., Zehnter, E., Wienand, P., & Baldamus, C. A., (1988). Pregnancy under cyclosporine administration after renal transplantation. *Dtsch. Med. Wochenschr., 113*, 260–263.

## 10.5.1.7   GOLD SODIUM THIOMALATE

**FDA Category: C**
***Risk Summary:*** It should be used with caution because the pregnancy experience in humans is limited and the reproduction studies in animals have shown low risk.

**Further Reading:**
- Cohen, D. L., Orzel, J., & Taylor, A., (1981). Infants of mothers receiving gold therapy. *Arthritis. Rheum., 24*, 104, 105.
- *Drug Information. Myochrysine.* Merck.
- Fuchs, U., & Lippert, T. H., (1986). Gold therapy and pregnancy. *Dtsch. Med. Wochenschr., 111*, 31–34.

## 10.5.1.8   LEFLUNOMIDE

**FDA Category: X**
***Risk Summary:*** It is an animal teratogen, and its use is contraindicated during pregnancy. It is advisable for the female patient planning to become pregnant to stop the drug for two years before the conception.

**Further Reading:**
- Chambers, C. D., Johnson, D. L., Robinson, L. K., Braddock, S. R., Xu, R., Lopez-Jimenez, J., Mirrasoul, N., Salas, E., Luo, Y. J., Jin, S., & Jones, K. L., (2010). and the Organizations of Teratology Information Specialists Collaborative Research Group. Birth outcomes in women who have taken leflunomide during pregnancy. *Arthritis. Rheum., 62*, 1494–1503.
- De Santis, M., Straface, G., Cavaliere, A., Carducci, B., & Caruso, A., (2005). Paternal and maternal exposure to leflunomide: Pregnancy and neonatal outcome. *Ann. Rheum. Dis., 64*, 1096–1097.
- *Drug Information. Arava.* Sanofi-Aventis.
- Neville, C. E., & McNally, J., (2007). Maternal exposure to leflunomide associated with blindness and cerebral palsy. *Rheumatology, 46*, 1506.

## 10.5.1.9  METHOTREXATE

**FDA Category: X**
*Risk Summary:* It is contraindicated during pregnancy because the administration of Methotrexate during organogenesis has been associated with the fetal aminopterin-methotrexate syndrome. Additionally, its use during the 2nd and 3rd Trimesters has been linked to fetal toxicity and mortality.

**Further Reading:**
- Bawle, E. V., Conard, J. V., & Weiss, L., (1998). Adult and two children with fetal methotrexate syndrome. *Teratology*, *57*, 51–55.
- Kozlowski, R. D., Steinbrunner, J. V., MacKenzie, A. H., Clough, J. D., Wilke, W. S., & Segal, A. M., (1990). Outcome of first-trimester exposure to low-dose methotrexate in eight patients with rheumatic disease. *Am. J. Med.*, *88*, 589–592.
- Powell, H. R., & Ekert, H., (1971). Methotrexate-induced congenital malformations. *Med. J. Aust.*, *2*, 1076–1077.

## 10.5.1.10  MYCOPHENOLATE MOFETIL

**FDA Category: D**
*Risk Summary:* The use of Mycophenolate Mofetil should be avoided in pregnant women because the pregnancy experience in humans has shown the risk of teratogenicity associated with the use of this drug.

**Further Reading:**
- *Drug Information. CellCept.* Roche Pharmaceuticals.
- Tjeertes, I. F. A., Bastiaans, D. E. T., van Ganzewinkel, C. J. L. M., Zegers, S. H. J., (2007). Neonatal anemia and hydrops fetalis after maternal mycophenolate mofetil use. *J. Perinatal.*, *27*, 62–64.
- Velinov, M., & Zellers, N., (2008). The fetal mycophenolate mofetil syndrome. *Clin. Dysmorphol.*, *17*, 77–78.

## 10.5.1.11  SULFASALAZINE

**FDA Category: B**
*Risk Summary:* Although Sulfasalazine has been assigned with the letter (B) by the FDA categorization, however, it should be used with caution because the available human data have shown a low risk of congenital malformations.

**Further Reading:**
- Craxi, A., & Pagliarello, F., (1980). Possible embryotoxicity of sulfasalazine. *Arch. Intern. Med., 140,* 1674.
- Hoo, J. J., Hadro, T. A., & Von Behren, P., (1988). Possible teratogenicity of sulfasalazine. *N. Engl. J. Med., 318,* 1128.
- Mogadam, M., Dobbins, W. O. III., Korelitz, B. I., & Ahmed, S. W., (1981). Pregnancy in inflammatory bowel disease: Effect of sulfasalazine and corticosteroids on fetal outcome. *Gastroenterology, 80,* 72–76.

## 10.5.2 BIOLOGICAL DMARDS

### 10.5.2.1 ABATACEPT

**FDA Category: C**
*Risk Summary:* It should be used with caution because the pregnancy experience in humans is limited and the reproduction studies in animals have shown low risk.

**Further Reading:**
- Goeb, V., Gossec, L., Goupille, P., Guillaume-Czitrom, S., Hachulla, E., Lequerre, T., Marolleau, J. P., Martinez, V., Masson, C., Mouthon, L., Puechal, X., Richette, P., Saraux, A., Schaeverbeke, T., Soubrier, M., Viguier, M., Vittecoq, O., Wendling, D., Mariette, X., & Sibilia, J., (2012). Abatacept therapy and safety management. *Joint Bone Spine, 72*(Suppl 1), 3–84.
- *Drug Information. Orencia.* Bristol-Myers Squibb.
- Ojeda-Uribe, M., Afif, N., Dahan, E., Sparsa, L., Haby, C., Sibilia, J., Ternant, D., & Ardizzone, M., (2013). Exposure to abatacept or rituximab in the first trimester of pregnancy of three women with autoimmune diseases. *Clin. Rheumatol.,* 2013 *32,* 695–700.
- Pham, T., Bachelez, H., Barthelot, J. M., Blacher, J., Claudepierre, P., Constantin, A., Fautrel, B., Gaujoux-Viala.

### 10.5.2.2 ADALIMUMAB

**FDA Category: B**
*Risk Summary:* The reproduction studies in animals have shown no evidence of fetal harm or impaired fertility. The pregnancy experience in humans is adequate to exhibit that the embryo-fetal risk is nonexistent or very low.

**Further Reading:**
- Dessinioti, C., Stefanaki, I., Stratigos, A. J., Kostaki, M., Katsambas, A., & Antoniou, C., (2011). Pregnancy during adalimumab use for psoriasis. *J. Eur. Acad. Dermatol. Venereol., 25*, 738–739.
- *Drug Information. Humira.* Abbott Laboratories.
- Vesga, L., Terdiman, J. P., & Mahadevan, U., (2005). Adalimumab use in pregnancy. *Gut., 54*, 890.

### 10.5.2.3 CERTOLIZUMAB

**FDA Category: B**
***Risk Summary:*** The reproduction studies in animals have shown no evidence of fetal harm or impaired fertility. The pregnancy experience in humans is limited.

**Further Reading:**
- *Drug Information. Cimzia.* UCB.
- Khanna, D., McMahon, M., & Furst, D. E., (2004). Safety of tumor necrosis factor-α antagonists. *Drug Saf., 27*, 307–324.
- Mahadevan, U., Cucchiara, S., Hyams, J. S., Steinwurz, F., Nuti, F., Travis, S. P. L., Sandborn, W. J., & Colombel, I. H., (2011). The London position statement of the World Congress of Gastroenterology on biological therapy for IBD with the European Crohn's and Colitis Organization: Pregnancy and pediatrics. *Am. J. Gastroenterol., 106*, 214–223.

### 10.5.2.4 ETANERCEPT

**FDA Category: B**
***Risk Summary:*** The reproduction studies in animals have shown no evidence of fetal harm or impaired fertility. The pregnancy experience in humans is limited.

**Further Reading:**
- *Drug Information. Enbrel.* Immunex.
- Murashima, A., Watanabe, N., Ozawa, N., Saito, H., & Yamaguchi, K., (2009). Etanercept during pregnancy and lactation in a patient

with rheumatoid arthritis: Drug levels in maternal serum, cord blood, breast milk, and the infant's serum. *Ann. Rheum. Dis., 68*, 1793–1794.
- Umeda, N., Ito, S., Hayashi, T., Goto, D., Matsumoto, I., & Sumida, T., (2010). A patient with rheumatoid arthritis who had a normal delivery under etanercept treatment. *Inter. Med., 49*, 187–189.

## 10.5.2.5   GOLIMUMAB

**FDA Category: B**
*Risk Summary:* It is better to be avoided during the 1st Trimester because the pregnancy experience in humans is limited and the reproduction studies in animals have shown low risk.

**Further Reading:**
- *Drug Information. Simponi.* Centocor Ortho Biotech.
- Khanna, D., McMahon, M., & Furst, D. E., (2004). Safety of tumor necrosis factor-α antagonists. *Drug Saf.,* 2004 *27*, 307–324.
- Martin, P. L., Oneda, S., & Treacy, G., (2007). Effects of an anti-TNF-α monoclonal antibody, administered throughout pregnancy and lactation, on the development of the macaque immune system. *Am. J. Reprod. Immunol., 58*, 138–149.

## 10.5.2.6   INFLIXIMAB

**FDA Category: B**
*Risk Summary:* The reproduction studies in animals have shown no evidence of fetal harm or impaired fertility. The pregnancy experience in humans is limited.

**Further Reading:**
- Antoni, C. E., Furst, D., Manger, B., Lichtenstein, G. R., Keenan, G. F., Healy, D. E., Jacobs, S. J., & Katz Erlangen, J. A., (2001). Outcome of pregnancy in women receiving Remicade (infliximab) for the treatment of Crohn's disease or rheumatoid arthritis (abstract). *Arthritis. Rheum., 44*(Suppl 9), S152.
- Burt, M. J., Frizelle, F. A., & Barbezar, G. O., (2003). Pregnancy and exposure to infliximab (anti-tumor necrosis factor-alpha monoclonal antibody). *J. Gastroenterol. Hepatol., 18*, 465, 466.

• *Drug Information. Remicade.* Centocor.

## 10.5.2.7   RITUXIMAB

**FDA Category: C**
***Risk Summary:*** It should be used with caution because the human pregnancy experience has shown a low risk.

**Further Reading:**
• *Drug Information. Rituxan.* Genentech.
• Friedrichs, B., Tiemann, M., Salwender, H., Verpoort, K., Wenger, M. K., & Schmitz, N., (2006). The effects of rituximab treatment during pregnancy on a neonate. *Haematologica., 91,* 1426, 1427.
• Klink, D. T., van Elburg, R. M., Schreurs, M. W. J., van & Well, T. J., (2008). Rituximab administration in third trimester of pregnancy suppresses neonatal B-cell development. *Clin. Dev. Immunol.,* 271–363.
• Ojeda-Uribe, M., Afif, N., Dahan, E., Sparsa, L., Haby, C., Sibilia, J., Ternant, D., & Ardizzone, M., (2013). Exposure to abatacept or rituximab in the first trimester of pregnancy of three women with autoimmune diseases. *Clin. Rheumatol., 32,* 695–700.

## 10.5.2.8   TOCILIZUMAB

**FDA Category: C**
***Risk Summary:*** The reproduction studies in animals have shown no evidence of fetal harm or impaired fertility. The pregnancy experience in humans is limited.

**Further Reading:**
• *Drug Information. Actemra,* Genentech.
• Mano, Y., Shibata, K., Sumigama, S., Hayakawa, H., Ino, K., Yamamoto, E., Kajiyama, H., Nawa, A., Kikkawa, F., (2009). Tocilizumab inhibits interleukin-6-mediated matrix metalloproteinase-2 and -9 secretions from human amnion cells in preterm premature rupture of membranes. *Gynecol. Obstet. Invest., 68,* 145–153.

- Rubbert-Roth, A., Goupile, P. M., Moosavi, S., & Hou, A., (2010). First experiences with pregnancies in RA patients receiving tocilizumab therapy (abstract). *Arthritis. Rheum.*, (Suppl), p. 384.

## 10.6   OTHER ANALGESICS

### 10.6.1   *ACETAMINOPHEN*

**FDA Category: C**
***Risk Summary:*** It should be used with caution because the continuous use of high doses of Acetaminophen during pregnancy has been linked with severe maternal anemia (possibly hemolytic), and fatal kidney disease in the newborn.

**Further Reading:**
- Accessdata.fda.gov. (2018). Available from: https://www.accessdata.fda.gov/drugsatfda_docs/label/2015/204767s000lbl.pdf (accessed on 31 January 2020)
- Char, V. C., Chandra, R., Fletcher, A. B., & Avery, G. B., (1975). Polyhydramnios and neonatal renal failure—a possible association with maternal acetaminophen ingestion. *J. Pediatr., 86*, 638–639.
- Feldkamp, M. L., Meyer, R. E., Krikov, S., & Botto, L. D., (2010). Acetaminophen use in pregnancy and risk of birth defects. Findings from the National Birth Defects Prevention Study. *Obstet. Gynecol., 115*, 109–115.
- Kang, E. M., Lundsberg, L. S., Illuzzi, J. L., & Bracken, M. B., (2009). Prenatal exposure to acetaminophen and asthma in children. *Obstet. Gynecol., 114*, 1295–1306.
- Rebordosa, C., Kogevinas, M., Horvath-Puho, E., Norgard, B., Morales, M., Czeizel, A. E., Vilstrup, H., Sorensen, H. T., Olsen, J., (2008). Acetaminophen use during pregnancy: Effects on risk for congenital abnormalities. *Am. J. Obstet. Gynecol., 198*, 178e1–7.

### 10.6.2   *ANTIPYRINE (PHENAZONE)*

**FDA Category: N**
***Risk Summary:*** It should be used only when the maternal benefit outweighs the fetal risk because there is very limited human pregnancy data, and animal studies are not relevant.

**Further Reading:**
- Lewis, P. J., & Friedman, L. A., (1979). Prophylaxis of neonatal jaundice with maternal antipyrine treatment. *Lancet, 1*, 300–302.
- Swanson, M., & Cook, R., (1977). *Drugs Chemicals and Blood Dyscrasias. Hamilton*, (pp. 88, 89). IL: Drug Intelligence Publications.

## 10.6.3 ZICONOTIDE

**FDA Category: C**
***Risk Summary:*** Although there is limited data from the human pregnancy experience, but the possible maternal benefit extremely outweighs the unknown or known embryo/fetal risk.

**Further Reading:**
- *Drug Information. Prialt.* Elan Pharmaceuticals.

## 10.7 DRUGS USED FOR GOUT

## 10.7.1 ALLOPURINOL

**FDA Category: C**
***Risk Summary:*** It should be used only when the maternal benefit outweighs the fetal risk because there is very limited human pregnancy data, and animal studies are not relevant.

**Further Reading:**
- *Drug Information. Zyloric.* GSK.
- Kaandorp, J. J., Benders, M. J. N. L., Rademaker, C. M. A., Torrance, H. L., & Oudijk, M. A., (2010). Antenatal allopurinol for reduction birth asphyxia induced brain damage (ALLO-Trial); a randomized double-blind placebo-controlled multicenter study. *BMC Pregnancy Child Birth, 10*, 8.
- Kozenko, M., Grynspan, D., Oluyomi-Obi, Sitar, D., Elliott, A. M., & Chodirker, B. N., (2011). Potential teratogenic effects of allopurinol: A case report. *Am. J. Med. Genet., 155*, 2247–2252.

## 10.7.2   COLCHICINE

**FDA Category: C**
***Risk Summary:*** Although the reproduction studies in animals have shown the risk of teratogenic effects, however, the pregnancy experience in humans did not found evidence of developmental toxicity or teratogenicity when Colchicine was used at recommended doses.

**Further Reading:**
- Diav-Citrin, O., Shechtman, S., Schwartz, V., Avgil-Tsadok, M., Finkel-Pekarsky, V., Wajnberg, R., et al., (2010). Pregnancy outcome after in utero exposure to colchicine. *Am. J. Obstet. Gynecol., 203,* 144, e1–8.
- Michael, O., Goldman, R. D., & Koren, G., (2003). and Motherisk Team. Safety of colchicine during pregnancy. *Can. Fam. Physician., 49,* 967–969.
- Rabinovitch, O., Zemer, D., Kukia, E., Sohar, E., & Mashlach, S., (1992). Colchicine treatment in conception and pregnancy: Two hundred thirty-one pregnancies in patients with familial Mediterranean fever. *Am. J. Reprod. Immunol., 28,* 245–246.

## 10.7.3   FEBUXOSTAT

**FDA Category: C**
***Risk Summary:*** It should be used with caution because the pregnancy experience in humans is limited and the reproduction studies in animals have shown low risk.

**Further Reading:**
- *Drug Information. Uloric.* Takeda Pharmaceuticals America.

## 10.7.4   PEGLOTICASE

**FDA Category: C**
***Risk Summary:*** It should be used with caution because the pregnancy experience in humans is limited and the reproduction studies in animals have shown low risk.

## Further Reading:

- *Drug Information. Krystexxa.* Savient Pharmaceuticals.
- Sundy, J. S., Ganson, N. J., Kelly, S. J., Scarlett, E. L., Rehrig, C. D., Huang, W., & Hershfield, M. S., (2007). Pharmacokinetics and phar-macodynamics of intravenous PEGylated recombinant mammalian urate oxidase in patients with refractory gout. *Arthritis. Rheum., 56,* 1021–1028.
- Yue, C. S., Huang, W., Alton, M., Maroli, A. N., Wright, D., & Marco, M. D., (2008). Population pharmacokinetic and pharmacodynamic analysis of pegloticase in subjects with hyperuricemia and treatment-failure gout. *J. Clin. Pharmacol., 48,* 708–718.

## *10.7.5 PROBENECID*

### FDA Category: N

*Risk Summary:* The reproduction studies in animals have shown no evidence of fetal harm or impaired fertility. The pregnancy experience in humans is limited.

### Further Reading:

- Cavenee, M. R., Farris, J. R., Spalding, T. R., Barnes, D. L., Castaneda, Y. S., Wendel, G. D. Jr., (1993). Treatment of gonorrhea in pregnancy. *Obstet. Gynecol., 81,* 33–38.
- *Drug Information.* Probenecid. Mylan Pharmaceuticals.
- Lee, F. I., & Loeffler, F. E., (1962). Gout and pregnancy. *J. Obstet. Gynaecol. Br. Commonw., 69,* 299.

## KEYWORDS

- **allopurinol**
- **colchicine**
- **disease-modifying anti-rheumatic drugs**
- **febuxostat**
- **pegloticase**
- **probenecid**

# CHAPTER 11

# Drugs Affecting the Urinary Tract

## 11.1  ANALGESICS

### 11.1.1  PENTOSAN

**FDA Category: B**
*Risk Summary:* The reproduction studies in animals have shown no evidence of fetal harm or impaired fertility. The pregnancy experience in humans is limited.

**Further Reading:**
- *Drug Information.* Elmiron. Ortho Women's Health & Urology, Ortho-McNeil Pharmaceutical, 2006.
- Rosenberg, M. T., Moldwin, R. M., & Stanford, E. J., (2004). Early diagnosis and management of interstitial cystitis. *Women's Health Primary Care, 7,* 456–463.

### 11.1.2  PHENAZOPYRIDINE

**FDA Category: B**
*Risk Summary:* The reproduction studies in animals have shown no evidence of fetal harm or impaired fertility. The pregnancy experience in humans is adequate to exhibit that the embryo-fetal risk is nonexistent or very low.

**Further Reading:**
- Heinonen, O. P., Slone, D., & Shapiro, S., (1977). *Birth Defects and Drugs in Pregnancy.* Littleton, MA: Publishing Sciences Group.
- Lee, M., Bozzo, P., Einarson, A., & Koren, G., (2008). Urinary tract infections in pregnancy. *Can Fam Physician, 54,* 853, 854.

## 11.2   ANTISPASMODICS

### 11.2.1   *DARIFENACIN*

**FDA Category: C**
*Risk Summary:* It should be used with caution because the pregnancy experience in humans is limited and the reproduction studies in animals have shown low risk.

**Further Reading:**
• *Drug Information. Enablex.* Novartis.

### 11.2.2   *FESOTERODINE*

**FDA Category: C**
*Risk Summary:* It should be used with caution because the pregnancy experience in humans is limited and the reproduction studies in animals have shown low risk.

**Further Reading:**
• *Drug Information. Toviaz.* Pfizer.

### 11.2.3   *FLAVOXATE*

**FDA Category: B**
*Risk Summary:* It should be used with caution because the pregnancy experience in humans is limited and the reproduction studies in animals have shown low risk.

**Further Reading:**
• *Drug Information. Urispas.* SmithKline Beecham Pharmaceuticals.
• Esposito, A., (1975). *Preliminary Studies on the Use of Flavoxate in Obstetrics and Gynaecology* (pp. 66–73). International Round Table Discussion on Flavoxate, Opatija, Yugoslavia (translation provided by BA Wallin, Smith Kline & French Laboratories, 1987).

## 11.2.4 MIRABEGRON

**FDA Category: B**
*Risk Summary:* It should be used with caution because the pregnancy experience in humans is limited and the reproduction studies in animals have shown low risk.

**Further Reading:**
- *Drug Information. Myrbetriq.* Astellas Pharma US.


## 11.2.5 OXYBUTYNIN

**FDA Category: B**
*Risk Summary:* It should be used with caution because the pregnancy experience in humans is limited and the reproduction studies in animals have shown low risk.

**Further Reading:**
- *Drug Information. Ditropan.* ALZA Pharmaceuticals.
- Edwards, J. A., Reid, Y. J., & Cozens, D. D., (1986). Reproductive toxicity studies with oxybutynin hydrochloride. *Toxicology, 40,* 31–44.
- Schardein, J. L., (1993). *Chemically Induced Birth Defects* (2nd edn., p. 645). New York, NY: Marcel Dekker.


## 11.2.6 SOLIFENACIN

**FDA Category: C**
*Risk Summary:* There is limited pregnancy experience in humans, and the reproduction studies in animals have shown moderate risk. Therefore, it is advisable to avoid its use until the human pregnancy experience is available.

**Further Reading:**
- *Drug Information. Vesicare.* Astellas Pharma US.

### 11.2.7   TOLTERODINE

**FDA Category: C**
***Risk Summary:*** It should be used with caution because the pregnancy experience in humans is limited and the reproduction studies in animals have shown low risk.

**Further Reading:**
- *Drug Information. Detrol.* Pharmacia & Upjohn.
- Pahlman, I., d'Argy, R., & Nilvebrant, L., (2001). Tissue distribution of tolterodine, a muscarinic receptor antagonist, and transfer into fetus and milk in mice. *Arzneimittelforschung, 51*, 125–133.

### 11.2.8   TROSPIUM

**FDA Category: C**
***Risk Summary:*** It should be used with caution because the pregnancy experience in humans is limited and the reproduction studies in animals have shown low risk.

**Further Reading:**
- *Drug Information. Sanctura.* Odyssey Pharmaceuticals.

### 11.3   URINARY ACIDIFIER

### 11.3.1   AMMONIUM CHLORIDE

**FDA Category: C**
***Risk Summary:*** The reproduction studies in animals have shown no evidence of fetal harm or impaired fertility. The pregnancy experience in humans is adequate to exhibit that the embryo-fetal risk is nonexistent or very low.

**Further Reading:**
- Goodlin, R. C., & Kaiser, I. H., (1957). The effect of ammonium chloride-induced maternal acidosis on the human fetus at term. I. pH, hemoglobin, blood gases. *Am. J. Med. Sci., 233*, 666–674.
- Heinonen, O. P., Slone, D., & Shapiro, S., (1977). *Birth Defects and Drugs in Pregnancy.* Littleton, MA: Publishing Sciences Group.

- Kaiser, I. H., & Goodlin, R. C., (1958). The effect of ammonium chloride-induced maternal acidosis on the human fetus at term. II. Electrolytes. *Am. J. Med. Sci., 235*, 549–554.

## 11.4  URINARY ALKALINIZERS

### *11.4.1  POTASSIUM CITRATE*

**FDA Category: B**
***Risk Summary:*** The reproduction studies in animals have shown no evidence of fetal harm or impaired fertility. The pregnancy experience in humans is limited.

**Further Reading:**
- *Drug Information. Potassium Citrate*. Upsher-Smith Laboratories.
- Mellin, G. W., (1964). Drugs in the first trimester of pregnancy and the fetal life of Homo sapiens. *Am. J. Obstet. Gynecol., 90*, 1169–1180.

## KEYWORDS

- **oxybutynin**
- **solifenacin**
- **tolterodine**
- **trospium**
- **urinary acidifier**
- **urinary alkalinizers**

# CHAPTER 12

# Dermatologic Drugs

## 12.1 TOPICAL ANTIBACTERIAL PREPARATIONS

### 12.1.1 BACITRACIN

**FDA Category: N**
*Risk Summary:* The reproduction studies in animals have shown no evidence of fetal harm or impaired fertility. The pregnancy experience in humans is adequate to exhibit that the embryo-fetal risk is very low. Therefore, it is safe to be used during pregnancy.

**Further Reading:**
- Heinonen, O. P., Slone, D., & Shapiro, S., (1977). *Birth Defects and Drugs in Pregnancy* (pp. 297, 301). Littleton, MA: Publishing Sciences Group.

### 12.1.2 CLINDAMYCIN

**FDA Category: B**
*Risk Summary:* The reproduction studies in animals have shown no evidence of fetal harm or impaired fertility. The pregnancy experience in humans is adequate to exhibit that the embryo-fetal risk is very low. Therefore, it is safe to be used during pregnancy.

**Further Reading:**
- Briggs, G., Freeman, R., Towers, C., & Forninash, A., (2017). *Drugs in Pregnancy and Lactation: A Reference Guide to Fetal and Neonatal Risk.* Philadelphia, Pa: Wolters Kluwer Health.

### 12.1.3   ERYTHROMYCIN

**FDA Category: B**
*Risk Summary:* The reproduction studies in animals have shown no evidence of fetal harm or impaired fertility. The pregnancy experience in humans is adequate to exhibit that the embryo-fetal risk is very low. Therefore, it is safe to be used during pregnancy.

**Further Reading:**
- Briggs, G., Freeman, R., Towers, C., & Forninash, A., (2017). *Drugs in Pregnancy and Lactation: A Reference Guide to Fetal and Neonatal Risk.* Philadelphia, Pa: Wolters Kluwer Health.

### 12.1.4   GENTAMICIN SULFATE

**FDA Category: N**
*Risk Summary:* Although there is limited data from the human pregnancy experience, but the possible maternal benefit extremely outweighs the unknown or known embryo/fetal risk.

**Further Reading:**
- Briggs, G., Freeman, R., Towers, C., & Forninash, A., (2017). *Drugs in Pregnancy and Lactation: A Reference Guide to Fetal and Neonatal Risk.* Philadelphia, Pa: Wolters Kluwer Health.

### 12.1.5   METRONIDAZOLE

**FDA Category: B**
*Risk Summary:* The reproduction studies in animals have shown no evidence of fetal harm or impaired fertility. The pregnancy experience in humans is limited. Therefore, it does not represent a significant risk to the embryo-fetus.

**Further Reading:**
- Briggs, G., Freeman, R., Towers, C., & Forninash, A., ()2017. *Drugs in Pregnancy and Lactation: A Reference Guide to Fetal and Neonatal Risk.* Philadelphia, Pa: Wolters Kluwer Health; 2017.
- *Drug Information. Metrogel.* Galderma Laboratories Inc.

## 12.1.6   MUPIROCIN

**FDA Category: B**
*Risk Summary:* The reproduction studies in animals have shown no evidence of fetal harm or impaired fertility. The pregnancy experience in humans is limited. Therefore, it does not represent a significant risk to the embryo-fetus.

**Further Reading:**
- *Drug Information. Bactroban.* GlaxoSmithKline.

## 12.1.7   NEOMYCIN

**FDA Category: N**
*Risk Summary:* Although there is limited data from the human pregnancy experience, but the possible maternal benefit extremely outweighs the unknown or known embryo/fetal risk.

**Further Reading:**
- *Drug Information.* Myciguent. Pharmacia and Upjohn.

## 12.1.8   POLYMYXIN B SULFATE

**FDA Category: C**
*Risk Summary:* The reproduction studies in animals have shown no evidence of fetal harm or impaired fertility. The pregnancy experience in humans is adequate to exhibit that the embryo-fetal risk is very low. Therefore, it is safe to be used during pregnancy.

**Further Reading:**
- Kazy, Z., Puho, E., & Czeizel, A. E., (2005). Parenteral polymyxin B treatment during pregnancy. *Reprod. Toxicol.,* 2005 *20*, 181–182.

## 12.1.9   RETAPAMULIN

**FDA Category: B**
*Risk Summary:* The reproduction studies in animals have shown no evidence of fetal harm or impaired fertility. The pregnancy experience in

humans is limited. Therefore, it does not represent a significant risk to the embryo-fetus.

**Further Reading:**
- *Drug Information. Altabax.* GlaxoSmithKline.

### 12.1.10  DAPSONE

**FDA Category: C**
***Risk Summary:*** It should be used with caution because the pregnancy experience in humans is limited and the reproduction studies in animals have shown low risk.

**Further Reading:**
- Briggs, G., Freeman, R., Towers, C., & Forninash, A., (2017. *Drugs in Pregnancy and Lactation: A Reference Guide to Fetal and Neonatal Risk.* Philadelphia, Pa: Wolters Kluwer Health; 2017.
- *Drug Information. Aczone.* QLT USA, Inc.

## 12.2  TOPICAL ANTIFUNGAL PREPARATIONS

### 12.2.1  BUTENAFINE

**FDA Category: C**
***Risk Summary:*** It should be used with caution because the pregnancy experience in humans is limited and the reproduction studies in animals have shown low risk.

**Further Reading:**
- *Drug Information. Mentax.* Mylan Pharmaceuticals.

### 12.2.2  CICLOPIROX

**FDA Category: B**
***Risk Summary:*** The reproduction studies in animals have shown no evidence of fetal harm or impaired fertility. The pregnancy experience in humans is limited. Therefore, it does not represent a significant risk to the embryo-fetus.

**Further Reading:**
- *Drug Information. Loprox.* MEDICIS, The Dermatology Company.


### 12.2.3   CLOTRIMAZOLE

**FDA Category: B**
*Risk Summary:* The reproduction studies in animals have shown no evidence of fetal harm or impaired fertility. The pregnancy experience in humans is adequate to exhibit that the embryo-fetal risk is very low. Therefore, it is safe to be used during pregnancy.

**Further Reading:**
- Czeizel, A. E., Toth, M., & Rockenbauer, M., (1999). No teratogenic effect after clotrimazole therapy during pregnancy. *Epidemiology, 10,* 437–440.
- *Drug Information. Lotrimin.* Schering.
- Svendsen, E., Lie, S., Gunderson, T. H., Lyngstad-Vik, I., & Skuland, J., (1978). Comparative evaluation of miconazole, clotrimazole, and nystatin in the treatment of candidal vulvovaginitis. *Curr. Ther. Res., 23,* 666–672.


### 12.2.4   ECONAZOLE

**FDA Category: N**
*Risk Summary:* The reproduction studies in animals have shown no evidence of fetal harm or impaired fertility. The pregnancy experience in humans is adequate to exhibit that the embryo-fetal risk is very low. Therefore, it is safe to be used during pregnancy.

**Further Reading:**
- Czeizel, A. E., Kazy, Z., & Vargha, P., (2003). A population-based case-control teratological study of vaginal econazole treatment during pregnancy. *Eur. J. Obstet. Gynecol., Reprod. Biol., 111,* 135–140.
- *Drug Information. Spectazole.* Ortho-McNeil Pharmaceuticals.
- Goormans, E., Beck, J. M., Declercq, J. A., Loendersloot, E. W., Roelofs, H. J. M., & van Zanten, A., (1985). Efficacy of econazole ('Gyno-Pevaryl' 150) in vaginal candidosis during pregnancy. *Curr. Med. Res. Opin., 9,* 371–377.

## 12.2.5   *KETOCONAZOLE*

**FDA Category: C**
*Risk Summary:* The reproduction studies in animals have shown no evidence of fetal harm or impaired fertility. The pregnancy experience in humans is limited. Therefore, it does not represent a significant risk to the embryo-fetus.

**Further Reading:**
- Divers, M. J., (1990). Ketoconazole treatment of Cushing's syndrome in pregnancy. *Am. J. Obstet. Gynecol., 163*, 1101.
- *Drug Information. Nizoral*. Janssen Pharmaceutics.
- Lind, J., (1985). Limb malformations in the case of hydrops fetalis with ketoconazole use during pregnancy (abstract). *Arch Gynecol., 237*(Suppl), 398.

## 12.2.6   *MICONAZOLE*

**FDA Category: C**
*Risk Summary:* The reproduction studies in animals have shown no evidence of fetal harm or impaired fertility. The pregnancy experience in humans is limited. Therefore, it does not represent a significant risk to the embryo-fetus.

**Further Reading:**
- *Drug Information. Monistat*. Ortho Pharmaceutical.
- Kazy, Z., Puho, E., & Czeizel, A. E., (2005). The possible association between the combination of vaginal metronidazole and miconazole treatment and poly-syndactyly population-based case-control teratologic study. *Reprod. Toxicol., 20*, 89–94.
- Wallenburg, H. C. S., & Wladimiroff, J. W., (1976). Recurrence of vulvovaginal candidosis during pregnancy. Comparison of miconazole vs nystatin treatment. *Obstet. Gynecol., 48*, 491–494.

## 12.2.7   *NAFTIFINE*

**FDA Category: B**
*Risk Summary:* It should be used with caution because the pregnancy experience in humans is limited and the reproduction studies in animals have shown low risk.

**Further Reading:**
- *Drug Information. Naftin.* Merz Pharmaceuticals.

## 12.2.8 NYSTATIN

**FDA Category: C (cream, ointment, and powder)**
**FDA Category: A (vaginal tablet)**
*Risk Summary:* The reproduction studies in animals have shown no evidence of fetal harm or impaired fertility. The pregnancy experience in humans is adequate to exhibit that the embryo-fetal risk is very low. Therefore, it is safe to be used during pregnancy.

**Further Reading:**
- Wallenburg, H. C. S., & Wladimiroff, J. W., (1976). Recurrence of vulvovaginal candidosis during pregnancy. Comparison of miconazole vs. nystatin treatment. *Obstet. Gynecol., 48*, 491–494.

## 12.2.9 OXICONAZOLE

**FDA Category: B**
*Risk Summary:* The reproduction studies in animals have shown no evidence of fetal harm or impaired fertility. The pregnancy experience in humans is limited. Therefore, it does not represent a significant risk to the embryo-fetus.

**Further Reading:**
- *Drug Information. Oxistat.* PharmaDerm.

## 12.2.10 TERBINAFINE

**FDA Category: B**
*Risk Summary:* It should be used with caution because the pregnancy experience in humans is limited and the reproduction studies in animals have shown low risk.

**Further Reading:**
- *Drug Information. Lamisil.* Novartis Pharmaceuticals.

## 12.2.11   TOLNAFTATE

**FDA Category: C**
*Risk Summary:* It should be used only when the maternal benefit outweighs the fetal risk because there is very limited human pregnancy data, and the animal studies are not relevant.

**Further Reading:**
• *Drug Information. Tinactin.* Southwood Pharmaceuticals Inc.

## 12.2.12   SULCONAZOLE

**FDA Category: C**
*Risk Summary:* Because of the potential risk to the fetus, it is advisable to use it only when safer alternatives are not available or have failed.

**Further Reading:**
• *Drug Information. Exelderm.* Bristol-Myers Squibb.
• Rosa, F. W., Baum, C., & Shaw, M., (1987). Pregnancy outcomes after first-trimester vaginitis drug therapy. *Obstet. Gynecol., 69,* 751–755.

## 12.3   TOPICAL ANTIVIRAL PREPARATIONS

### 12.3.1   ACYCLOVIR

**FDA Category: B**
*Risk Summary:* The reproduction studies in animals have shown no evidence of fetal harm or impaired fertility. The pregnancy experience in humans is adequate to exhibit that the embryo-fetal risk is very low. Therefore, it is safe to be used during pregnancy.

**Further Reading:**
• *Drug Information.* Valtrex. Glaxo Wellcome.
• Mills, J. L., & Carter, T. C., (2010). Acyclovir exposure and birth defects—an important advance, but more are needed. *JAMA, 304,* 905–906.

- Pasternak, B., & Hviid, A., (2010). Use of acyclovir, valacyclovir, and famciclovir in the first trimester of pregnancy and the risk of birth defects. *JAMA*, *304*, 859–866.

## 12.3.2  FAMCICLOVIR

**FDA Category: B**
*Risk Summary:* It should be used with caution because the pregnancy experience in humans is limited and the reproduction studies in animals have shown low risk.

**Further Reading:**
- *Drug Information. Famvir.* Novartis Pharmaceuticals.
- Mubareka, S., Leung, V., Aoki, F. Y., & Vinh, D. C., (2010). Famciclovir: A focus on efficacy and safety. *Expert. Opin. Drug Saf.*, *9*, 643–658.

## 12.3.3  PENCICLOVIR

**FDA Category: B**
*Risk Summary:* The reproduction studies in animals have shown no evidence of fetal harm or impaired fertility. The pregnancy experience in humans is limited. Therefore, it does not represent a significant risk to the embryo-fetus.

**Further Reading:**
- *Drug Information. Denavir.* New American Therapeutics.
- Pasternak, B., & Hviid, A., (2010). Use of acyclovir, valacyclovir, and famciclovir in the first trimester of pregnancy and the risk of birth defects. *JAMA, 304*, 859–866.

## 12.3.4  VALACYCLOVIR

**FDA Category: B**
*Risk Summary:* The reproduction studies in animals have shown no evidence of fetal harm or impaired fertility. The pregnancy experience in

humans is limited. Therefore, it does not represent a significant risk to the embryo-fetus.

**Further Reading:**
- *Drug Information. Valtrex.* Glaxo Wellcome.
- Pasternak, B., & Hviid, A., (2010). Use of acyclovir, valacyclovir, and famciclovir in the first trimester of pregnancy and the risk of birth defects. *JAMA, 304,* 859–866.
- Sheffield, J. S., Hill, J. B., Hollier, L. M., Laibl, V. R., Roberts, S. W., Sanchez, P. J., Wendel, G. D. Jr., (2006). Valacyclovir prophylaxis to prevent recurrent herpes at delivery. *Obstet. Gynecol.,108,* 141–147.

## 12.4   TOPICAL IMMUNOMODULATORS

### 12.4.1   IMIQUIMOD

**FDA Category: C**
*Risk Summary:* It should be used with caution because the human pregnancy experience has shown a low risk.

**Further Reading:**
- Audisio, T., Roca, F. C., & Piatti, C., (2008). Topical imiquimod therapy for external anogenital warts in pregnant women. *Int. J. Gynaecol. Obstet., 110,* 275–286.
- Ciavattini, A., Tsiroglou, D., Vichi, M., Di Giuseppe, J., Cecchi, S., & Tranquilli, A. L., (2012). Topical imiquimod 5% cream therapy for external anogenital warts in pregnant women: Report of four cases and review of the literature. *J. Matern Fetal Neonatal. Med., 25,* 873–876.
- *Drug Information. Aldara.* 3M Pharmaceuticals.

### 12.4.2   TACROLIMUS

**FDA Category: C**
*Risk Summary:* It should be used with caution because the human pregnancy experience has shown a low risk.

**Further Reading:**
- *Drug Information. Prograf.* Astellas & Pharma, U. S., ().
- Jabiry-Zieniewicz, Z., Kaminski, P., Pietrzak, B., Cyganek, A., Bobrowska, K., Ziotkowski, J., Otdakowska-Jedynak, U., Zieniewicz, K., Paczek, L., Jankowska, I., Wielgos, M., & Krawczyk, M., (2006). Outcome of four high-risk pregnancies in female liver transplant recipients on tacrolimus immunosuppression. *Transplant Proc., 38*, 255–257.

### 12.4.3 PIMECROLIMUS

**FDA Category: C**
*Risk Summary:* It should be used with caution because the human pregnancy experience has shown a low risk.

**Further Reading:**
- *Drug Information. Elidel.* Novartis Pharmaceuticals.
- Scott, G., Osborne, S. A., Greig, G., Hartmann, S., Ebelin, M. E., Burtin, P., Rappersberger, K., Komar, M., & Wolff, K., (2003). Pharmacokinetics of pimecrolimus, a novel nonsteroid anti-inflammatory drug, after single and multiple oral administration. *Clin. Pharmacokinet., 42*, 1305–1314.

## 12.5 ECTOPARASITICIDES

### 12.5.1 PERMETHRIN

**FDA Category: B**
*Risk Summary:* The reproduction studies in animals have shown no evidence of fetal harm or impaired fertility. The pregnancy experience in humans is adequate to exhibit that the embryo-fetal risk is very low. Therefore, it is safe to be used during pregnancy.

**Further Reading:**
- *Drug Information.* Elimite. Allergan.
- Kennedy, D., Hurst, V., Konradsdottir, E., & Einarson, A., (2005). Pregnancy outcome following exposure to permethrin and use of teratogen information. *Am. J. Perinatol., 22*, 87–90.

## 12.5.2  LINDANE

**FDA Category: C**
*Risk Summary:* It should be used with caution because the pregnancy experience in humans is limited and the reproduction studies in animals have shown low risk.

**Further Reading:**
- *Drug Information*. Lindane Lotion USP 1%. Alpharma.
- Palmer, A. K., Bottomley, A. M., Worden, A. N., Frohberg, H., & Bauer, A., (1978). Effect of lindane on pregnancy in the rabbit and rat. *Toxicology, 10,* 239–247.

## 12.5.3  CROTAMITON

**FDA Category: C**
*Risk Summary:* The reproduction studies in animals have shown no evidence of fetal harm or impaired fertility. The pregnancy experience in humans is limited. Therefore, it does not represent a significant risk to the embryo-fetus.

**Further Reading:**
- *Drug Information. Eurax*. Ranbaxy Pharmaceuticals.

## 12.5.4  BENZYL ALCOHOL

**FDA Category: B**
*Risk Summary:* The reproduction studies in animals have shown no evidence of fetal harm or impaired fertility. The pregnancy experience in humans is limited. Therefore, it does not represent a significant risk to the embryo-fetus.

**Further Reading:**
- Craig, D. B., & Habib, G. G., (1977). Flaccid paraparesis following obstetrical epidural anesthesia: Possible role of benzyl alcohol. *Anesth. Analg., 56,* 219–221.
- *Drug Information. Ulesfia*. Shionogi Pharma.

## 12.6   AGENTS FOR PIGMENTATION

### 12.6.1   HYDROQUINONE

**FDA Category: C**
*Risk Summary:* It should be used with caution because the human pregnancy experience has shown a low risk.

**Further Reading:**
- *Drug Information*. Claripel Cream. Stiefel Laboratories.
- Garcia, A., & Fulton, J. E. Jr., (1996). The combination of glycolic acid and hydroquinone or kojic acid for the treatment of melasma and related conditions. *Dermatol. Surg., 22*, 443–447.
- Guevara, I. L., & Pandya, A. G., (2003). Safety and efficacy of 4% hydroquinone combined with 10% glycolic acid, antioxidants, and sunscreen in the treatment of melasma. *Int. J. Dermatol., 42*, 966–972.

### 12.6.2   METHOXSALEN

**FDA Category: C**
*Risk Summary:* The reproduction studies in animals have shown no evidence of fetal harm or impaired fertility. The pregnancy experience in humans is adequate to exhibit that the embryo-fetal risk is very low. Therefore, it is safe to be used during pregnancy.

**Further Reading:**
- *Drug Information*. Oxsoralen. ICN Pharmaceuticals.
- Garbis, H., Eléfant, E., Bertolotti, E., Robert, E., Serafini, M. A., & Prapas, N., (1995). Pregnancy outcome after periconceptional and first-trimester exposure to methoxsalen photochemotherapy. *Arch Dermatol., 131*, 492, 493.

### 12.6.3   MONOBENZONE

**FDA Category: C**
*Risk Summary:* It should be used only when the maternal benefit outweighs the fetal risk because there is very limited human pregnancy data, and the animal studies are not relevant.

**Further Reading:**
- Briggs, G., Freeman, R., Towers, C., & Forninash, A., (2017). *Drugs in Pregnancy and Lactation: A Reference Guide to Fetal and Neonatal Risk.* Philadelphia, Pa: Wolters Kluwer Health.

## 12.7 ACNE PREPARATIONS

### 12.7.1 ADAPALENE

**FDA Category: C**
**Risk Summary:** It is better to be avoided during the 1st Trimester because the pregnancy experience in humans is limited and the reproduction studies in animals have shown low risk.

**Further Reading:**
- Autret, E., Berjot, M., Jonville-Bera, A. P., Aubry, M. C., & Moraine, C., (1997). Anophthalmia and agenesis of optic chiasma associated with adapalene gel in early pregnancy. *Lancet, 350,* 339.
- *Drug Information. Differin.* Galderma Laboratories.

### 12.7.2 ISOTRETINOIN

**FDA Category: X**
**Risk Summary:** It is contraindicated during pregnancy due to the tremendous risk of congenital malformations associated with its use.

**Further Reading:**
- Rizzo, R., Lammer, E. J., Parano, E., Pavone, L., & Argyle, J. C., (1991). Limb reduction defects in humans associated with prenatal isotretinoin exposure. *Teratology, 44,* 599–604.
- Rosa, F. W., (1983). Teratogenicity of isotretinoin. *Lancet, 2,* 513.
- Willhite, C. C., Hill, R. M., & Irving, D. W., (1986). Isotretinoin-induced craniofacial malformations in humans and hamsters. *J. Craniofac. Genet. Dev. Biol., 2*(Suppl),193–209.

### 12.7.3 TAZAROTENE

**FDA Category: X**
***Risk Summary:*** It is contraindicated during pregnancy due to the tremendous risk of congenital malformations associated with its use.

**Further Reading:**
- *Drug Information. Tazorac.* Allergan.

### 12.7.4 TRETINOIN

**FDA Category: C**
***Risk Summary:*** It is better to be avoided during the 1st Trimester because the pregnancy experience in humans has shown a low risk of teratogenicity associated with the use of Tretinoin.

**Further Reading:**
- *Drug Information. Renova,* Retin-A. Ortho Dermatological.
- Martinez-Frias, M. L., & Rodriguez-Pinilla, E., (1999). First-trimester exposure to topical tretinoin: Its safety is not warranted. *Teratology, 60,* 5.
- Selcen, D., Seidman, S., & Nigro, M. A., (2000). Otocerebral anomalies associated with topical tretinoin use. *Brain Dev., 22,* 218–220.

## 12.8 TOPICAL PREPARATIONS FOR PSORIASIS

### 12.8.1 ACITRETIN

**FDA Category: C**
***Risk Summary:*** Although Acitretin has been given the letter (C), according to the FDA categorization, but it is better to absolutely avoid the use of Acitretin during pregnancy due to the tremendous risk of congenital malformations associated with its use.

**Further Reading:**
- Barbero, P., Lotersztein, V., Bronberg, R., Perez, M., & Alba, L., (2004). Acitretin embryopathy: A case report. Birth Defects Res A Clin Mol Teratol 2004 *70,* 831–3.

- De Die-Smulders, C. E. M., Sturkenboom, M. C. J. M., Veraart, J., Van Katwijk, C., Sastrowijoto, P., & Van Der Linden, E., (1995). Severe limb defects and craniofacial anomalies in a fetus conceived during acitretin therapy. *Teratology, 52,* 215–219.
- *Drug Information. Soriatane.* Roche Laboratories.

## 12.8.2   CALCIPOTRIENE

**FDA Category: C**
*Risk Summary:* The reproduction studies in animals have shown no evidence of fetal harm or impaired fertility. The pregnancy experience in humans is limited. Therefore, it does not represent a significant risk to the embryo-fetus.

**Further Reading:**
- *Drug Information. Dovonex Cream.* LEO Pharma.
- Lebwohl, M., (2005). A clinician's paradigm in the treatment of psoriasis. *J. Am. Acad Dermatol., 53,* S59–69.
- Tauscher, A. E., Fleischer, A. B. Jr., Phelps, K. C., & Feldman, S. R., (2002). Psoriasis and pregnancy. *J. Cutan. Med. Surg., 6,* 561–570.

## 12.8.3   CALCITRIOL

**FDA Category: C**
*Risk Summary:* The reproduction studies in animals have shown no evidence of fetal harm or impaired fertility. The pregnancy experience in humans is adequate to exhibit that the embryo-fetal risk is very low. Therefore, it is safe to be used during pregnancy.

**Further Reading:**
- *Drug Information.* Rocaltrol. Roche Laboratories.

## 12.8.4   TAZAROTENE

**FDA Category: X**
*Risk Summary:* It is contraindicated during pregnancy due to the tremendous risk of congenital malformations associated with its use.

**Further Reading:**
*   *Drug Information. Tazorac.* Allergan.

## 12.9   SELECTED TOPICAL CORTICOSTEROIDS

### 12.9.1   *BETAMETHASONE*

**FDA Category: C**
***Risk Summary:*** Although there is limited data from the human pregnancy experience, but the possible maternal benefit extremely outweighs the unknown or known embryo/fetal risk.

**Further Reading:**
*   Czeizel, A. E., & Rockenbauer, M., (1997). Population-based case-control study of teratogenic potential of corticosteroids. *Teratology, 56,* 335–340.
*   Helal, K. J., Gordon, M. C., Lightner, C. R., & Barth, W. H. Jr., (2000). Adrenal suppression induced by betamethasone in women at risk for premature delivery. *Obstet. Gynecol., 96,* 287–290.

### 12.9.2   *CLOBETASOL PROPIONATE*

**FDA Category: C**
***Risk Summary:*** Although there is limited data from the human pregnancy experience, but the possible maternal benefit extremely outweighs the unknown or known embryo/fetal risk.

**Further Reading:**
*   Accessdata.fda.gov. (2018). Available from: https://www.accessdata. fda.gov/drugsatfda_docs/label/2015/204767s000lbl.pdf(accessed on 31 January 2020).
*   Czeizel, A. E., & Rockenbauer, M., (1997). Population-based case-control study of teratogenic potential of corticosteroids. *Teratology, 56,* 335–340.

### 12.9.3   DEXAMETHASONE

**FDA Category: C**
*Risk Summary:* Although there is limited data from the human pregnancy experience, but the possible maternal benefit extremely outweighs the unknown or known embryo/fetal risk.

**Further Reading:**
- Czeizel, A. E., & Rockenbauer, M., (1997). Population-based case-control study of teratogenic potential of corticosteroids. *Teratology, 56*, 335–340.
- Osathanondh, R., Tulchinsky, D., Kamali, H., Fencl, M., & Taeusch, H. W. Jr., (1977). Dexamethasone levels in treated pregnant women and newborn infants. *J. Pediatr., 90*, 617–620.

### 12.9.4   FLUOCINOLONE

**FDA Category: C**
*Risk Summary:* It should be used with caution because the pregnancy experience in humans is limited and the reproduction studies in animals have shown low risk.

**Further Reading:**
- Czeizel, A. E., & Rockenbauer, M., (1997). Population-based case-control study of teratogenic potential of corticosteroids. *Teratology, 56*, 335–340.
- *Drug Information.* Synalar Cream 0.025%. MEDICIS, The Dermatology Company.
- *Drug Information.* Synalar Solution 0.01%. MEDICIS, The Dermatology Company.

### 12.9.5   FLUOCINONIDE

**FDA Category: C**
*Risk Summary:* It should be used with caution because there is a risk of suppression of the HPA axis (hypothalamic-pituitary-adrenal axis).

**Further Reading:**
- Czeizel, A. E., & Rockenbauer, M., (1997). Population-based case-control study of teratogenic potential of corticosteroids. *Teratology*, *56*, 335–340.
- *Drug Information. Vanos*. MEDICIS, The Dermatology Company.


## 12.9.6  HYDROCORTISONE

**FDA Category: C**
*Risk Summary:* It should be used with caution because there is a risk of suppression of the HPA axis.

**Further Reading:**
- Czeizel, A. E., & Rockenbauer, M., (1997). Population-based case-control study of teratogenic potential of corticosteroids. *Teratology*, *56*, 335–340.


## 12.9.7  MOMETASONE

**FDA Category: C**
*Risk Summary:* The reproduction studies in animals have shown no evidence of fetal harm or impaired fertility. The pregnancy experience in humans is limited. Therefore, it does not represent a significant risk to the embryo-fetus.

**Further Reading:**
- Czeizel, A. E., & Rockenbauer, M., (1997). Population-based case-control study of teratogenic potential of corticosteroids. *Teratology*, *56*, 335–340.
- Joint Committee of the American College of Obstetricians and Gynecologists (ACOG) and the American College of Allergy, Asthma, and Immunology (ACAAI) (2000). Position statement. The use of newer asthma and allergy medications during pregnancy. *Ann. Allergy Asthma Immunol., 84*, 475–480.

## 12.9.8  TRIAMCINOLONE

**FDA Category: C**
*Risk Summary:* It should be used with caution because there is a risk of intrauterine growth retardation.

**Further Reading:**
- Czeizel, A. E., & Rockenbauer, M., (1997). Population-based case-control study of teratogenic potential of corticosteroids. *Teratology.,* *56,* 335–340.
- Katz, V. L., Thorp, J. M. Jr., & Bowes, W. A. Jr., (1990). Severe symmetric intrauterine growth retardation associated with the topical use of triamcinolone. *Am. J. Obstet. Gynecol., 162,* 396–397.

## 12.10  KERATOLYTIC AND DESTRUCTIVE AGENTS

### 12.10.1  SALICYLIC ACID

**FDA Category: C**
*Risk Summary:* The reproduction studies in animals have shown no evidence of fetal harm or impaired fertility. The pregnancy experience in humans is limited. Therefore, it does not represent a significant risk to the embryo-fetus.

**Further Reading:**
- Murase, J. E., Heller, M. M., & Butler, D. C., (2014). Safety of dermatologic medications in pregnancy and lactation: Part I. Pregnancy. *J. Am. Acad Dermatol., 70,* 401, e1–14, quiz 415.

### 12.10.2  PROPYLENE GLYCOL

**FDA Category: N**
*Risk Summary:* The reproduction studies in animals have shown no evidence of fetal harm or impaired fertility. The pregnancy experience in humans is limited. Therefore, it does not represent a significant risk to the embryo-fetus.

**Further Reading:**
- Murase, J. E., Heller, M. M., & Butler, D. C., (2014). Safety of dermatologic medications in pregnancy and lactation: Part I. Pregnancy. *J. Am. Acad Dermatol., 70*, 401, e1–14, quiz 415.
- Taub, A. F., (2007). Procedural treatments for acne vulgaris. *Dermatol. Surg., 33*, 1005–1026.

### *12.10.3 PODOPHYLLUM*

**FDA Category: X**
*Risk Summary:* It is contraindicated due to the severe maternal myelotoxicity and neurotoxicity.

**Further Reading:**
- American College of Obstetricians and Gynecologists (1994). *Genital Human Papillomavirus Infections.* Technical Bulletin, No. 193.
- Didcock, K. A., Picard, C. W., & Robson, J. M., (1952). The action of podophyllotoxin on pregnancy. *J Physiol. (London), 117*, 65P–66P. As cited in: Schardein, J. L., (1993). *Chemically Induced Birth Defects* (2nd edn., p. 491). New York, NY: Marcel Dekker.
- Murase, J. E., Heller, M. M., & Butler, D. C., (2014). Safety of dermatologic medications in pregnancy and lactation: Part I. Pregnancy. *J. Am. Acad Dermatol., 70*, 401, e1–14, quiz 415.

### *12.10.4 PODOFILOX*

**FDA Category: C**
*Risk Summary:* It should be used with caution because the pregnancy experience in humans is limited and the reproduction studies in animals have shown low risk.

**Further Reading:**
- *Drug Information. Condylox.* Oclassen Pharmaceuticals.
- Murase, J. E., Heller, M. M., & Butler, D. C., (2014). Safety of dermatologic medications in pregnancy and lactation: Part I. Pregnancy. *J. Am. Acad Dermatol., 70*, 401, e1–14, quiz 415.

### 12.10.5   SINECATECHINS

**FDA Category: C**
*Risk Summary:* It should be used with caution because the pregnancy experience in humans is limited and the reproduction studies in animals have shown low risk.

**Further Reading:**
- *Drug Information*. Veregen. Fougera.
- Murase, J. E., Heller, M. M., & Butler, D. C., (2014). Safety of dermatologic medications in pregnancy and lactation: Part I. Pregnancy. *J. Am. Acad Dermatol., 70*, 401, e1–14, quiz 415.

## 12.11   TRICHOGENIC AGENTS

### 12.11.1   MINOXIDIL

**FDA Category: C**
*Risk Summary:* There is limited pregnancy experience in humans, and the reproduction studies in animals have shown moderate risk. Therefore, it is advisable to avoid its use until the human pregnancy experience is available.

**Further Reading:**
- *Drug Information*. Rogaine. RxMed: Pharmaceutical Information.
- Smorlesi, C., Caldarella, A., Caramelli, L., Di Lollo, S., & Moroni, F., (2003). Topically applied minoxidil may cause fetal malformation: A case report. *Birth Defects Res. A Clin. Mol. Teratol., 67*, 997–1001.

### 12.11.2   BIMATOPROST

**FDA Category: C**
*Risk Summary:* The reproduction studies in animals have shown no evidence of fetal harm or impaired fertility. The pregnancy experience in humans is limited. Therefore, it does not represent a significant risk to the embryo-fetus.

**Further Reading:**
- *Drug Information. Lumigan*. Allergan.

## KEYWORDS

- **bimatoprost**
- **podofilox**
- **podophyllum**
- **salicylic acid**
- **sinecatechins**
- **trichogenic agents**

# CHAPTER 13

# Diagnostic Agents

## 13.1 DIATRIZOATE

**FDA Category: C**
*Risk Summary:* The reproduction studies in animals have shown no evidence of fetal harm or impaired fertility. The pregnancy experience in humans is limited. Therefore, it does not represent a significant risk to the embryo-fetus.

**Further Reading:**
- *Drug Information. Hypaque Sodium.* Amersham Health.
- Webb, J. A. W., Thomsen, H. S., & Morcos, S. K., (2005). The use of iodinated and gadolinium contrast media during pregnancy and lactation. *Eur. Radiol., 15*, 1234–1240.

## 13.2 EVANS BLUE

**FDA Category: N**
*Risk Summary:* The reproduction studies in animals have shown no evidence of fetal harm or impaired fertility. The pregnancy experience in humans is limited. Therefore, it does not represent a significant risk to the embryo-fetus.

**Further Reading:**
- Morrison, L., & Wiseman, H. J., (1972). Intra-amniotic injection of Evans blue dye. *Am. J. Obstet. Gynecol., 113*, 1147.
- Quinlivan, W. L. G., Brock, J. A., & Sullivan, H., (1970). Blood volume changes and blood loss associated with labor. I. Correlation of changes in blood volume measured by [131]I-albumin and Evans blue dye, with measured blood loss. *Am. J. Obstet. Gynecol., 106*, 843–849.

## 13.3   FLUORESCEIN SODIUM

**FDA Category: C**
*Risk Summary:* It should be used with caution because the human pregnancy experience has shown a low risk.

**Further Reading:**
- Burnett, C. M., & Goldenthal, E. I., (1986). The teratogenic potential in rats and rabbits of D and C Yellow no. 8. *Food Chem. Toxicol., 24,* 819–823.
- Kearns, G. L., Williams, B. J., & Timmons, O. D., (1985). Fluorescein phototoxicity in a premature infant. *J. Pediatr., 107,* 796–798.

## 13.4   GADOBENATE DIMEGLUMINE

**FDA Category: C**
*Risk Summary:* There is limited pregnancy experience in humans, and the reproduction studies in animals have shown moderate risk. Therefore, it is advisable to avoid its use until the human pregnancy experience is available.

**Further Reading:**
- Chen, M. M., Coakley, F. V., Kaimal, A., & Laros, R. K. Jr., (2008). Guidelines for computed tomography and magnetic resonance imaging use during pregnancy and lactation. *Obstet. Gynecol., 112,* 333–340.
- *Drug Information. Multihance.* Bracco Diagnostics.
- Garcia-Bournissen, F., Shrim, A., & Koren, G., (2006). Safety of gadolinium during pregnancy. *Can. Fam. Physician, 52,* 309–310.

## 13.5   GADOBUTROL

**FDA Category: C**
*Risk Summary:* There is limited pregnancy experience in humans, and the reproduction studies in animals have shown moderate risk. Therefore, it is advisable to avoid its use until the human pregnancy experience is available.

**Further Reading:**
- *Drug Information.* Gadavist. Bayer HealthCare Pharmaceuticals.

- Garcia-Bournissen, F., Shrim, A., & Koren, G., (2006). Safety of gadolinium during pregnancy. *Can. Fam. Physician, 52*, 309–310.
- Webb, J. A. W., Thomsen, H. S., & Morcos, S. K., (2005). Members of Contrast Media Safety Committee of the European Society of Urogenital Radiology (ESUR). The use of iodinated and gadolinium contrast media during pregnancy and lactation. *Eur. Radiol., 15*, 1234–1240.

## 13.5 GADOBUTROL

**FDA Category: C**
***Risk Summary:*** There is limited pregnancy experience in humans, and the reproduction studies in animals have shown moderate risk. Therefore, it is advisable to avoid its use until the human pregnancy experience is available.

**Further Reading:**
- Chen, M. M., Coakley, F. V., Kaimal, A., & Laros, R. K. Jr., (2008). Guidelines for computed tomography and magnetic resonance imaging use during pregnancy and lactation. *Obstet. Gynecol., 112*, 333–340.
- *Drug Information. Omniscan*. GE Healthcare.
- Garcia-Bournissen, F., Shrim, A., & Koren, G., (2006). Safety of gadolinium during pregnancy. *Can. Fam. Physician, 2006 52*, 309–310.

## 13.6 GADOFOSVESET

**FDA Category: C**
***Risk Summary:*** There is limited pregnancy experience in humans, and the reproduction studies in animals have shown moderate risk. Therefore, it is advisable to avoid its use until the human pregnancy experience is available.

**Further Reading:**
- Chen, M. M., Coakley, F. V., Kaimal, A., & Laros, R. K. Jr., (2008). Guidelines for computed tomography and magnetic resonance imaging use during pregnancy and lactation. *Obstet. Gynecol., 112*, 333–340.
- *Drug Information. Ablavar*. Lantheus Medical Imaging.
- Garcia-Bournissen, F., Shrim, A., & Koren, G., (2006). Safety of gadolinium during pregnancy. *Can. Fam. Physician, 2006 52*, 309–310.

## 13.7  GADOPENTETATE DIMEGLUMINE

**FDA Category: C**
***Risk Summary:*** There is limited pregnancy experience in humans, and the reproduction studies in animals have shown moderate risk. Therefore, it is advisable to avoid its use until the human pregnancy experience is available.

**Further Reading:**
*   Barkhof, F., Heijboer, R. J. J., & Algra, P. R., (1992). Inadvertent IV administration of gadopentetate dimeglumine during early pregnancy. *AJR Am. J. Roentgenol.,158,* 1171.
*   *Drug Information. Magnevist.* Bayer HealthCare Pharmaceuticals.
*   Garcia-Bournissen, F., Shrim, A., & Koren, G., (2006). Safety of gadolinium during pregnancy. *Can. Fam. Physician,* 2006 *52,* 309–310.

## 13.8  GADOTERIDOL

**FDA Category: C**
***Risk Summary:*** There is limited pregnancy experience in humans, and the reproduction studies in animals have shown moderate risk. Therefore, it is advisable to avoid its use until the human pregnancy experience is available.

**Further Reading:**
*   Chen, M. M., Coakley, F. V., Kaimal, A., & Laros, R. K. Jr., (2008). Guidelines for computed tomography and magnetic resonance imaging use during pregnancy and lactation. *Obstet. Gynecol., 112,* 333–340.
*   *Drug Information. Prohance.* Bracco Diagnostics.
*   Garcia-Bournissen, F., Shrim, A., & Koren, G., (2006). Safety of gadolinium during pregnancy. *Can. Fam. Physician, 52,* 309–310.

## 13.9  GADOVERSETAMIDE

**FDA Category: C**
***Risk Summary:*** There is limited pregnancy experience in humans, and the reproduction studies in animals have shown moderate risk. Therefore, it is advisable to avoid its use until the human pregnancy experience is available.

**Further Reading:**
- Chen, M. M., Coakley, F. V., Kaimal, A., & Laros, R. K. Jr., (2008). Guidelines for computed tomography and magnetic resonance imaging use during pregnancy and lactation. *Obstet. Gynecol., 112,* 333–340.
- *Drug Information.* OptiMARK. Mallinckrodt.
- Garcia-Bournissen, F., Shrim, A., & Koren, G., (2006). Safety of gadolinium during pregnancy. *Can. Fam. Physician, 52,* 309–310.

## 13.10  INDIGO CARMINE

**FDA Category: N**
*Risk Summary:* It should be used only when the maternal benefit outweighs the fetal risk because there is very limited human pregnancy data, and the animal studies are not relevant.

**Further Reading:**
- Fribourg, S., (1981). Safety of intraamniotic injection of indigo carmine. *Am. J. Obstet. Gynecol., 140,* 350–351.
- Horger, E. O. III., & Moody, L. O., (1984). Use of indigo carmine for twin amniocentesis and its effect on bilirubin analysis. *Am. J. Obstet. Gynecol., 150,* 858–860.

## 13.11  IOCETAMIC ACID

**FDA Category: B**
*Risk Summary:* The reproduction studies in animals have shown no evidence of fetal harm or impaired fertility. The pregnancy experience in humans is limited. Therefore, it does not represent a significant risk to the embryo-fetus.

**Further Reading:**
- Webb, J. A. W., Thomsen, H. S., & Morcos, S. K., (2005). The use of iodinated and gadolinium contrast media during pregnancy and lactation. *Eur. Radiol., 15,* 1234–1240.

## 13.12   IODIPAMIDE

**FDA Category: C**
*Risk Summary:* The reproduction studies in animals have shown no evidence of fetal harm or impaired fertility. The pregnancy experience in humans is limited. Therefore, it does not represent a significant risk to the embryo-fetus.

**Further Reading:**
• Webb, J. A. W., Thomsen, H. S., & Morcos, S. K., (2005). The use of iodinated and gadolinium contrast media during pregnancy and lactation. *Eur. Radiol., 15*, 1234–1240.

## 13.13   IODOXAMATE

**FDA Category: N**
*Risk Summary:* The reproduction studies in animals have shown no evidence of fetal harm or impaired fertility. The pregnancy experience in humans is limited. Therefore, it does not represent a significant risk to the embryo-fetus.

**Further Reading:**
• Webb, J. A. W., Thomsen, H. S., & Morcos, S. K., (2005). The use of iodinated and gadolinium contrast media during pregnancy and lactation. *Eur. Radiol., 15*, 1234–1240.

## 13.14   IOFLUPANE 123I

**FDA Category: C**
*Risk Summary:* It is contraindicated during pregnancy due to the potentially tremendous risks with its use.

**Further Reading:**
• Djang, D. S. W., Janssen, M. J. R., Bohnen, N., Booij, J., Henderson, T. A., Herholz, K., Minoshima, S., Rowe, C. C., Sabri, O., Seibyl, J., Van Berckel, B. N. M., & Wanner, M., (2012). SNM practice guideline for dopamine transporter imaging with [123]I-ioflupane SPECT 1.0. *J. Nucl. Med., 53*, 154–163.
• *Drug Information. DaTscan.* GE Healthcare, Medi-Physics.

## 13.15   IOHEXOL

**FDA Category: B**
*Risk Summary:* The reproduction studies in animals have shown no evidence of fetal harm or impaired fertility. The pregnancy experience in humans is adequate to exhibit that the embryo-fetal risk is very low. Therefore, it is safe to be used during pregnancy.

**Further Reading:**
- Bourjeily, G., Chalhoub, M., Phornphutkul, C., Alleyne, T. C., Wood-field, C. A., & Chen, K. K., (2010). Neonatal thyroid function: Effect of a single exposure to iodinated contrast medium in utero. *Radiology, 256*, 744–750.
- Kochi, M. H., Kaloudis, E. V., Ahmed, W., & Moore, W. H., (2012). Effect of in utero exposure of iodinated intravenous contrast on neonatal thyroid function. *J. Comput. Assist. Tomogr., 36*, 165–169.

## 13.16   IOPAMIDOL

**FDA Category: B**
*Risk Summary:* The reproduction studies in animals have shown no evidence of fetal harm or impaired fertility. The pregnancy experience in humans is limited. Therefore, it does not represent a significant risk to the embryo-fetus.

**Further Reading:**
- Chen, M. M., Coakley, F. V., Kaimal, A., & Laros, R. K. Jr.,(2008). Guidelines for computed tomography and magnetic resonance imaging use during pregnancy and lactation. *Obstet. Gynecol., 112*, 333–340.
- *Drug Information. Isovue.* Bracco Diagnostics.

## 13.17   IOPANOIC ACID

**FDA Category: B**
*Risk Summary:* The reproduction studies in animals have shown no evidence of fetal harm or impaired fertility. The pregnancy experience in humans is limited. Therefore, it does not represent a significant risk to the embryo-fetus.

**Further Reading:**
- Holmdahl, K. H., (1956). Cholecystography during lactation. *Acta Radiol., 45*, 305–7.

## 13.18   IOTHALAMATE

**FDA Category: B**
*Risk Summary:* The reproduction studies in animals have shown no evidence of fetal harm or impaired fertility. The pregnancy experience in humans is limited. Therefore, it does not represent a significant risk to the embryo-fetus.

**Further Reading:**
- Webb, J. A. W., Thomsen, H. S., & Morcos, S. K., (2005). The use of iodinated and gadolinium contrast media during pregnancy and lactation. *Eur. Radiol., 15*, 1234–1240.

## 13.19   IPODATE

**FDA Category: B**
*Risk Summary:* The reproduction studies in animals have shown no evidence of fetal harm or impaired fertility. The pregnancy experience in humans is limited. Therefore, it does not represent a significant risk to the embryo-fetus.

**Further Reading:**
- Webb, J. A. W., Thomsen, H. S., & Morcos, S. K., (2005). The use of iodinated and gadolinium contrast media during pregnancy and lactation. *Eur. Radiol., 15*, 1234–1240.

## 13.20   METHYLENE BLUE

**FDA Category: C**
*Risk Summary:* It is better to be avoided during the 2nd and 3rd Trimesters because the pregnancy experience in humans suggests risks of hyperbilirubinemia, hemolytic anemia, and methemoglobinemia in the newborn.

**Further Reading:**
- Fish, W. H., & Chazen, E. M., (1992). Toxic effects of methylene blue on the fetus. *Am. J. Dis. Child, 146,* 1412–1413.
- Troche, B. I., (1989). The methylene-blue baby. *N Engl. J. Med., 320,* 1756–1757.
- Vincer, M. J., Allen, A. C., Evans, J. R., Nwaesei, C., & Stinson, D. A., (1987). Methylene-blue-induced hemolytic anemia in a neonate. *CMAJ, 136,* 503–504.

## 13.21 TECHNETIUM TC-99M

**FDA Category: C**

***Risk Summary:*** The reproduction studies in animals have shown no evidence of fetal harm or impaired fertility. The pregnancy experience in humans is limited. Therefore, it does not represent a significant risk to the embryo-fetus.

**Further Reading:**
- *Drug Information. Technetium Tc 99m* Sestamibi Injection.
- Schaefer, C., Meister, R., Wentzeck, R., & Weber-Schoendorfer, C., (2009). Fetal outcome after technetium scintigraphy in early pregnancy. *Reprod. Toxicol., 28,* 161–166.

## KEYWORDS

- **iohexol**
- **iopamidol**
- **iopanoic acid**
- **iothalamate**
- **ipodate**
- **methylene blue**

# CHAPTER 14

# Vitamins and Dietary Supplements

## 14.1  VITAMINS

### 14.1.1  B-CAROTENE

**FDA Category: C**
*Risk Summary:* The reproduction studies in animals have shown no evidence of fetal harm or impaired fertility. The pregnancy experience in humans is adequate to exhibit that the embryo-fetal risk is very low. Therefore, it is safe to be used during pregnancy.

**Further Reading:**
- Nishimura, H., & Tanimura, T., (1978). *Clinical Aspects of the Teratogenicity of Drugs* (p. 252). New York, NY: American Elsevier.
- Polifka, J. E., Dolan, C. R., Donlan, M. A., & Friedman, J. M., (1996). Clinical teratology counseling and consultation report: High dose β-carotene use during early pregnancy. *Teratology, 54,* 103–107.

### 14.1.2  CALCITRIOL

**FDA Category: C**
*Risk Summary:* The reproduction studies in animals have shown no evidence of fetal harm or impaired fertility. The pregnancy experience in humans is adequate to exhibit that the embryo-fetal risk is very low. Therefore, it is safe to be used during pregnancy.

**Further Reading:**
- *Drug Information. Rocaltrol.* Roche Laboratories.

### 14.1.3   DEXPANTHENOL

**FDA Category: C**
***Risk Summary:*** It should be used only when the maternal benefit outweighs
the fetal risk because there is very limited human pregnancy data, and the
animal studies are not relevant.

**Further Reading:**
- *Drug Information. Ilopan.* Adria Laboratories.
- Hanck, A. B., & Goffin, H., (1982). Dexpanthenol (Ro 01-4709) in
  the treatment of constipation. *Acta Vitaminol. Enzymol., 4,* 87–97.

### 14.1.4   FOLIC ACID

**FDA Category: A**
***Risk Summary:*** The reproduction studies in animals have shown no evidence
of fetal harm or impaired fertility. The pregnancy experience in humans is
adequate to exhibit that the embryo-fetal risk is very low. Therefore, it is
recommended to be used during pregnancy.

**Further Reading:**
- Dansky, L. V., Rosenblatt, D. S., & Andermann, E., (1992). Mecha-
  nisms of teratogenesis: Folic acid and antiepileptic therapy. *Neurology,
  42*(Suppl 5), 32–42.
- MRC Vitamin Study Research Group (1991). Prevention of neural
  tube defects: Results of the Medical Research Council vitamin study.
  *Lancet, 338,* 131–137.

### 14.1.5   LEUCOVORIN (FOLINIC ACID)

**FDA Category: C**
***Risk Summary:*** The reproduction studies in animals have shown no evidence
of fetal harm or impaired fertility. The pregnancy experience in humans is
adequate to exhibit that the embryo-fetal risk is very low. Therefore, it is safe
to be used during pregnancy.

**Further Reading:**
- American Hospital Formulary Service, (1997). *Drug Information* (pp. 2890–2893). Bethesda, MD: American Society of Health-System Pharmacists.
- Scott, J. M., (1957). Folinic acid in megaloblastic anemia of pregnancy. *Br. Med. J., 2*, 270–272.

## 14.1.6 NIACINAMIDE

**FDA Category: N**
*Risk Summary:* The reproduction studies in animals have shown no evidence of fetal harm or impaired fertility. The pregnancy experience in humans is adequate to exhibit that the embryo-fetal risk is very low. Therefore, it is recommended to be used during pregnancy.

**Further Reading:**
- Hart, B. F., & McConnell, W. T., (1943). Vitamin B factors in toxic psychosis of pregnancy and the puerperium. *Am. J. Obstet. Gynecol., 46*, 283.
- Kaminetzky, H. A., Baker, H., Frank, O., & Langer, A., (1974). The effects of intravenously administered water-soluble vitamins during labor in normovitaminemic and hypovitaminemic gravidas on maternal and neonatal blood vitamin levels at delivery. *Am. J. Obstet. Gynecol., 120*, 697–703.

## 14.1.7 PANTOTHENIC ACID

**FDA Category: C**
*Risk Summary:* The reproduction studies in animals have shown no evidence of fetal harm or impaired fertility. The pregnancy experience in humans is adequate to exhibit that the embryo-fetal risk is very low. Therefore, it is safe to be used during pregnancy.

**Further Reading:**
- Cohenour, S. H., & Calloway, D. H., (1972). Blood, urine, and dietary pantothenic acid levels of pregnant teenagers. *Am. J.* Clin Nutr., *25*, 512–517.

- Kaminetsky, H. A., Baker, H., Frank, O., & Langer, A., (1974). The effects of intravenously administered water-soluble vitamins during labor in normovitaminemic and hypovitaminemic gravidas on maternal and neonatal blood vitamin levels at delivery. *Am. J. Obstet. Gynecol., 120*, 697–703.

### 14.1.8   VITAMIN A

**FDA Category: X (at doses above the U.S. recommended daily allowance (RDA))**
*Risk Summary:* Doses exceeding 8000 IU/day should be avoided by women who are pregnant or who may become pregnant because of the associated risk of teratogenicity.

**Further Reading:**
- Dudas, I., & Czeizel, A. E., (1992). Use of 6,000 IU vitamin A during early pregnancy without teratogenic effect. *Teratology, 45*, 335, 336.
- Lungarotti, M. S., Marinelli, D., Mariani, T., & Calabro, A., (1987). Multiple congenital anomalies associated with apparently normal maternal intake of vitamin A: A phenocopy of the isotretinoin syndrome? *Am. J. Med. Genet., 27*, 245–248.
- Teratology Society Publications [Internet]. Teratology.org. (2018). Available from: http://teratology.org/pubs/vitamina.htm (accessed on 31 January 2020).

### 14.1.9   VITAMIN B1

**FDA Category: A (at doses within the U.S. RDA)**
**FDA Category: C (at doses above the U.S. RDA)**
*Risk Summary:* The reproduction studies in animals have shown no evidence of fetal harm or impaired fertility. The pregnancy experience in humans is adequate to exhibit that the embryo-fetal risk is very low. Therefore, it is safe to be used during pregnancy.

**Further Reading:**
- Reading, C., (1976). Down's syndrome, leukemia, and maternal thiamine deficiency. *Med. J. Aust., 1*, 505.

- Roecklein, B., Levin, S. W., Comly, M., & Mukherjee, A. B., (1985). Intrauterine growth retardation induced by thiamine deficiency and pyrithiamine during pregnancy in the rat. *Am. J. Obstet. Gynecol., 151,* 455–460.

## 14.1.10 VITAMIN B2

**FDA Category: A (at doses within the U.S. RDA)**

**FDA Category: C (at doses above the U.S. RDA)**

***Risk Summary:*** The reproduction studies in animals have shown no evidence of fetal harm or impaired fertility. The pregnancy experience in humans is adequate to exhibit that the embryo-fetal risk is very low. Therefore, it is safe to be used during pregnancy.

**Further Reading:**

- Ronnholm, K. A. R., (1986). Need for riboflavin supplementation in small prematures fed human milk. *Am. J. Clin. Nutr., 43,* 1–6.
- Thomas, M. R., Sneed, S. M., Wei, C., Nail, P. A., Wilson, M., & Sprinkle, E. E. III., (1980). The effects of vitamin C, vitamin B6, vitamin B12, folic acid, riboflavin, and thiamin on the breast milk and maternal status of well-nourished women at 6 months postpartum. *Am. J. Clin. Nutr., 33,* 2151–2156.

## 14.1.11 VITAMIN B3

**FDA Category: C**

***Risk Summary:*** The reproduction studies in animals have shown no evidence of fetal harm or impaired fertility. The pregnancy experience in humans is adequate to exhibit that the embryo-fetal risk is very low. Therefore, it is safe to be used during pregnancy.

**Further Reading:**

- Hart, B. F., & McConnell, W. T., (1943). Vitamin B factors in toxic psychosis of pregnancy and the puerperium. *Am. J. Obstet. Gynecol., 46,* 283.

## 14.1.12    *VITAMIN B6*

**FDA Category: A**
*Risk Summary:* The reproduction studies in animals have shown no evidence of fetal harm or impaired fertility. The pregnancy experience in humans is adequate to exhibit that the embryo-fetal risk is very low. Therefore, it is safe to be used during pregnancy.

**Further Reading:**
- Sahakian, V., Rouse, D., Sipes, S., Rose, N. B., & Niebyl, J., (1991). Vitamin B6 is an effective therapy for nausea and vomiting of pregnancy: A randomized double-blind placebo-controlled study. *Obstet. Gynecol., 78*, 33–36.
- Thomas, M. R., Sneed, S. M., Wei, C., Nail, P. A., Wilson, M., & Sprinkle, E. E. III., (1980). The effects of vitamin C, vitamin B6, vitamin B12, folic acid, riboflavin, and thiamin on the breast milk and maternal status of well-nourished women at 6 months postpartum. *Am. J. Clin. Nutr., 33*, 2151–2156.

## 14.1.13    *VITAMIN B12*

**FDA Category: C**
*Risk Summary:* The reproduction studies in animals have shown no evidence of fetal harm or impaired fertility. The pregnancy experience in humans is adequate to exhibit that the embryo-fetal risk is very low. Therefore, it is safe to be used during pregnancy.

**Further Reading:**
- Schorah, C. J., Smithells, R. W., & Scott, J., (1980). Vitamin B12 and anencephaly. *Lancet, 1*, 880.
- Sklar, R., (1986). Nutritional vitamin B12 deficiency in a breastfed infant of a vegan-diet mother. *Clin. Pediatr., 25*, 219–221.

## 14.1.14    *VITAMIN C*

**FDA Category: A (at doses within the U.S. RDA)**
**FDA Category: C (at doses above the U.S. RDA)**
*Risk Summary:* The reproduction studies in animals have shown no evidence of fetal harm or impaired fertility. The pregnancy experience in humans is

adequate to exhibit that the embryo-fetal risk is very low. Therefore, it is safe to be used during pregnancy.

**Further Reading:**
- Bates, C. J., Prentice, A. M., Prentice, A., Lamb, W. H., & Whitehead, R. G., (1983). The effect of vitamin C supplementation on lactating women in Keneba, a West African rural community. *Int. J. Vitam Nutr. Res., 53,* 68–76.
- Byerley, L. O., & Kirksey, A., (1985). Effects of different levels of vitamin C intake on the vitamin C concentration in human milk and the vitamin C intake of breastfed infants. *Am. J. Clin. Nutr.,* 1985 *41,* 665–671.
- Vobecky, J. S., Vobecky, J., Shapcott, D., & Munan, L., (1974). Vitamin C and outcome of pregnancy. *Lancet, 1,* 630.

## 14.1.15   *VITAMIN D*

**FDA Category: C**
*Risk Summary:* The reproduction studies in animals have shown no evidence of fetal harm or impaired fertility. The pregnancy experience in humans is adequate to exhibit that the embryo-fetal risk is very low. Therefore, it is safe to be used during pregnancy.

**Further Reading:**
- Hollis, B. W., & Wagner, C. L., (2004). Assessment of dietary vitamin D requirements during pregnancy and lactation. *Am. J. Clin. Nutr., 79,* 717–276.
- Mulligan, M. L., Felton, S. K., Riek, A. E., & Bernal-Mizrachi, C., (2010). Implications of vitamin D deficiency in pregnancy and lactation. *Am. J. Obstet. Gynecol., 202,* 429, e1–9.

## 14.1.16   *VITAMIN E*

**FDA Category: A (at doses within the U.S. RDA)**
**FDA Category: C (at doses above the U.S. RDA)**
*Risk Summary:* The reproduction studies in animals have shown no evidence of fetal harm or impaired fertility. The pregnancy experience in humans is

adequate to exhibit that the embryo-fetal risk is very low. Therefore, it is safe to be used during pregnancy.

**Further Reading:**
- Boskovic, R., Gargaun, L., Oren, D., Djulus, J., & Koren, G., (2005). Pregnancy outcome following high doses of vitamin E supplementation. *Reprod. Toxicol., 20*, 85–88.
- Hook, E. B., Healy, K. M., Niles, A. M., & Skalko, R. G., (1974). Vitamin E: Teratogen or anti-teratogen? *Lancet, 1*, 809.

## *14.1.17   VITAMIN K*

**FDA Category: C**
*Risk Summary:* The reproduction studies in animals have shown no evidence of fetal harm or impaired fertility. The pregnancy experience in humans is adequate to exhibit that the embryo-fetal risk is very low. Therefore, it is safe to be used during pregnancy.

**Further Reading:**
- Payne, N. R., & Hasegawa, D. K., (1984). Vitamin K deficiency in newborns: A case report in α-1-antitrypsin deficiency and a review of factors predisposing to hemorrhage. *Pediatrics, 73*, 712–716.
- Shearer, M. J., Rahim, S., Barkhan, P., & Stimmler, L., (1982). Plasma vitamin K1 in mothers and their newborn babies. *Lancet, 2*, 460–463.

## 14.2   DIETARY SUPPLEMENTS

### *14.2.1   CHONDROITIN*

**FDA Category: N**
*Risk Summary:* The reproduction studies in animals have shown no evidence of fetal harm or impaired fertility. The pregnancy experience in humans is limited. Therefore, it does not represent a significant risk to the embryo-fetus.

**Further Reading:**
- Chondroitin (2004). *The Review of Natural Products*. St. Louis, MO: Wolters Kluwer Health.

- Chondroitin Sulfate (2003). *Natural Medicines Comprehensive Database* (pp. 345–347). Stockton, CA: Therapeutic Research Faculty.

## 14.2.2  GLUCOSAMINE

**FDA Category: N**
*Risk Summary:* The reproduction studies in animals have shown no evidence of fetal harm or impaired fertility. The pregnancy experience in humans is limited. Therefore, it does not represent a significant risk to the embryo-fetus.

**Further Reading:**
- Glucosamine (2004). The Review of Natural Products. St. Louis, MO: Wolters Kluwer Health.
- Sivojelezova, A., Einarson, A., & Koren, G., (2005). A prospective cohort study evaluating pregnancy outcomes and risk perceptions of pregnant women following glucosamine use during pregnancy (abstract). *Birth Defects Res. (Part A), 73*, 395.

## 14.2.3  OMEGA-3

**FDA Category: C**
*Risk Summary:* The reproduction studies in animals have shown no evidence of fetal harm or impaired fertility. The pregnancy experience in humans is adequate to exhibit that the embryo-fetal risk is very low. Therefore, it could be considered, relatively, safe to be used during pregnancy.

**Further Reading:**
- Coletta, J. M., Bell, S. J., & Roman, A. S., (2010). Omega-3 fatty acids and pregnancy. *Rev. Obstet. Gynecol., 3*, 163–171.
- Makrides, M., & Gibson, R. A., (2000). Long-chain polyunsaturated fatty acid requirements during pregnancy and lactation. *Am. J. Clin. Nutr., 71*(1 Suppl), 307S–311S.
- Morse, N. L., (2012). Benefits of docosahexaenoic acid, folic acid, vitamin D and iodine on fetal and infant brain development and function following maternal supplementation during pregnancy and lactation. *Nutrients, 4*, 799–840.

**KEYWORDS**

- dietary supplements
- glucosamine
- omega-3
- pantothenic acid
- recommended daily allowance
- vitamin B12

# CHAPTER 15

# Medicinal Herbs

## 15.1  ARNICA

**FDA Category: N**
*Risk Summary:* It is contraindicated during pregnancy due to its uterine stimulant action.

**Further Reading:**
- Arnica, (2010). *The Review of Natural Products*. St. Louis, MO: Wolters Kluwer Health, 2010.
- Miller, A. D., Ly, B. T., & Clark, R. F., (2009). Neonatal hemolysis associated with the nursing mother's ingestion of arnica tea (abstract). *Clin. Toxicol., 47*, 726.

## 15.2  BLACK SEED/KALANJI

**FDA Category: N**
*Risk Summary:* It should be used only when the maternal benefit outweighs the fetal risk because there is very limited human pregnancy data, and the animal studies are not relevant.

**Further Reading:**
- Black Seed (2008). *Natural Medicines Comprehensive Database* (10th edn., pp. 191–192). Stockton, CA: Therapeutic Research Faculty.
- Briggs, G., Freeman, R., Towers, C., & Forninash, A., (2017). *Drugs in Pregnancy and Lactation: A Reference Guide to Fetal and Neonatal Risk*. Philadelphia, Pa: Wolters Kluwer Health.

## 15.3   BLUE COHOSH

**FDA Category: N**

*Risk Summary:* Blue cohosh should be avoided in pregnant women because of its uterine stimulant action and the risk of teratogenicity associated with the use of this herb.

**Further Reading:**
- Blue Cohosh (2000). In: *PDR for Herbal Medicines* (2ⁿᵈ edn., pp. 109, 110). Montvale, NJ: Medical Economics.
- Briggs, G., Freeman, R., Towers, C., & Forninash, A., (2017). Drugs in Pregnancy and Lactation: A Reference Guide to Fetal and Neonatal Risk. Philadelphia, Pa: Wolters Kluwer Health.
- Jones, T. K., & Lawson, B. M., (1998). Profound neonatal congestive heart failure caused by maternal consumption of blue cohosh herbal medication. *J. Pediatr., 132,* 550–552.

## 15.4   CAFFEINE

**FDA Category: C**

*Risk Summary:* The reproduction studies in animals have shown no evidence of fetal harm or impaired fertility. The pregnancy experience in humans is adequate to exhibit that the embryo-fetal risk is very low. Therefore, it is safe to be used during pregnancy-if used in moderation.

**Further Reading:**
- Linn, S., Schoenbaum, S. C., Monson, R. R., Rosner, B., Stubble-field, P. G., & Ryan, K. J., (1982). No association between coffee consumption and adverse outcomes of pregnancy. *N Engl. J. Med., 306,* 141–145.
- Mills, J. L., Holmes, L. B., Aarons, J. H., Simpson, J. L., Brown, Z. A., Jovanovic-Peterson, L. G., Conley, M. R., Graubard, B. I., Knopp, R. H., & Metzger, B. E., (1993). Moderate caffeine use and the risk of spontaneous abortion and intrauterine growth retardation. *JAMA, 269,* 593–597.

## 15.5 CHAMOMILE

**FDA Category: N**
*Risk Summary:* It should be used only when the maternal benefit outweighs the fetal risk because there is very limited human pregnancy data, and the animal studies are not relevant.

**Further Reading:**
- Chamomile (2007). *The Review of Natural Products*. St. Louis, MO: Wolters Kluwer Health, 2007.
- Johns, T., & Sibeko, L., (2003). Pregnancy outcomes in women using herbal therapies. *Birth Defects Res.* (Part B), *68*, 501–504.

## 15.6 ECHINACEA

**FDA Category: N**
*Risk Summary:* It should be used only when the maternal benefit outweighs the fetal risk because there is very limited human pregnancy data, and the animal studies are not relevant.

**Further Reading:**
- Gallo, M., Sarkar, M., Au, W., Pietrzak, K., Comas, B., Smith, M., Jaeger, T. V., Einarson, A., & Koren, G., (2000). Pregnancy outcome following gestational exposure to echinacea. A prospective controlled study. *Arch Intern. Med., 160*, 3141–3143.
- Zink, T., & Chaffin, J., (1998). Herbal 'health' products: What family physicians need to know. *Am. Fam. Physician, 58*, 1133–1140.

## 15.7 EVENING PRIMROSE OIL

**FDA Category: N**
*Risk Summary:* The reproduction studies in animals have shown no evidence of fetal harm or impaired fertility. The pregnancy experience in humans is limited. In general, it does not represent a significant risk to the embryo-fetus. However, it should be kept in mind that Evening Primrose Oil has the ability to induce labor.

**Further Reading:**
- Evening Primrose Oil (2006). The Review of Natural Products. St. Louis, MO: Wolters Kluwer Health.
- Ty-Torredes, K. A., (2006). The effect of oral evening primrose oil on Bishop score and cervical length among term gravidas (abstract). *Am. J. Obstet. Gynecol., 195,* S30.

## 15.8 FEVERFEW

**FDA Category: N**
*Risk Summary:* It should be avoided during pregnancy because the human pregnancy experience is very limited and the animal reproduction studies have shown the risk of embryo lethality.

**Further Reading:**
- Briggs, G., Freeman, R., Towers, C., & Forninash, A., (2017). Drugs in Pregnancy and Lactation: A Reference Guide to Fetal and Neonatal Risk. Philadelphia, Pa: Wolters Kluwer Health.
- Feverfew. Natural Medicines Comprehensive Database. 10th ed. Stockton, CA: Therapeutic Research Faculty, 2008:584–5.

## 15.9 GARLIC

**FDA Category: N**
*Risk Summary:* The reproduction studies in animals have shown no evidence of fetal harm or impaired fertility. The pregnancy experience in humans is adequate to exhibit that the embryo-fetal risk is very low. Therefore, it is safe to be used during pregnancy. However, consumption of large amounts of garlic during pregnancy should be avoided because of the potential for inducing uterine contractions.

**Further Reading:**
- Briggs, G., Freeman, R., Towers, C., & Forninash, A., (2017). Drugs in Pregnancy and Lactation: A Reference Guide to Fetal and Neonatal Risk. Philadelphia, Pa: Wolters Kluwer Health.
- Garlic (1999). *Natural Medicines Comprehensive Database* (pp366–368.). Stockton, CA: Therapeutic Research Faculty.

## 15.10   GINGER

**FDA Category: N**
*Risk Summary:* The reproduction studies in animals have shown no evidence of fetal harm or impaired fertility. The pregnancy experience in humans is adequate to exhibit that the embryo-fetal risk is very low. Therefore, it is safe to be used during pregnancy.

**Further Reading:**
- Portnoi, G., Chng, L. A., Karimi-Tabesh, L., Koren, G., Tan, M. P., & Einarson, A., (2003). Prospective comparative study of the safety and effectiveness of ginger for the treatment of nausea and vomiting in pregnancy. *Am. J. Obstet. Gynecol., 189*, 1374–1377.
- Smith, C., Crowther, C., Willson, K., Hotham, N., & McMillian, V., (2004). A randomized controlled trial of ginger to treat nausea and vomiting of pregnancy. *Obstet. Gynecol., 103*, 639–645.

## 15.11   GINKGO BILOBA

**FDA Category: N**
*Risk Summary:* It should be used with caution because the pregnancy experience in humans is limited and the reproduction studies in animals have shown low risk.

**Further Reading:**
- Briggs, G., Freeman, R., Towers, C., & Forninash, A., (2017). Drugs in Pregnancy and Lactation: A Reference Guide to Fetal and Neonatal Risk. Philadelphia, Pa: Wolters Kluwer Health.
- Ginkgo Biloba Leaf Extract (1998). In: Blumenthal, M., (ed.) *The Complete German Commission E Monographs* (pp. 136–138). Therapeutic Guide to Herbal Medicines. Austin, TX: American Botanical Council.

## 15.12   GINSENG

**FDA Category: N**
*Risk Summary:* It should be used with caution because the pregnancy experience in humans is limited and the reproduction studies in animals have shown low risk.

**Further Reading:**

- Ginseng, Panax (2001). *The Review of Natural Products*. St. Louis, MO: Facts and Comparisons.
- Koren, G., Randor, S., Martin, S., & Danneman, D., (1990). Maternal ginseng use associated with neonatal androgenization. *JAMA, 264*, 2866.

## 15.13   KUDZU

**FDA Category: N**

*Risk Summary:* The reproduction studies in animals have shown no evidence of fetal harm or impaired fertility. The pregnancy experience in humans is limited. Therefore, it does not represent a significant risk to the embryo-fetus.

**Further Reading:**

- Jaroenporn, S., Malaivijitnond, S., Wattanasirmkit, K., Watanabe, G., Taya, K., & Cherdshewasart, W., (2007). Assessment of fertility and reproductive toxicity in adult female mice after long-term exposure to Pueraria mirifica herb. *J. Reprod. Dev., 53*, 995–1005.
- Kudzu (2008). In: *The Review of Natural Products*. St. Louis, MO: Wolters Kluwer Health.

## 15.14   NUTMEG

**FDA Category: N**

*Risk Summary:* The reproduction studies in animals have shown no evidence of fetal harm or impaired fertility. The pregnancy experience in humans is limited. Therefore, it does not represent a significant risk to the embryo-fetus.

**Further Reading:**

- Briggs, G., Freeman, R., Towers, C., & Forninash, A., (2017). Drugs in Pregnancy and Lactation: A Reference Guide to Fetal and Neonatal Risk. Philadelphia, Pa: Wolters Kluwer Health.
- Lavy, G., (1987). Nutmeg intoxication in pregnancy; A case report. *J. Reprod. Med., 32*, 63–64.

## 15.15   PASSION FLOWER

**FDA Category: N**
*Risk Summary:* Passion fruit should be avoided in pregnant women because Passion fruit has the ability of inducing abortions due to its uterine stimulant properties.

**Further Reading:**
- Passionflower (1999). In: *The Review of Natural Products*. St. Louis, MO: Facts and Comparisons.
- Robbers, J. E., & Tyler, V. E., (2000). *Tyler's Herbs of Choice* (pp. 159, 160). The Therapeutic Use of Phytomedicinals. Binghamton, NY: Haworth Press.

## 15.16   PEPPERMINT

**FDA Category: N**
*Risk Summary:* The reproduction studies in animals have shown no evidence of fetal harm or impaired fertility. The pregnancy experience in humans is limited. Therefore, it does not represent a significant risk to the embryo-fetus.

**Further Reading:**
- Ernst, E., (2002). Herbal medicinal products during pregnancy: Are they safe? *Br. J. Obstet. Gynaecol., 109,* 227–235.
- Peppermint (2006). *The Review of Natural Products*. Facts and Comparisons. St. Louis, MO: Wolters Kluwer Health.

## 15.17   PUMPKIN SEED

**FDA Category: N**
*Risk Summary:* The reproduction studies in animals have shown no evidence of fetal harm or impaired fertility. The pregnancy experience in humans is limited. Therefore, it does not represent a significant risk to the embryo-fetus.

**Further Reading:**
- Jellin, J. M., (2008). Pumpkin. *Natural Medicines Comprehensive Database* (10th edn., pp. 1219, 1220). Stockton, CA: Therapeutic Research Faculty.
- Pumpkin, (2004). In: Der Marderosian, A., & Beutler, J. A., (eds.), *The Review of Natural Products*. St. Louis, MO: Wolters Kluwer Health.

## 15.18   RASPBERRY LEAF

**FDA Category: N**

*Risk Summary:* The reproduction studies in animals have shown no evidence of fetal harm or impaired fertility. The pregnancy experience in humans is limited. Therefore, it does not represent a significant risk to the embryo-fetus.

**Further Reading:**
- Raspberry Leaf, (2003). In: *Natural Medicines Comprehensive Database* (5th edn., pp. 1105, 1106). Stockton, CA: Therapeutic Research Faculty.
- Simpson, M., Parsons, M., Greenwood, J., & Wade, K., (2001). Raspberry leaf in pregnancy: Its safety and efficacy in labor. *J. Midwifery Women's Health, 46,* 51–59.

## 15.19   SAFFLOWER

**FDA Category: N**

*Risk Summary:* The reproduction studies in animals have shown no evidence of fetal harm or impaired fertility. The pregnancy experience in humans is adequate to exhibit that the embryo-fetal risk is very low. Therefore, it is safe to be used during pregnancy.

**Further Reading:**
- Nobakht, M., Fattahi, M., Hoormand, M., Milanian, I., Rahbar, N., & Mahmoudian, M., (2000). A study on the teratogenic and cytotoxic effects of safflower extract. *J. Ethnopharmacol., 73,* 453–459.
- Safflower, (2009). In: *The Review of Natural Products*. St. Louis, MO: Wolters Kluwer Health.

## 15.20 SALVIA DIVINORUM

**FDA Category: N**
*Risk Summary:* It is better to be avoided during pregnancy because there is very limited human pregnancy data, and the animal studies are not relevant.

**Further Reading:**
- Butelman, E. R., Prisinzano, T. E., Deng, H., Rus, S., & Kreek, M. J., (2009). Unconditioned behavioral effects of the powerful k-opioid hallucinogen salvinorin A in nonhuman primates: Fast onset and entry into the cerebrospinal fluid. *J. Pharmacol. Exp. Ther., 328*, 588–597.
- Prezekop, P., & Lee, T., (2009). Persistent psychosis associated with Salvia divinorum use. *Am. J.* Psychiatry, *166*, 832.
- Salvia Divinorum (2010). In: *The Review of Natural Products*. St. Louis, MO: Wolters Kluwer Health.

## 15.21 ST. JOHN'S WORT

**FDA Category: N**
*Risk Summary:* The reproduction studies in animals have shown no evidence of fetal harm or impaired fertility. The pregnancy experience in humans is limited. Therefore, it does not represent a significant risk to the embryo-fetus.

**Further Reading:**
- Moretti, M. E., Maxson, A., Hanna, F., & Koren, G., (2009). Evaluating the safety of St. John's wort in human pregnancy. *Reprod. Toxicol., 28*, 96–99.
- Rayburn, W. F., Christensen, H. D., & Gonzalez, C. L., (2000). Effect of antenatal exposure to Saint John's wort (Hypericum) on neurobehavior of developing mice. *Am. J. Obstet. Gynecol., 183*, 1225–1231.
- St. John's Wort (1997). In: *The Review of Natural Products*. St. Louis, MO: Facts and Comparisons.

## 15.22 VALERIAN

**FDA Category: N**
*Risk Summary:* It is better to be avoided during pregnancy because there is very limited human pregnancy data, and the animal studies are not relevant.

**Further Reading:**
- Garges, H. P., Varia, I., & Doraiswamy, P. M., (1998). Cardiac complications and delirium associated with valerian root withdrawal. *JAMA,280*, 1566–1567.
- Valerian (1991). *The Lawrence Review of Natural Products: Facts and Comparisons*. St. Louis, MO: J.B. Lippincott.

## 15.23  YOHIMBINE

**FDA Category: N**

*Risk Summary:* It is better to be avoided during pregnancy because there is very limited human pregnancy data, and the animal studies are not relevant.

**Further Reading:**
- Al-Majed, A. A., Al-Yahya, A. A., Al-Bekairi, A. M., Al-Shabanah, O. A., & Qureshi, S., (2006). Reproductive, cytological and biochemical toxicity of Yohimbe in male Swiss albino mice. *Asian J. Androl.,* 8, 469–476.
- Bovet-Nitti, F., & Bovet, D., (1959). Action of some sympatholytic agents on pregnancy in the rat. *Proc. Soc. Exp. Biol. Med., 100,* 555–557.

## KEYWORDS

- **nutmeg**
- **peppermint**
- **pumpkin seed**
- **raspberry leaf**
- **Salvia divinorum**
- **valerian**

# Index

Buprenorphine, 342, 343
Bupropion, 233, 234, 264
Butenafine, 382
Butorphanol, 343

## C

Cabergoline, 193, 194
Caffeine, 260, 296, 424
Calcipotriene, 185, 394
Calcitriol, 184, 394, 413
Calcium
  carbonate, 309
  channel blockers, 104, 105
  receptor agonist, 189
  regulation hormones, 188
Camphor, 272
Candesartan cilexetil, 111
Captopril, 107, 108
Carbachol, 285
Carbamazepine, 5, 223
Carbapenems, 29
Carbenicillin, 20
Carbidopa/levodopa, 256
Carbimazole, 175–177
Carbinoxamine, 209
Carbonic anhydrase inhibitor, 125
Carboprost, 190
Cardiac defects, 237, 242, 346
Cardiovascular, 81, 115, 200, 228, 288, 330
Carglumic acid, 193, 194
Carisoprodol, 278
Carteolol, 294
Carvedilol, 104, 295
Casanthranol, 327
Cascara sagrada, 328
Caspofungin, 53
Castor oil, 328
Cefaclor, 22, 23
Cefadroxil, 21
Cefazolin, 21, 22, 28, 32
Cefdinir, 24
Cefepime, 28, 29
Cefixime, 25
Cefoperazone, 25, 29
Cefotaxime, 26
Cefotetan, 23
Cefoxitin, 23
Cefprozil, 24

Ceftaroline fosamil, 29
Ceftazidime, 21, 27
Ceftibuten, 27
Cefuroxime, 24
Celecoxib, 346, 347
Cephalexin, 22
Cephalosporins, 21–29
Certolizumab, 365
Cetirizine, 210
Cevimeline, 286
Chamomile, 425
Chenodiol, 326
Chloral hydrate, 264
Chloramphenicol, 46, 47
Chlordiazepoxide, 265
Chloroquine, 69, 70, 360
Chlorothiazide, 122
Chlorpheniramine, 210
Chlorpromazine, 247
Chlorpropamide, 155, 156
Chlorthalidone, 123, 124
Chlorzoxazone, 278
Cholecalciferol, 182
Cholesterol, 125–129
Cholestyramine, 130, 131
Cholinergic drugs, 285
Cholinesterase inhibitors, 262
Chondroitin, 420
Ciclesonide, 206
Ciclopirox, 382
Cilostazol, 138
Cimetidine, 320, 321
Cinacalcet, 189
Ciprofloxacin, 44
Citalopram, 236
Clarithromycin, 35
Clavulanic acid, 19, 20
Cleft palate, 165–167, 208, 227, 252
Clemastine, 210
Clidinium, 289
Clindamycin, 36, 37, 379
Clobazam, 223, 224
Clobetasol propionate, 395
Clomiphene, 169
Clomipramine, 242
Clonazepam, 224
Clonidine, 114
Clopidogrel, 137, 138, 140

Glycopeptides, 31
Glycopyrrolate, 288, 290
Gold sodium thiomalate, 362
Golimumab, 366
Gram-negative pathogens, 38–40
Granisetron, 315
Gray baby syndrome, 46
Growth
 hormone related agents, 191
 restriction, 11–13, 85, 131, 164, 186, 194,
  228, 233, 259, 293, 295, 307, 346,
Guaifenesin, 216
Guanethidine, 297
Guanfacine, 297

# H

H2-receptor antagonists, 320
Haloperidol, 246, 289
Halothane, 274, 275, 277
Hematopoietic drugs, 145
Hemin, 147
Hemolysis, 42, 71, 423
Hemolytic, 42, 368, 410, 411
 anemia, 42, 410, 411
Hemorheologic drug, 151
Hemorrhage, 130, 149, 230, 346, 420
Hemorrheologic drug, 149
Hemostatic drugs, 148, 151
Hepatotoxicity, 34, 233, 326
Herb, 424, 428
Hereditary angioedema, 151, 167, 168
HMG-coa inhibitors, 125
Holoprosencephaly, 280
Homatropine, 290
HPA axis, 396, 397
Human
 data, 9, 32, 36, 49, 54, 55, 58, 75, 83, 89,
  90, 100, 118, 149, 264, 279, 293, 301,
  310, 312, 320, 363
 pregnancy
  data, 192, 264, 431, 432
  experience, 35, 48, 50, 58–61, 66–69,
   72–74, 89, 92, 94, 96, 100, 104, 106,
   113, 116, 118, 139, 140, 142, 143,
   145, 146, 150, 163, 164, 206, 213,
   231, 251–253, 283, 295, 296, 303,
   310, 318, 319, 360, 369, 375, 380,
   381, 395, 396, 400, 404–406, 426

Hydralazine, 117
Hydrocephalus, 136, 192
Hydrochlorothiazide, 122
Hydrocodone, 197, 337
Hydrocortisone, 165, 166, 397
Hydroflumethiazide, 123
Hydromorphone, 337
Hydroquinone, 391
Hydroxychloroquine, 70, 360, 361
Hydroxyprogesterone, 172
Hydroxyzine, 214
Hyperbilirubinemia, 41, 410
Hyperlipidemia, 125–128
Hypertension, 88, 102, 103, 108, 109,
 117–125, 297, 298, 300, 335, 347–351,
 353–358
Hyperthyroidism, 175–177, 189
Hypothalamic-pituitary-adrenal axis, 396
Hypothyroidism, 90
Hypovolemia, 117–125

# I

Ibandronate, 186
Ibuprofen, 350
Ibutilide, 91
Icatibant, 150
Iloperidone, 250
Imipenem-cilastatin, 29
Imipramine, 243, 244
Imiquimod, 388
Immunocompromised patients, 56, 57
Immunosuppression, 359, 389
Indacaterol, 199
Indigo carmine, 407
Indomethacin, 351
Induce labor, 425
Infliximab, 319, 366
Inhaled corticosteroids, 163, 164, 167, 205–208
Insulin
 aspart, 153
 detemir, 154
 glargine, 154, 155
 lispro, 155
Intestinal atresia, 306
Intrauterine
 death, 242
 growth